VOLUME ONE HUNDRED AND FORTY FIVE

ADVANCES IN IMMUNOLOGY

Advances in Immunology in China - Part B

ASSOCIATE EDITORS

VOLUME ONE HUNDRED AND FORTY FIVE

ADVANCES IN IMMUNOLOGY

Advances in Immunology in China - Part B

Edited by

CHEN DONG
Institute for Immunology and School of Medicine, Tsinghua University; Beijing Key Lab for Immunological Research on Chronic Diseases, Beijing, China

ZHENGFAN JIANG
Key Laboratory of Cell Proliferation and Differentiation of the Ministry of Education, School of Life Sciences, Peking University, Beijing, China

ELSEVIER

ACADEMIC PRESS
An imprint of Elsevier

Academic Press is an imprint of Elsevier
50 Hampshire Street, 5th Floor, Cambridge, MA 02139, United States
525 B Street, Suite 1650, San Diego, CA 92101, United States
The Boulevard, Langford Lane, Kidlington, Oxford OX5 1GB, United Kingdom
125 London Wall, London, EC2Y 5AS, United Kingdom

First edition 2020

Notices
Knowledge and best practice in this field are constantly changing. As new research and experience broaden our understanding, changes in research methods, professional practices, or medical treatment may become necessary.

Practitioners and researchers must always rely on their own experience and knowledge in evaluating and using any information, methods, compounds, or experiments described herein. In using such information or methods they should be mindful of their own safety and the safety of others, including parties for whom they have a professional responsibility.

To the fullest extent of the law, neither the Publisher nor the authors, contributors, or editors, assume any liability for any injury and/or damage to persons or property as a matter of products liability, negligence or otherwise, or from any use or operation of any methods, products, instructions, or ideas contained in the material herein.

ISBN: 978-0-12-817878-2
ISSN: 0065-2776

For information on all Academic Press publications
visit our website at https://www.elsevier.com/books-and-journals

Publisher: Zoe Kruze
Acquisitions Editor: Ashlie M. Jackman
Editorial Project Manager: Joanna Collett
Production Project Manager: Vijayaraj Purushothaman
Cover Designer: Alan Studholme

Typeset by SPi Global, India

Contents

Contributors

Shasha Chen
School of Medicine and Institute for Immunology, Beijing Key Lab for Immunological Research on Chronic Diseases, Tsinghua University, Beijing, China

Zhongjun Dong
School of Medicine and Institute for Immunology, Beijing Key Lab for Immunological Research on Chronic Diseases, Tsinghua University, Beijing, China

Chengjiang Gao
State Key Laboratory of Microbial Technology, Key Laboratory of Infection and Immunity of Shandong Province & Department of Immunology, the School of Basic Medical Sciences, Shandong University, Jinan, Shandong, China

Tao Gong
Hefei National Laboratory for Physical Sciences at Microscale, CAS Key Laboratory of Innate Immunity and Chronic Disease, School of Basic Medical Sciences, Division of Life Science and Medicine, University of Science and Technology of China, Hefei, China

Xiaoyu Hu
Institute for Immunology and School of Medicine; Beijing Key Laboratory for Immunological Research on Chronic Diseases, Tsinghua University, Beijing, China

Liangliang Ji
Institute for Immunology and School of Medicine; Beijing Key Laboratory for Immunological Research on Chronic Diseases; Tsinghua-Peking Center for Life Sciences, School of Life Sciences, Tsinghua University, Beijing, China

Hua Jiang
Hefei National Laboratory for Physical Sciences at Microscale, CAS Key Laboratory of Innate Immunity and Chronic Disease, School of Basic Medical Sciences, Division of Life Science and Medicine, University of Science and Technology of China, Hefei, China

Zhengfan Jiang
Key Laboratory of Cell Proliferation and Differentiation of the Ministry of Education, School of Life Sciences; Peking-Tsinghua Center for Life Sciences, Peking University, Beijing, China

Lan Kang
Institute for Immunology and School of Medicine; Beijing Key Laboratory for Immunological Research on Chronic Diseases; Joint Graduate Program of Peking-Tsinghua-NIBS, School of Life Sciences, Tsinghua University, Beijing, China

Dan Li
School of Medicine and Institute for Immunology, Beijing Key Lab for Immunological Research on Chronic Diseases, Tsinghua University, Beijing, China

Qiaozhen Li
School of Medicine and Institute for Immunology, Beijing Key Lab for Immunological Research on Chronic Diseases, Tsinghua University, Beijing, China

Shaonan Liang
Institute for Immunology and School of Medicine; Beijing Key Laboratory for Immunological Research on Chronic Diseases, Tsinghua University, Beijing, China

Mengze Lv
Key Laboratory of Cell Proliferation and Differentiation of the Ministry of Education, School of Life Sciences; Peking-Tsinghua Center for Life Sciences, Peking University, Beijing, China

Hui Peng
Division of Molecular Medicine, Hefei National Laboratory for Physical Sciences at Microscale, The CAS Key Laboratory of Innate Immunity and Chronic Disease, School of Life Sciences; Institute of Immunology, University of Science and Technology of China, Hefei, Anhui, China

Hong-Bing Shu
Department of Infectious Diseases, Medical Research Institute, Zhongnan Hospital of Wuhan University, Wuhan University, Wuhan, China

Zhigang Tian
Division of Molecular Medicine, Hefei National Laboratory for Physical Sciences at Microscale, The CAS Key Laboratory of Innate Immunity and Chronic Disease, School of Life Sciences; Institute of Immunology, University of Science and Technology of China, Hefei, Anhui, China

Chenguang Wang
Key Laboratory of Cell Proliferation and Differentiation of the Ministry of Education, School of Life Sciences; Peking-Tsinghua Center for Life Sciences, Peking University, Beijing, China

Yuande Wang
School of Medicine and Institute for Immunology, Beijing Key Lab for Immunological Research on Chronic Diseases, Tsinghua University, Beijing, China

Xiaoming Wei
Key Laboratory of Cell Proliferation and Differentiation of the Ministry of Education, School of Life Sciences; Peking-Tsinghua Center for Life Sciences, Peking University, Beijing, China

Qing Yang
Department of Infectious Diseases, Medical Research Institute, Zhongnan Hospital of Wuhan University, Wuhan University, Wuhan, China

Rui Zhang
Key Laboratory of Cell Proliferation and Differentiation of the Ministry of Education, School of Life Sciences; Peking-Tsinghua Center for Life Sciences, Peking University, Beijing, China

Yi Zheng
State Key Laboratory of Microbial Technology, Key Laboratory of Infection and Immunity of Shandong Province & Department of Immunology, the School of Basic Medical Sciences, Shandong University, Jinan, Shandong, China

Jing Zhou
Division of Molecular Medicine, Hefei National Laboratory for Physical Sciences at Microscale, The CAS Key Laboratory of Innate Immunity and Chronic Disease, School of Life Sciences; Institute of Immunology, University of Science and Technology of China, Hefei, Anhui, China

Rongbin Zhou
Hefei National Laboratory for Physical Sciences at Microscale, CAS Key Laboratory of Innate Immunity and Chronic Disease, School of Basic Medical Sciences, Division of Life Science and Medicine; CAS Centre for Excellence in Cell and Molecular Biology, University of Science and Technology of China, Hefei, China

CHAPTER ONE

Deciphering the pathways to antiviral innate immunity and inflammation

Qing Yang, Hong-Bing Shu*

Department of Infectious Diseases, Medical Research Institute, Zhongnan Hospital of Wuhan University, Wuhan University, Wuhan, China

*Corresponding author: e-mail address: shuh@whu.edu.cn

Contents

Abstract

The antiviral innate immune and inflammatory responses are critical for host defense against viral infection. How these antiviral responses are initiated and regulated has been intensively investigated. Viral nucleic acids are sensed by pattern-recognition receptors (PRRs), which trigger various signaling pathways by utilizing distinct adaptor

Advances in Immunology, Volume 145
ISSN 0065-2776
https://doi.org/10.1016/bs.ai.2019.11.001

proteins, kinases and regulatory proteins. These pathways lead to activation of the transcriptional factors NF-κB and IRF3 and ultimate induction of antiviral effector proteins including type I interferons (IFNs), TNF and IL-1β, which are critical mediators of antiviral innate immune and inflammatory responses. For the past 20 years, our groups at Peking University and Wuhan University have made restless efforts in deciphering the molecular mechanisms of antiviral innate immune and inflammatory responses. Here, we summarize the major discoveries from our groups, including the identifications of the critical adaptors VISA/MAVS and MITA/STING, regulatory mechanisms of these adapter-mediated signaling, and regulation of TNF- and IL1β-triggered inflammatory responses.

1. Introduction

The mammalian immune defense against viral infection is consisted of innate and adaptive immune arms. The innate immune response is the first-line of host defense against viral infection, which is initiated upon sensing of viral conserved structural components called pathogen-associated molecular patterns (PAMPs) by pattern recognition receptors (PRRs) of host cells. The sensing of viral PAMPs by PRRs activates a series of signaling events, leading to induction of downstream antiviral effector proteins including type I interferons (IFNs) and proinflammatory cytokines (Akira, Uematsu, & Takeuchi, 2006; Hu & Shu, 2018, 2019). These effector proteins are not only essential for innate antiviral responses, but are also important for the maturation and activation of antigen-presenting cells, such as dendritic cells (DCs), which promote adaptive immune response to fully clear the invaded viruses and infected cells (Janeway, 1989).

The most important PAMPs of viruses are viral nucleic acids, which are sensed by several different PRRs. The best characterized PRRs in antiviral responses include the Toll-like receptor (TLR) family members and the RIG-I-like receptors (RLRs) (Akira, 2006; Osorio & Reis e Sousa, 2011). In addition, other PRRs which do not fall into these families also exist. The most known example is the cyclic GMP-AMP synthase (cGAS), which acts as a sensor for cytosolic viral DNA (Li et al., 2013; Sun, Wu, Du, Chen, & Chen, 2013). The different types of PRRs are located in distinct cellular compartments, including the plasma membrane, endosome, cytosol and nucleus (Takeuchi & Akira, 2010). These features account for the capacities of the cell to sense viral PAMPs from extracellular environment or various intracellular compartments.

Upon detection of viral nucleic acids, the PRRs initiate signaling events that involve distinct adaptor proteins, kinases and transcription factors, leading to induction of downstream antiviral effector proteins and innate immune responses (Takeuchi & Akira, 2010). Furthermore, these PRR-mediated innate immune responses are tightly and delicately regulated in a spatial and temporal manner by multiple post-translational modifications of the signaling components, including phosphorylation, polyubiquitination, sumoylation, acetylation and glutamylation (Liu, Qian, & Cao, 2016). These mechanisms ensure the optimal activation of innate immune responses and their timely termination to avoid tissue damages and/or autoimmune diseases.

Proinflammatory cytokines, such as TNF and IL1β, are important downstream effector proteins induced by viral infection. These cytokines bind to their respective receptors and further induce downstream inflammatory genes, leading to inflammatory responses. Signaling of TNF- and IL1β-triggered inflammation is also heavily regulated by post-translational modifications to avoid immune damage and autoimmune diseases.

Dr. Shu has worked on inflammatory and innate immune responses for 24 years. During his post-doctoral training with Dr. David Goeddel at Tularik Inc. at South San Francisco, Dr. Shu deciphered the early molecular events of TNF-triggered NF-κB activation and apoptosis. After establishing his own laboratory at National Jewish Medical and Research Center (now National Jewish Health) at Denver in 1998, Dr. Shu's group identified two new members of the TNF family, which they called TNF- and ApoL-related leukocyte expressed ligand 1 (TALL-1, also called Blys, BAFF, THANK) and TALL-2 (also called APRIL). They also identified B cell maturation protein (BCMA) is a receptor of TALL-1. In addition, they deciphered the signaling mechanisms triggered by TALL-1 and another TNF family member called TRAIL. In 2000, Dr. Shu joined Peking University as a Changjiang Professor and then in 2005, moved to Wuhan University to serve as the dean of College of Life Sciences. Since the establishment of our laboratories firstly at Peking University in 2000 and then at Wuhan University in 2005, our group has made restless efforts in deciphering the molecular mechanisms of antiviral innate immune and inflammatory responses. After returning to China, Dr. Shu's group has mostly focused on mechanisms of antiviral innate immune responses and regulation of TNF- and IL1β-triggered inflammation. In this review, we summarize the major discoveries from our groups in China, including the identifications of the critical adaptor proteins virus-induced signaling adaptor

(VISA)/mitochondrial antiviral signaling (MAVS) and mediator of IRF3 activation (MITA)/stimulator of interferon genes (STING), regulatory mechanisms of VISA/MAVS-, MITA/STING- and TRIF-mediated signaling, and regulation of TNF- and IL1β-triggered inflammatory responses.

2. RLR-VISA-mediated innate immune response

Two members of the RLR family, RIG-I and MDA5, act as the major cytoplasmic viral sensors. RLRs are consisted of two N-terminal tandemly linked caspase activation and recruitment domains (CARDs), a DEAD box helicase domain and a C-terminal regulatory domain (CTD) (Takeuchi & Akira, 2010). RIG-I prefers to recognizes viral 5′-ppp double-strand (ds) RNA and short dsRNA, while MDA5 preferentially detects long dsRNA (Gitlin et al., 2006; Hornung et al., 2006; Pichlmair et al., 2006). Various studies have shown that RIG-I is responsible for sensing infection of Sendai virus (SeV), vesicular stomatitis virus (VSV), Newcastle disease virus (NDV), and influenza virus, while MDA5 appears to mostly detect infection of picornaviruses, such as encephalomyocarditis virus (EMCV) (Kato et al., 2006). Infection of some RNA viruses, such as Dengue virus (DENV), can be sensed by both RIG-I and MDA5 (Loo et al., 2008). In the past 20 years, we have made tremendous efforts to decipher the mechanisms and regulations of RLR-mediated innate immune response (Fig. 1).

2.1 Identification of the key adaptor protein VISA and its associated components

It has been well established that sensing of viral RNA by RLRs activates the kinases TBK1/IKKε and IKK, leading to activation of the transcription factors IRF3 and NF-κB (Hiscott et al., 2003). However, how RLRs activate two distinct downstream pathways was not known until our discovery of VISA in 2005 (Xu et al., 2005). In expression screens for proteins that activate NF-κB, we identified VISA. VISA is a 540 aa protein, which contains an N-terminal CARD domain and a C-terminal transmembrane (TM) domain. Overexpression of VISA potently activates NF-κB and IRF3, suggesting a critical role of VISA in innate immune responses. Knockdown of VISA dramatically inhibits SeV-induced transcription of downstream antiviral genes, suggesting that VISA is essential for innate immune response to RNA virus. Biochemical experiments indicate that upon binding of viral RNA, RIG-I is recruited to VISA through their respective CARD domains. After that, VISA recruits several TRAF family

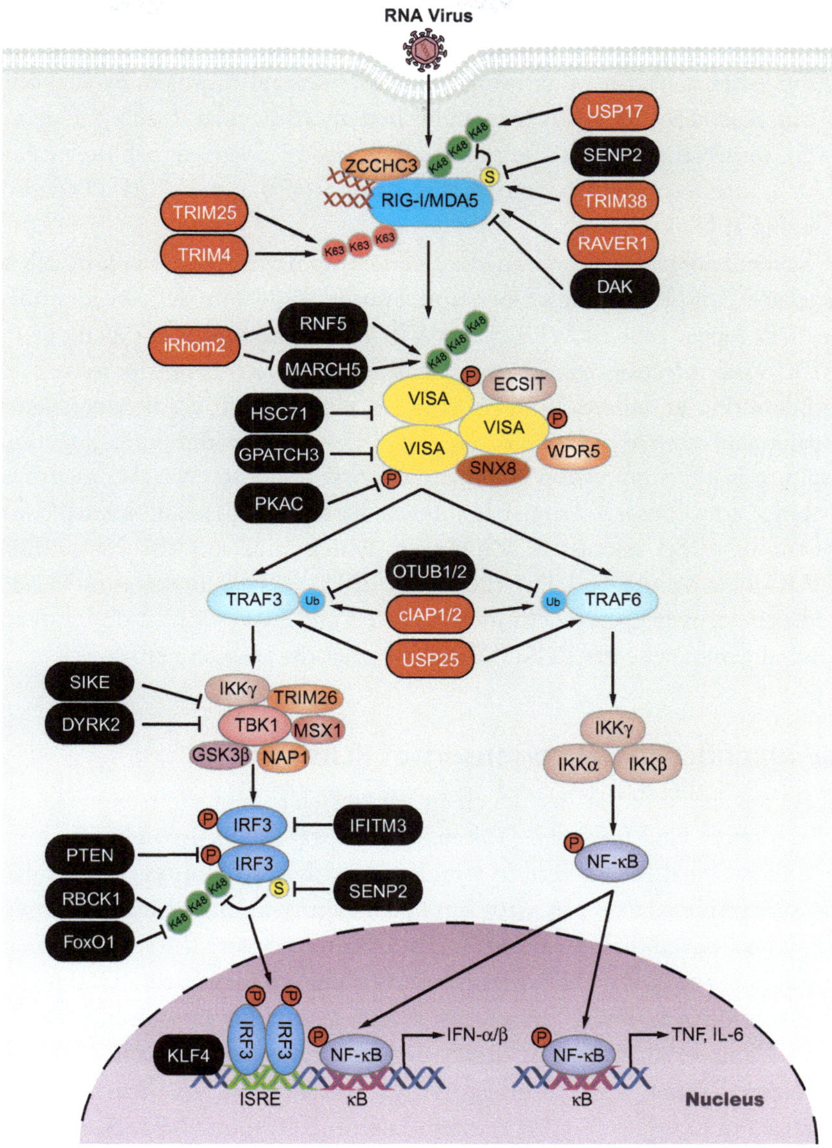

Fig. 1 Molecular mechanisms and regulation of RLR-VISA-mediated innate immune response. Viral RNA in the cytosol is recognized by the RLR family members RIG-I and MDA5. These receptors signal through the VISA/MAVS-TRAFs complex to activate both TBK1-IRF3 and IKKα/β/γ-NF-κB axes for production of type I IFNs and inflammatory cytokines. RLR-mediated signaling is regulated by distinct components and posttranslational modifications as indicated in the figure to ensure proper innate antiviral response.

proteins TRAF2/3/6 to activate downstream kinases IKK and TBK1/IKKε, leading to induction of downstream antiviral genes (Xu et al., 2005). After a lengthy reviewing process at several journals, by the time of our discovery of VISA was published in Molecular Cell (Xu et al., 2005), three other groups also reported the same protein, which they called MAVS, interferon-beta promoter stimulator 1 (IPS-1) and CARD adaptor inducing IFN-β (Cardif).

Several molecules have been identified as important components in VISA-associated complex. Using a biochemical purification approach, we identified the WD repeat protein WDR5 as a VISA-associated protein (Wang et al., 2010). Viral infection triggers translocation of WDR5 from the nucleus to mitochondria at where WDR5 interacts with VISA. WDR5-deficiency impairs the assembly of VISA-associated complexes after viral infection, resulting in the suppression of innate antiviral response. We also identified evolutionarily conserved signaling intermediate (ECSIT) as an essential component of VISA-associated complexes, which mediates the recruitment of RIG-I or MDA5 to VISA (Lei et al., 2015). Overexpression of ECSIT promotes virus-triggered activation of IRF3 and expression of downstream antiviral genes, whereas ECSIT-deficiency has the opposite effects.

2.2 Identification of co-sensors of RLRs

RLRs are expressed at low levels in various cells, and their expression is induced after viral infection (Takeuchi & Akira, 2010). In addition, it has been shown that RLRs bind to viral RNA with low affinities. How innate immune response to RNA virus can be efficiently mounted was unknown. We hypothesized that co-sensors might exist to promote the recognition of viral RNA by RLRs. By expression screening, we identified ZCCHC3, a CCHC-type zinc-finger protein, as a co-receptor for RIG-I and MDA5 (Lian, Zang, et al., 2018). ZCCHC3-deficiency causes reduction of type I IFNs and other antiviral effectors in response to RNA virus infection in vitro and in vivo. ZCCHC3 interacts with RIG-I and MDA5, and regulates their activities in two different manners. In one hand, ZCCHC3 binds to dsRNA and promotes the RNA binding activities of RIG-I and MDA5. In the other hand, ZCCHC3 enhances the recruitment of the E3 ubiquitin ligase TRIM25 to RIG-I and MDA5 to facilitate their K63-linked polyubiquitination and activation. Though RIG-I and MDA5 are structurally related and mediate similar signaling pathways, we found that ribonucleoprotein PTB-binding 1 (RAVER1) could act as a specific co-activator for MDA5 (Chen et al., 2013). RAVER1 specially enhances RNA binding of MDA5 but not RIG-I. Viral RNA or its analog triggers the association of RAVER1 with MDA5 in cells. Overexpression of RAVER1 enhances MDA5- but not RIG-I-mediated activation of the IFN-β promoter, whereas RAVER1-deficiency inhibits MDA5- but not RIG-I-mediated induction of downstream antiviral genes.

2.3 Identification of TBK1-activating components

TBK1 is a kinase that mediates IRF3 activation of viral infection, therefore plays a key role in innate antiviral response. We identified several proteins that modulate TBK1 activity. Glycogen synthase kinase 3β (GSK3β) is a serine/threonine kinase that is involved in various biological processes, including such as metabolism, cell cycle, transcription regulation, vesicular transport, neuronal function, oncogenesis, and development (Jope & Johnson, 2004). Viral infection induces the association of GSK3β with TBK1. Importantly, GSK3β facilitates TBK1 self-association and autophosphorylation at S172, which is critical for virus-induced IRF3 activation and IFN-β induction. Interestingly, the effects of GSK3β on virus-induced signaling are independent of its kinase activity. Deficiency of GSK3β impairs virus-induced IRF3 activation, transcription of antiviral genes, as well as cellular antiviral response (Lei et al., 2010). Our findings suggest a critical role of GSK3β in innate antiviral response.

Muscle segment homeobox1 (MSX1) is another important modulator of assembly of TBK1-associated complexes (Chen, Hu, Xu, Liu, & Shu, 2016). Viral infection induces translocation of MSX1 from the nucleus to mitochondria, at where it modulates the formation of TBK1-associated complexes. MSX1-deficiency impairs virus-triggered activation of TBK1 and IRF3, expression of downstream antiviral genes, and cellular antiviral responses.

The E3 ubiquitin ligase tripartite motif 26 (TRIM26) was also identified as an important regulator of TBK1 (Ran et al., 2016). TRIM26 is constitutively associated with TBK1. Viral infection induces autoubiquitination of TRIM26. The polyubiquitin chains of TRIM26 links NEMO to TBK1, and promotes the subsequent recruitment of TBK1 to VISA-associated complexes. Knockdown of TRIM26 impairs virus-triggered activation of IRF3 and NF-κB, induction of IFN-β, and cellular antiviral response.

2.4 Regulatory mechanisms of the RLR-VISA axis

The RLR-VISA axis is temporally and spatially regulated by a series of distinct mechanisms to achieve the optimal outcomes of innate immune responses to RNA viruses. Each components of the RLR-VISA axis are regulated by both similar and distinct mechanisms, which contributes to the complications and delicate of innate immune responses to RNA viruses.

2.4.1 Regulation of RLR activities

Various studies have shown that RLRs are regulated by post-translational modifications. It has been reported that RIG-I and MDA5 are dephosphorylated by the phosphatase PP1 and conjugated with K63-linked polyubiquitin chains by TRIM25, RNF135, TRIM4 and/or TRIM65 (Gack et al., 2007; Lang et al., 2017; Oshiumi et al., 2010; Yan, Li, Mao, Hu, & Shu, 2014).

Both RIG-1 and MDA5 are also critically regulated by sumoylation and desumuoylation. We found that the TRIM family member TRIM38 acts as a SUMO E3 ligase for dynamic sumoylation of RIG-I at K43/K865 and MDA5 at K96/K888 before and after viral infection (Hu, Liao, Yang, Xie, & Shu, 2017). The sumoylation of MDA5 and RIG-I suppresses their K48-linked polyubiquitination and degradation in uninfected or early-infected cells. Sumoylation of the CARD domains of MDA5 and RIG-I is also required for their dephosphorylation by PP1 and activation upon viral infection. At the late phase of viral infection, both MDA5 and RIG-I are desumoylated by deSUMOylating enzyme Sentrin/SUMO-specific protease 2 (SENP2), resulting in their K48-linked polyubiquitination and degradation. These findings suggest that dynamic sumoylation and desumoylation of MDA5 and RIG-I modulate efficient innate immunity to RNA virus and its timely termination.

Deubiquitination may also play a role in regulating RLR activities. We found that the deubiquitinating enzyme ubiquitin-specific protease 17 (USP17) promotes RIG-I- and MDA5-mediated induction of type I IFN through deubiquitinating RIG-I and MDA5 (Chen et al., 2010). Knockdown of USP17 results in an increase in ubiquitination levels of RIG-I and MDA5. Consistently, USP17-deficiency inhibits RNA virus-induced expression of the type I IFNs and cellular antiviral responses. Although RIG-I and MDA5 are regulated by many common regulators and mechanisms, they can also be regulated differentially. We identified a functionally unknown dihydroacetone kinase (DAK) as a specific MDA5-associated protein (Diao et al., 2007). DAK is associated with MDA5 but not RIG-I under physiological conditions. Knockdown of endogenous DAK increased cytoplasmic dsRNA- or SeV-triggered activation of the IFN-β.

2.4.2 Regulation of VISA-mediated signaling

VISA acts as a central adaptor in the RLR-mediated innate antiviral pathways. It has been demonstrated that VISA is activated by forming prion-like aggregates (Hou et al., 2011), and disassembly of VISA aggregates or VISA-associated complexes is an important strategy for host cells to terminate innate antiviral response. We found that sorting nexin 8 (SNX8) promotes antiviral response by facilitating VISA aggregation (Guo, Wei, Shu, & Yang, 2019), while heat shock cognate 71 (HSC71) regulates cellular antiviral response by impairing the formation of VISA aggregates (Liu et al., 2013). Overexpression of HSC71 results in inhibition of virus-triggered transcription of *IFNB1* gene and cellular antiviral response, while knock-down of HSC71 has opposite effects. G patch domain-containing protein 3 (GPATCH3) was also reported to disrupt the assembly of VISA-associated complexes. Viral infection triggers recruitment of GPATCH3 to VISA, which impairs the assembly of VISA/TRAF6/TBK1 signalosomes and subsequent innate antiviral response (Nie et al., 2017).

Regulation of VISA stability is also a critical mechanism to ensure its optimal activation. Several E3 ubiquitin ligases, including MARCH5, RNF5 and AIP4, have been reported to mediate VISA degradation (Yoo et al., 2015; You et al., 2009; Zhong et al., 2010; Zhou, You, Chen, & Jiang, 2012). How these E3 ligases are orchestrated in regulation of VISA stability before and after viral infection remains enigmatic until recently. We found that iRhom2 acts as a checkpoint for the ER-associated degradation (ERAD) or mitochondria-associated degradation (MAD) of VISA, which ensures proper innate immune response to RNA virus (Luo et al., 2017). In un-infected and early-infected cells, iRhom2 mediates auto-ubiquitination and degradation of the E3 ubiquitin ligase RNF5 and impairs the assembly of VISA-RNF5-GP78 complexes, thereby ERAD of VISA. In the late phase of viral infection, iRhom2 mediates proteasome-dependent degradation of the E3 ubiquitin ligase MARCH5 and impairs MAD of VISA. Maintenance of VISA stability by iRhom2 ensures efficient innate antiviral response at the early phase of viral infection.

The stability of VISA is also regulated by phosphorylation of its CARD domain. We identified the protein kinase A catalytic (PKAC) subunits α and β as negative regulators of VISA-mediated signaling in a redundant manner (Yan et al., 2017). Viral infection triggers increase of cellular cAMP levels and subsequent activation of PKACs, which then phosphorylates VISA at T54. This phosphorylation abrogates virus-induced aggregation of VISA and primes it for K48-linked polyubiquitination and degradation by the

E3 ligase MARCH5, resulting in attenuation of expression of downstream antiviral genes. Consistently, PKACs-deficiency promotes innate immune response to RNA viral infection in vitro and in vivo.

2.4.3 Regulation of the TRAF proteins

Several TRAF proteins, including TRAF2, TRAF3 and TRAF6, have been demonstrated to link VISA to downstream kinases (Park, 2018). Ubiquitination and deubiquitination of the TRAF proteins have emerged as critical post-translational regulatory mechanisms for the VISA-mediated signaling. We found that virus-triggered ubiquitination of TRAF3 and TRAF6 by cIAP1 and cIAP2 is essential for type I IFN induction and cellular antiviral response (Mao et al., 2010), while deubiquitination of TRAF3/6 by OTUB1 and OTUB2 exhibits the opposite effects (Li et al., 2010). In addition, we found that USP25 is induced upon viral infection, which is associated with TRAF3 and TRAF6 and inhibits proteasome-dependent or independent degradation of TRAF3 and TRAF6. Consistently, USP25-deficient cells produces lower levels of type I IFNs upon viral infection and USP25-deficient mice are more susceptible to H5N1 or HSV-1 infection (Lin et al., 2015).

2.4.4 Regulation of the TBK1/IKKε kinases

TBK1 and IKKε are two structurally conserved kinases that function in almost all signaling IRF3/7 activating pathways. Regulation of the activities of these two kinases has also been reported. We identified a protein termed suppressor of IKKε (SIKE) that interacts with IKKε and TBK1 (Huang et al., 2005). SIKE is associated with TBK1 under physiological conditions and viral infection triggers dissociation of SIKE from TBK1. Overexpression of SIKE disrupts the interactions of IKKε or TBK1 with IRF-3, and inhibits virus-triggered IRF3 activation and cellular antiviral response, whereas knockdown of SIKE exhibits the opposite effects. We also identified dual-specificity tyrosine-(Y)-phosphorylation-regulated kinase 2 (DYRK2) as a negative regulator of virus-triggered innate immune response by promoting phosphorylation of TBK1 at S527 and its subsequent degradation of by the NLRP4-DTX4 E3 ligase complex (An et al., 2015).

2.4.5 Regulation of IRF3 activity

Upon viral infection, IRF3 undergoes phosphorylation at S396 by TBK1, and subsequent dimerization as well as translocation into the nucleus for antiviral gene induction. Multiple mechanisms have been reported to regulate the subcellular location, DNA binding activity, and stability of IRF3 (Taniguchi, Ogasawara, Takaoka, & Tanaka, 2001; Taniguchi & Takaoka, 2002). Phosphatase and tensin homolog (PTEN) was identified as an IRF3-interacting protein and dephosphorylates IRF3 at S97, which is essential for IRF3 import into the nucleus (Li et al., 2016).

We also found that Krüppel-like factor 4 (KLF4) negatively regulates virus-triggered signaling by inhibiting the recruitment of IRF3 to the *IFNB* promoter (Luo, Lian, Zhong, Shu, & Li, 2016). KLF4 is localized in both the cytosol and nucleus, and viral infection triggers translocation of KLF4 from cytosol to nucleus, where it binds to the promoter of *IFNB* gene and impairs the recruitment of IRF3 to the *IFNB* gene promoter in response to viral infection, leading to suppression of innate antiviral response.

Degradation of IRF3 is also an important strategy for host cells to timely terminate the production of type I IFNs in response to viral infection. We found that IFITM3 plays important roles in regulating RNA virus-triggered production of IFN-β by mediating autophagic degradation of IRF3 (Jiang et al., 2018). In addition to autophagic degradation, IRF3 can also be degraded by the ubiquitin-proteasomal pathway. We found that the E3 ubiquitin ligase RBCC protein interacting with PKC1 (RBCK1) catalyzes the ubiquitination and degradation of IRF3 after viral infection (Zhang et al., 2008). In addition, FoxO1 also negatively regulates cellular antiviral response by promoting degradation of IRF3 (Lei et al., 2013). Following viral infection, FoxO1 is associated with IRF3 and promotes K48-linked polyubiquitination and degradation of IRF3 in the cytosol. The E3 ligase responsible for FoxO1-mediated IRF3 polyubiquitination is currently unknown.

Previously, it has been demonstrated that sumoylation of IRF3 regulates its stability and activation (Kubota et al., 2008). We identified SENP2 as a negative regulator of virus-triggered IFN-β induction by deSUMOylating IRF3 and conditioning it for ubiquitination and degradation (Ran et al., 2011). Both the SUMOylation and K48-linked ubiquitination of IRF3 occur at K70 and K87, and these processes are competitive. SENP2 causes IRF3 deSUMOylation, K48-linked ubiquitination and degradation, thereby negatively regulates innate antiviral response.

3. cGAS-MITA-mediated innate immune response

Upon DNA virus infection, viral DNA is sensed by cellular receptors to initiate innate immune response. It has been demonstrated that DAI

(Takaoka et al., 2007), DDX41 (Zhang et al., 2011), IFI16 (Unterholzner et al., 2010), Sox2 (Xia et al., 2015) and LSM14A (Li et al., 2012) can detect viral DNA at various cellular localizations to initiate innate immune response. However, it is believed that the mostly used DNA sensor in host cells is cGAS, a 522 aa protein containing an N-terminal unstructured and highly positively charged domain and a C-terminal nucleotidyltransferase (NTase) domain (Sun et al., 2013). Both the N- and C-terminal domains of cGAS bind to DNA (Du & Chen, 2018; Tao et al., 2017; Zhang, Lei, et al., 2014). Once binding to DNA, the catalytic pocket of cGAS undergoes a structural rearrangement, leading to the synthesis of 2′3′-cGAMP from ATP and GTP with one phosphodiester bond between the 2′- hydroxyl of GMP and 5′-phosphate of AMP and another between the 3′-hydroxyl of AMP and 5′-phosphate of GMP (Ablasser et al., 2013; Gao, Ascano, Wu, et al., 2013; Sun et al., 2013). In the past dozen of years, we have investigated how innate immune response to DNA virus is efficiently mount and timely terminated, including discovery of the critical adaptor protein MITA/STING (Fig. 2).

3.1 Identification of MITA

In 2008, we performed expression cloning experiments and identified MITA as a critical mediator of virus-triggered type I IFN induction (Zhong et al., 2008). This protein was also reported by another group, which was named as STING (Ishikawa, Ma, & Barber, 2009). MITA is a 379 aa protein consisting of several transmembrane domains at its N-terminus. MITA is expressed in various cell types and tissues. MITA recruits TBK1 and IRF3 upon viral infection. In the MITA-associated complex, MITA is firstly phosphorylated by TBK1, which is required for IRF3 phosphorylation by TBK1. Knockdown of MITA inhibits type I IFNs triggered by synthetic RNA and DNA (Ishikawa et al., 2009; Zhong et al., 2008). Various studies have well established that MITA mediates innate immune responses to DNA in the cytosol originated from pathogens, derived from aberrant self-DNA or leaked from mitochondria (Luo & Shu, 2018; Ran, Shu, & Wang, 2014). Upon sensing of cytosolic DNA by cGAS, the synthesized cGAMP binds to MITA. This causes cellular trafficking and activation of MITA, leading to activation of IRF3 and induction of downstream antiviral genes (Dobbs et al., 2015). It has also been demonstrated that MITA acts as an sensor for cyclic di-AMP (*c*-di-AMP) and cyclic di-GMP (*c*-di-GMP) derived from bacteria like *Listeria monocytogenes*

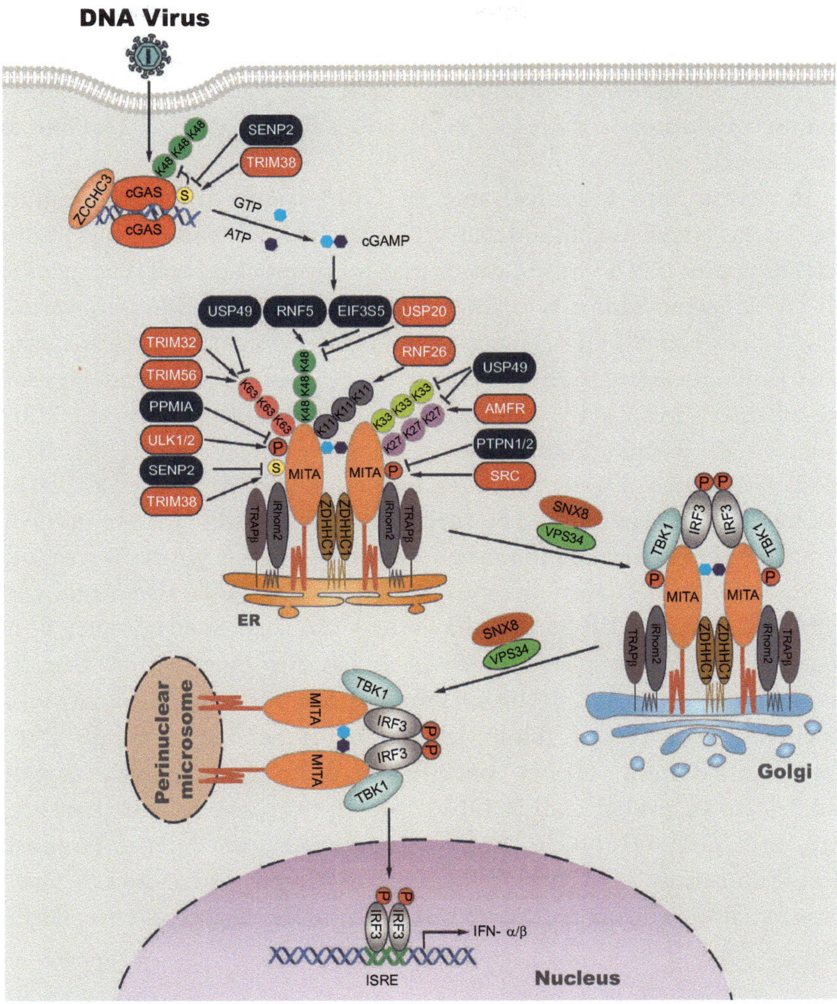

Fig. 2 Molecular mechanisms and regulation of cGAS-MITA-mediated innate immune response. After binding to DNA, cGAS utilizes ATP and GTP as substrates to synthesize cGAMP, which binds to the ER-located MITA. MITA is then translocated via the Golgi apparatus to perinuclear punctate structures. This step requires the iRhom2-TRAP complex. During the translocation process, TBK1 and IRF3 are recruited to the MITA complexes, leading to the phosphorylation and activation of IRF3 as well as to the eventual induction of type I IFNs. The cGAS-MITA axis is heavily regulated by various posttranslational modifications, such as polyubiquitination, sumoylation, and phosphorylation as indicated in the figure. These posttranslational modifications are important for regulating the stability and activation of components involved in the cGAS-MITA axis, ensuring efficient onset of the innate immune response to DNA and its timely termination to avoid host damage.

(Andrade et al., 2016; Burdette et al., 2011; Ergun, Fernandez, Weiss, & Li, 2019; Moretti et al., 2017; Yin et al., 2012), or small molecules such as DMXAA (5,6-dimethylxanthenone-4-acetic acid, Vadimezan) that exhibits immune modulatory activities (Gao, Ascano, Zillinger, et al., 2013; Prantner et al., 2012).

In addition to a critical role in DNA-triggered innate immune response, it is well established that MITA also plays important roles in host defense against RNA viruses, which may be virus or host cell type specific. MITA-deficiency impairs innate innate immune responses to various RNA viruses including Sendai virus (SeV), vesicular stomatitis virus (VSV), dengue virus (DENV), West Nile virus (WNV), and Japanese encephalitis virus (JEV) (Aguirre et al., 2012; Ishikawa et al., 2009; Ishikawa & Barber, 2008; Nazmi, Mukhopadhyay, Dutta, & Basu, 2012; Ni, Ma, & Damania, 2018; Sun et al., 2009; You et al., 2013; Zhong et al., 2008, 2009). The mechanisms responsible for the involvement of MITA in innate immune responses to RNA viruses is not fully understood. It has been demonstrated that MITA is associated with VISA and recruits TBK1 and IRF3 to the VISA-associated complex upon viral infection (Zhong et al., 2008). It has also been shown that the involvement of MITA in innate immune responses to RNA viruses is independent of RIG-I (Holm et al., 2012; Schoggins et al., 2011, 2014). In addition, DENV infection leads to mitochondria damage and release of mitochondrial DNA into the cytosol, which then activates the cGAS–STING pathway to potentiate host defense responses (Sun, Sundstrom, et al., 2017). MITA has also been proposed to play a role for host sensing of virus-cell membrane fusion events (Holm et al., 2012).

3.2 Modulation of the cGAS-MITA axis

Similar as RLRs, cGAS is lowly expressed in cells and binds to dsDNA with low affinity (Civril et al., 2013; Li et al., 2013). We found that ZCCHC3 can also serve as a co-receptor of cGAS (Lian, Wei, et al., 2018). ZCCHC3 binds to dsDNA and promotes the binding of cGAS to dsDNA following viral infection. ZCCHC3-deficiency inhibits dsDNA-triggered induction of downstream effector genes. ZCCHC3-deficient mice are more susceptible to lethal HSV-1 or vaccinia virus (VACV) infection.

Sensing of DNA by cGAS causes synthesis of cGAMP, which acts as a second messenger molecule and binds to the ER-associated transmembrane adaptor protein MITA/STING (Ishikawa et al., 2009; Zhang et al., 2008).

In un-infected cells, MITA is retained at the ER by the $Ca2^{+}$ sensor STIM1 via direct interaction (Srikanth et al., 2019). STIM1-deficiency causes spontaneous activation of MITA and enhanced expression of type I IFNs under resting conditions in cells and mice (Srikanth et al., 2019). After binding to cGAMP, MITA undergoes structural rearrangement and oligomerization (Zhang et al., 2019). MITA then interacts with the Sec5/TRAPβ/Sec61β translocon complex, resulting in translocation of the MITA-associated complex to ER-Golgi intermediate compartments (ERGICs). At the ERGIC, the TBK1 kinase and the transcriptional factor IRF3 are recruited to MITA via two distinct motifs. In this complex, TBK1 firstly catalyzes phosphorylation of MITA at S366 and then IRF3 at S396, leading to IRF3 dimerization and translocation into the nucleus for induction of downstream effector genes (Dobbs et al., 2015; Ishikawa et al., 2009). Furthermore, MITA is translocated to perinuclear punctate structures, where it undergoes lysosome-dependent degradation, which contributes to the termination of innate immune response (Konno, Konno, & Barber, 2013).

How MITA undergoes oligomerization and trafficking from the ER to ERGIC have been investigated in past years. The ER-associated protein ZDHHC1 is one of the critical proteins for MITA oligomerization (Zhou et al., 2014). ZDHHC1 is constitutively associated with MITA, which is important for the oligomerization of MITA and recruitment of downstream signaling components TBK1 and IRF3. Consistently, ZDHHC1-deficient mice produce less type I IFNs and other cytokines and exhibit higher lethality in response to HSV-1 infection.

The inactive rhomboid protein 2 (iRhom2) also plays an important role in modulating MITA activity (Luo, Li, et al., 2016). iRhom2 is constitutively associated with MITA and acts in two distinct processes to regulate MITA activity. iRhom2 mediates the interaction of MITA with the translocon-associated protein TRAPβ, which facilitates trafficking of MITA from the ER via ERGIC to perinuclear punctate structures. iRhom2 also recruits the deubiquitination enzyme EIF3S5 to maintain the stability of STING via removal of its K48-linked polyubiquitin chains. Consistently, iRhom2-deficiency impairs DNA virus- and cytosolic DNA-triggered induction of downstream antiviral genes, and iRhom2-deficient mice are more susceptible to lethal HSV-1 infection. In addition to iRhom2, SNX8 has been reported to recruit the class III phosphatylinositol 3-kinase VPS34 to MITA and facilitate trafficking of MITA from the ER to perinuclear punctate structures (Wei et al., 2018). Consistently, $Snx8^{-/-}$ mice exhibits lower serum cytokine levels and higher viral titers in the brains, resulting in higher lethality in response to HSV-1 infection.

3.3 Regulation of the cGAS-MITA axis by distinct mechanisms

The cGAS-MITA pathways are heavily regulated by various mechanisms, particularly post-translational modifications including sumoylation, glutarylation, ubiquitination and phosphorylation (Fig. 2). These regulator mechanisms contribute to dynamic regulation of innate immune response to DNA virus.

3.3.1 Regulation of cGAS by sumoylation

cGAS activity is critically regulated by post-translational modifications. We found that cGAS is sumoylated at K217 in uninfected cells and further sumoylated at K464 in the early phase of DNA viral infection by TRIM38 (Hu et al., 2016). Sumoylation of cGAS at K217 suppresses its K48-linked polyubiquitination at K271 by physical hindrance to maintain the stability of cGAS in uninfected cells, while sumoylation of cGAS at K464 prevents its K48-linked polyubiquitination at the same residue to prevent its degradation by the ubiquitin-proteasomal pathway in the early phase of viral infection. The maintenance of cGAS stability in uninfected and early-infected cells is important for efficient mount of innate antiviral response in the early phase of infection. In the late phase of infection, the SUMO moieties of cGAS at K217 and K464 are removed by the desumoylating enzyme SENP2, leading to K48-linked polyubiquitination and proteasomal degradation of cGAS and thereby attenuation of innate antiviral response (Hu et al., 2016; Hu & Shu, 2017).

3.3.2 Regulation of MITA activity by divergent mechanisms

Post-translational regulation of MITA has also been heavily investigated in the past years. It has been demonstrated that phosphorylation of MITA at S358 primes for its recruitment of TBK1 (Zhong et al., 2008), while TBK1-mediated phosphorylation of MITA at Ser366 is critical for the recruitment of IRF3 to MITA upon viral infection (Liu et al., 2015). Conversely, the phosphatase PPM1A dephosphorylates MITA to suppress its activation in response to viral infection (Li et al., 2015). ULK1/2 has also been reported to catalyze the phosphorylation of MITA at S366, leading to suppression of MITA activity (Konno et al., 2013). Mutation of S366 to either alanine (A) or aspartate (D) abolishes MITA-mediated induction of type I IFNs (Konno et al., 2013). It is possible that MITA is phosphorylated by TBK1 or ULK1/2 at different phases of viral infection, and the same phosphorylation modification on different MITA modification/

complex context results in different functional outcomes (Hu et al., 2016). Recent studies suggest that MITA is also phosphorylated at Y245 by the tyrosine kinase SRC, which is critical for its dimerization and stability (Xia, Yi, Wu, Shang, & Shu, 2019). In the late phase of DNA virus infection, the tyrosine phosphatases PTPN1 and PTPN2 dephosphorylate MITA Y245, which results in its degradation by an ubiquitin-independent 20S proteasome pathway and attenuation of innate immune response to DNA (Xia et al., 2019).

Several different types of polyubiquitin modifications, including K63-, K48-, K11-, and K27-linked polyubiquitination, regulate MITA protein level and activity before and/or after viral infection (Shu & Wang, 2014). Interestingly, MITA K150 has been reported to be modified by all these different types of polyubiquitination, probably at different phases of viral infection. After viral infection, TRIM32 and TRIM56 catalyze K63-linked polyubiquitination of MITA (Zhang, Hu, Wang, & Shu, 2012), whereas AMFR promotes its K27-linked polyubiquitination (Wang et al., 2014). These types of polyubiquitination are important for its recruitment of TBK1, therefore contributes to the onset of innate antiviral response. The E3 ligase RNF5 catalyzes K48-linked polyubiquitination and proteasomal degradation of MITA to negatively regulate the innate antiviral response at the late phase of infection (Zhong et al., 2009). It has also been shown that the E3 ligase RNF26 promotes K11-linked polyubiquitination of MITA K150, a residue also targeted by RNF5 for K48-linked polyubiquitination (Qin et al., 2014). Therefore, RNF26 protects MITA from RNF5-mediated K48-linked polyubiquitination and degradation, which contributes to quick and efficient type I IFN and proinflammatory cytokine induction after viral infection (Qin et al., 2014).

Recently, several deubiquitination enzymes have been reported to deconjugate the polyubiquitin moieties of MITA. USP13 and USP49 have been reported to remove K27/33- and K63-linked polyubiquitin chains of MITA, respectively, to inhibit its activation (Sun, Zhang, et al., 2017), while USP20 removes K48-linked polyubiquitin chains from MITA to promote its stability and activation (Zhang et al., 2016). How these polyubiquitination and deubiquitination processes are spatially and temporally coordinated needs further investigation.

Viral infection also induces sumoylation of MITA at K337 by TRIM38, which is crucial for its oligomerization and activation as well as for maintenance of stability by inhibiting chaperone-mediated autophagy, leading to an optimal innate antiviral response (Hu et al., 2016). Phosphorylation of

MITA at S366 after viral infection facilitates recruitment of SENP2 for its desumoylation in the late phase of viral infection, leading to lysosomal degradation of MITA and negative regulation of the innate antiviral response (Hu et al., 2016).

MITA level can be regulated by ways not directly related to its post-translational modifications. We found the processing body-associated protein LSm14A regulates MITA level in a cell-specific manner (Liu, Qian, & Cao, 2016; Liu, Yang, et al., 2016). By generating LSm14A-deficient mice, we found that LSm14A plays a critical and specific role in the induction of antiviral cytokines in dendritic cells (DCs) but not in macrophages and fibroblasts. LSm14A-deficiency specifically downregulates MITA level in DCs by impairing its nuclear mRNA precursor processing. Induction of antiviral cytokines triggered by HSV-1 and murine herpesvirus 68 is impaired in *Lsm14a*$^{-/-}$ DCs. These findings reveal a nuclear mRNA precursor processing and cell-specific regulatory mechanism of MITA-mediated antiviral immune response.

3.4 HCMV immune evasion of the cGAS-MITA axis

Since the cGAS-MITA axis plays critical roles in innate immune response to DNA virus, various DNA viruses have evolved strategies to counteract this axis for evading the host immunity (Ma & Damania, 2016). Our studies on how human cytomegalovirus (HCMV) evades the cGAS-MITA axis provide excellent examples for viral evasion strategies (Fig. 3).

Using expression screens, we identified multiple HCMV proteins that can efficiently inhibit the cGAS-MITA axis. HCMV UL31 interacts directly with cGAS and disassociates viral DNA from cGAS, leading to inhibition of cGAS enzymatic activity and reduction of cGAMP production. Therefore, wild-type HCMV replicates more efficiently than UL31-deficient HCMV, and this phenotype is reversed in cGAS-deficient cells (Huang et al., 2018).

HCMV UL42 targets both cGAS and MITA for immune evasion (Fu, Guo, et al., 2019). UL42 inhibits DNA binding, oligomerization and enzymatic activity of cGAS as well as impairs translocation of MITA from the ER to perinuclear punctate structures, which is required for MITA activation. Consistently, UL42-deficiency enhances HCMV-induced production of type I IFNs and downstream antiviral genes. Consequently, wild-type HCMV replicates more efficiently than UL42-deficient HCMV.

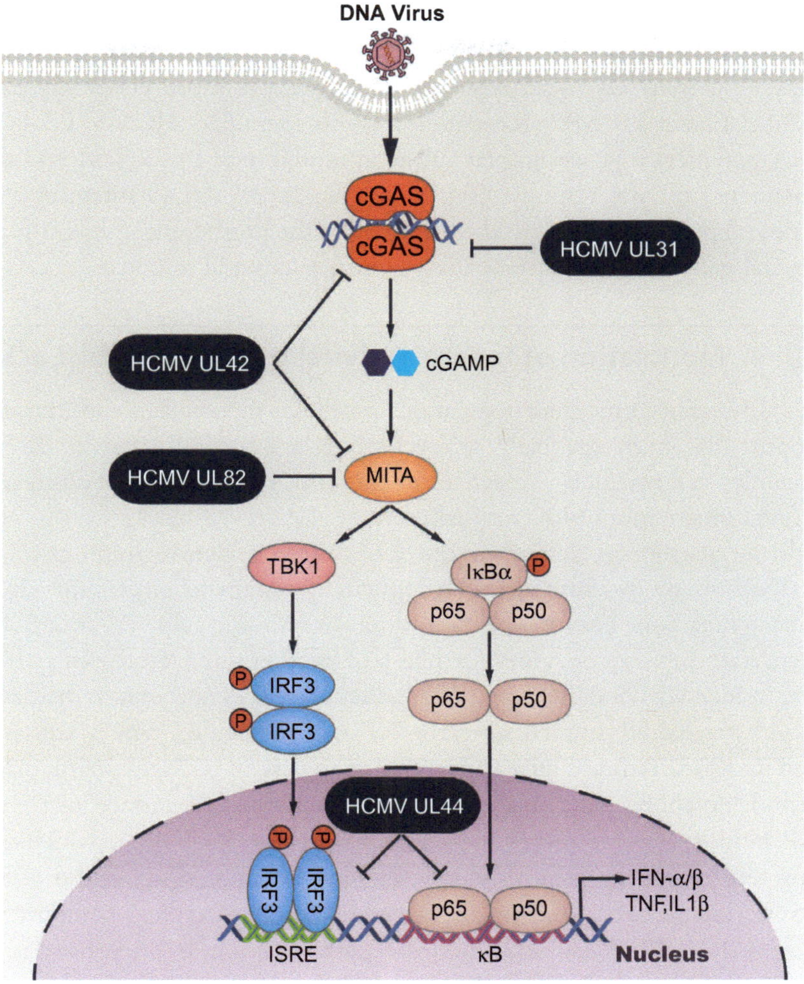

Fig. 3 Immune evasion of HCMV by antagonizing cGAS-MITA axis. The activities of cGAS and MITA are regulated by various HCMV proteins, including inhibition of DNA binding, oligomerization or enzymatic activity of cGAS, and impairment of translocation, oligomerization, TBK1 and IRF3 recruitment of MITA, resulting in impairment of production of type I IFNs and other antiviral genes.

HCMV tegument protein UL82 has also been reported to interact with MITA and impair MITA-mediated signaling by two different mechanisms (Fu et al., 2017). In one hand, UL82 inhibits the trafficking of MITA from the ER to perinuclear punctate structures by disrupting the MITA-iRhom2-TRAPβ translocation complex. In the other hand, UL82 impairs the recruitment of TBK1 and IRF3 to the MITA-associated complexes.

Consistently, the levels of downstream antiviral genes induced by UL82-deficient HCMV are higher than those induced by wild-type HCMV. Conversely, wild-type HCMV replicates more efficiently than UL82-deficient HCMV. Recently, we also identified HCMV UL44, a DNA polymerase processing factor, as an inhibitor of IRF3- and NF-κB-dependent antiviral response (Fu, Su, et al., 2019). UL44 interacts with IRF3 and p65, and it inhibits their binding to the promoters of downstream antiviral genes, resulting attenuation of innate antiviral response.

4. Modulation of innate antiviral response by bile acids

In recent years, inter-regulation of cellular metabolism and immune response has been gradually appreciated (Ganeshan & Chawla, 2014). Recently, we revealed a mechanism on how bile acid metabolism and antiviral innate immunity cross-talk (Hu et al., 2019) (Fig. 4).

In an attempt to determine the relationship of innate immunity and metabolism, we performed RNA-sequencing assays to screen for virus-induced metabolic enzymes or transporters in immune cells. We found that several rate-limiting enzymes for bile acid synthesis and their transporters were induced by viral infection. The induction of these proteins is mediated by virus-triggered immediate-early NF-κB activation, which causes a rapid increase of intracellular concentration of certain bile acids, particularly chenodeoxycholic acid (CDCA). The accumulated intracellular bile acids bind to Takeda G protein-coupled receptor 5 (TGR5), which is a G protein-coupled receptor, which subsequently induces activation of the tyrosine kinase SRC, leading to phosphorylation of critical components of the RIG-I-VISA and cGAS-MITA pathways. These phosphorylation events are essential for fully induction of downstream antiviral genes triggered by viral nucleic acids. Knockout of *Tgr5* results in lower levels of serum cytokines, higher levels of viral titers, and lower survival rates post HSV-1 and EMCV infection. Furthermore, CDCA treatment enhances innate immune response and protects from virus-induced lethality in wild-type but not TGR5-deficient mice (Hu et al., 2019). Our findings for the first time establish a physiological role of intracellular bile acids and a link between innate immunity and bile acid metabolism.

5. TLR3-TRIF-mediated innate immune response

TLRs recognize a set of pathogenic components and play critical roles in host defenses against certain microbes. So far, 10 TLRs have been

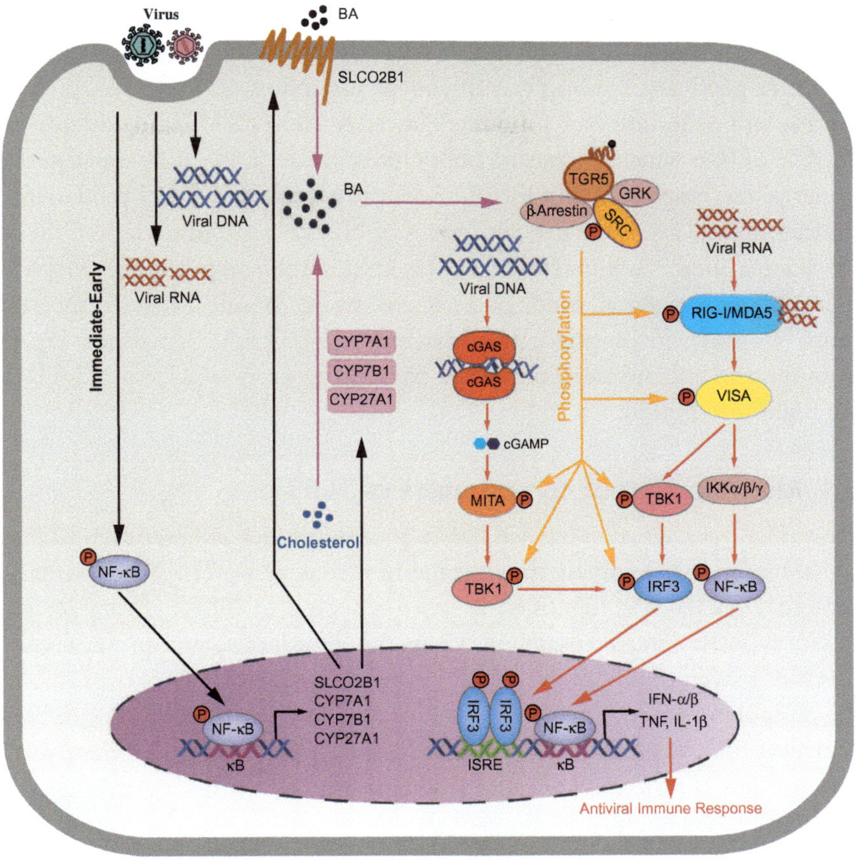

Fig. 4 Regulation of antiviral innate immunity by bile acids. Viral infection triggers an immediate-early NF-κB activation, which induces expression of bile acid transporter and rate-limiting biosynthesis enzymes, leading to accumulation of intracellular bile acids. The accumulated intracellular bile acids activate a TGR5-β-arrestin-SRC pathway, leading to SRC-mediated tyrosine phosphorylation of key components of the nucleic acid-triggered innate immune response pathways, which is essential for fully activation of these pathways.

reported in humans (TLR1-10), while there are 12 known TLRs in mice (TLR1-9, TLR11-13) (Kawai & Akira, 2006). TLRs contain an extracellular domain to which ligands bind, a transmembrane domain, and a conserved cytoplasmic Toll/IL-1R (TIR) domain which acts as a platform for the recruitment of downstream TIR domain-containing adaptor proteins and other signaling components upon ligand stimulation (Kawai & Akira, 2006). Among the TLRs, TLR3 recognizes extracellular and endosomal viral dsRNA as well as its synthetic analog poly(I:C). Upon activation, TLR3 recruits TIR domain-containing adaptor

(TRIF, also called TICAM-1). TRIF in turn recruits TRAF2/6 and two kinase complexes, IKK and TBK1 complexes, to activate NF-κB and IRF3, respectively, leading to subsequent induction of TNF, IL-1β, type I IFNs and other effector proteins (Kawai & Akira, 2006). In addition to TLR3, TLR4, which recognizes lipopolysaccharide (LPS) of Gram-negative bacteria, also employs TRIF for IRF3 activation and type I IFN production. Furthermore, TLR4 initiates two waves of NF-κB activation via MyD88 at the plasma membrane and TRIF at the endosomes, respectively, which is quite unique among all kinds of TLRs (Kawai & Akira, 2006). In the past years, we have investigated the mechanisms of TLR3/4-mediated innate immune and inflammatory responses, particularly on how TLR3 and TRIF are regulated (Fig. 5).

5.1 Identification of co-receptors of TLR3

How TLR3 recognizes viral dsRNA in the endosomes and recruits TIRF to signal has been extensively investigated in recent years. The RNA binding protein Mex3B was identified as a co-receptor of TLR3 (Yang et al., 2016). Mex3B interacts with TLR3 in the endosomes, and promotes the dsRNA binding activity of TLR3. Furthermore, Mex3B also promotes the proteolytic processing of TLR3 in response to viral RNA binding, which is critical for the activation of TLR3. Consistently, Mex3b-deficient mice produce less IFN-β and are more resistant to inflammatory death triggered by poly(I:C) injection.

Zinc-finger FYVE domain-containing protein ZFYVE1, a guanylate-binding protein (GBP), has been reported to promote the ligand binding of TLR3 (Zhong et al., 2019). ZFYVE1 is also associated with TLR3 at the endosomes, and promotes the binding affinity of TLR3 to poly(I:C). Zfyve1-deficient mice are less susceptible to poly(I:C)-induced inflammatory death than the wild-type mice. Further studies are needed to reveal the relationship of MEX3B and ZFYVE1 in regulating TLR3-mediated response.

5.2 Modulation of TRIF activity by WDFY1

As a critical adaptor in TLR3/4-mediated signaling, TRIF is modulated by various mechanisms. Recently, we found that the WD repeat and FYVE-domain-containing protein WDFY1 is important for recruitment of TRIF to TLR3/4 (Hu, Zhang, et al., 2015). Overexpression of WDFY1 or ZCCHC3 promotes TLR3- and TLR4-mediated induction of type I IFNs and inflammatory cytokines, whereas WDFY1- or ZCCHC3-deficiency exhibits the opposite effects.

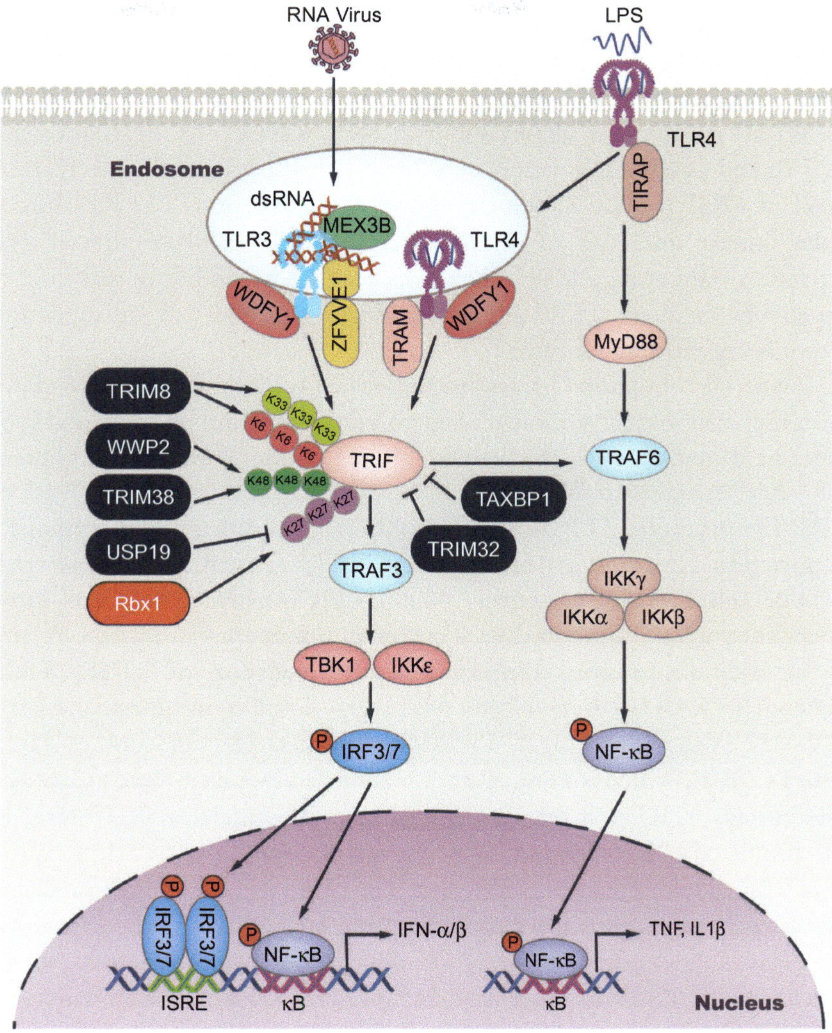

Fig. 5 Molecular mechanisms and regulation of TLR3/4-mediated innate immune signaling. After RNA binding at the endosome, TLR3 is cleaved to form active proteins, which recruits the adaptor TRIF and other signaling components, leading to activation of the transcription factors NF-κB and IRF3 and eventual induction of effectors of innate immune response. After LPS binding at the plasma membrane, TLR4 recruits MyD88 and other signaling components to activate NF-κB, followed by endocytosis of TLR4 to endosomes, at where TLR4 signals through TRIF for NF-κB and IRF3 activation, leading to the ultimate induction of effectors of innate immune responses. These processes are regulated by various proteins and mechanisms as illustrated in the figure.

5.3 Regulation of TRIF by ubiquitination

TRIF is dynamically modified by ubiquitination and deubuquitination, which plays a critical role in regulating its activity. Recently, we found that the RING E3 ubiquitin ligase complex Cullin-3–Rbx1–KCTD10 mediates K27-linked polyubiquitination of TRIF, which is critical for the recruitment of TRIF to TLR3 following poly(I:C) stimulation. The K27-linked polyubiquitin moieties of TRIF is removed by USP19 after TLR3 activation (Wu et al., 2019). Gene knockout studies indicates that USP19 negatively regulates TLR3-mediated innate immune and inflammatory responses in vitro and in vivo.

Two E3 ubiquitin ligases including WWP2 and TRIM38 have been reported to catalyze K48-linked polyubiquitination of TRIF and promote its degradation via the well established ubiquitin-proteasome system (Hu, Xie, et al., 2015; Yang et al., 2013). Deficiency of either WWP2 or TRIM38 promotes TLR3-mediated immune and inflammatory responses in mice (Hu, Xie, et al., 2015; Yang et al., 2013). These findings suggest that WWP2 and TRIM38 negatively inhibit TLR3-mediated response. How their functions are distinguished is currently unknown.

In addition to ubiquitin-proteasomal degradation of TRIF, TRIF undergoes TAX1BP1-mediated selectively autophagic degradation by TRIM32 (Yang et al., 2017). TRIM32 promotes the interaction of TRIF with LC3B-II, which is a critical component for autophagosome formation. Interestingly, TRIM38 but not TRIM32 down-regulates TRIF level in un-stimulated cells, whereas TRIM32 promotes ligand-induced degradation of TRIF. Therefore, TRIM38 and TRIM32 regulate TRIF-mediated signaling through distinct mechanisms (Yang et al., 2017).

TRIF is also modified by K6- and K33-linked polyubiquitination, which is mediated by TRIM8. These modifications of TRIF impair its recruitment of TBK1, leading to the suppression of TLR3/4-mediated innate immune responses (Ye et al., 2017).

6. TNF/IL-1β-triggered inflammatory responses

In addition to induction of antiviral genes, such as type I IFNs and ISGs, viral infection also triggers expression of proinflammatory cytokines, such as TNF and IL-1β. These proinflammatory cytokines further activate NF-κB and induce a group of downstream inflammatory genes, leading to inflammatory responses to clear invaded pathogens and infected cells.

After binding of TNF to TNF receptor 1 (TNFR1), the receptor recruits TRADD, TRAF2/5, cIAP1/2 and RIP1 to form a large receptor-associated complex, and then RIP1 undergoes K63-linked poly-ubiquitination probably mediated by TRAFs and cIAPs (Bianchi & Meier, 2009). IL-1β binds to IL-1 receptor (IL-1R), followed by recruitment of the IL-1R accessory protein (IL-1RAcP) and the adaptor protein MyD88, which in turn recruits IRAK1/4 and TRAF6 to the receptor complex, leading to K63-linked autoubiquitination of TRAF6 (Kuno & Matsushima, 1994). The polyubiquitin chains of RIP1 and TRAF6 can recruit the TAK1-TAB1-TAB2/3 complex via the ubiquitin-binding activity of TAB2/3, which causes TAK1 autophosphorylation and activation. TAK1 then activates NF-κB and AP1 via IKK and MAPK, respectively, leading to the ultimate induction of various proinflammatory cytokines, chemokines and other effector genes (Wisniewski & Vilcek, 1997). In the past years, we have revealed distinct regulatory mechanisms of TNF- and IL-1β-triggered inflammatory responses (Liu et al., 2012; Wu, Xu, Zhai, & Shu, 2003; Zhang et al., 2014; Zhang, Xu, Han, & Shu, 2004), and a few examples are introduced below (Fig. 6).

6.1 Regulation of IL-1 receptor complex

Several studies have suggested that ubiquitination is a central rhythm of regulation of IL-1β–induced NF-κB activation pathways. Several members of membrane-associated RING-CH-type finger (MARCH) ubiquitin ligase family have been shown to ubiquitinate and down-regulate trans-membrane proteins such as MHC-I, and ICAM-1 (Lin, Li, & Shu, 2019; Liu, Mintern, & Villadangos, 2019). In expression screens, we identified MARCH8 as a negative regulator of IL-1b-triggered signaling. MARCH8 interacts with IL1RAP and mediates its K48-linked polyubiquitination at K512 and degradation. Consistently, overexpression of MARCH8 inhibits IL-1β-induced NF-κB and MAPK activation, whereas knockdown of MARCH8 has the opposite effects (Chen, Li, Zhang, Zhou, & Shu, 2012). We further identified MARCH3 is also a negative regulator of IL-1β-triggered signaling. MARCH3 is associated with IL-1RI in resting cells, and IL-1β stimulation triggers dephosphorylation of MARCH3 by CDC25A and activation of its E3 ligase activity, leading to MARCH3-mediated K48-linked polyubiquitination of IL-1RI at K409 and its lysosomal-dependent degradation. MARCH3-deficient mice produces higher levels of serum inflammatory cytokines and are more sensitive to

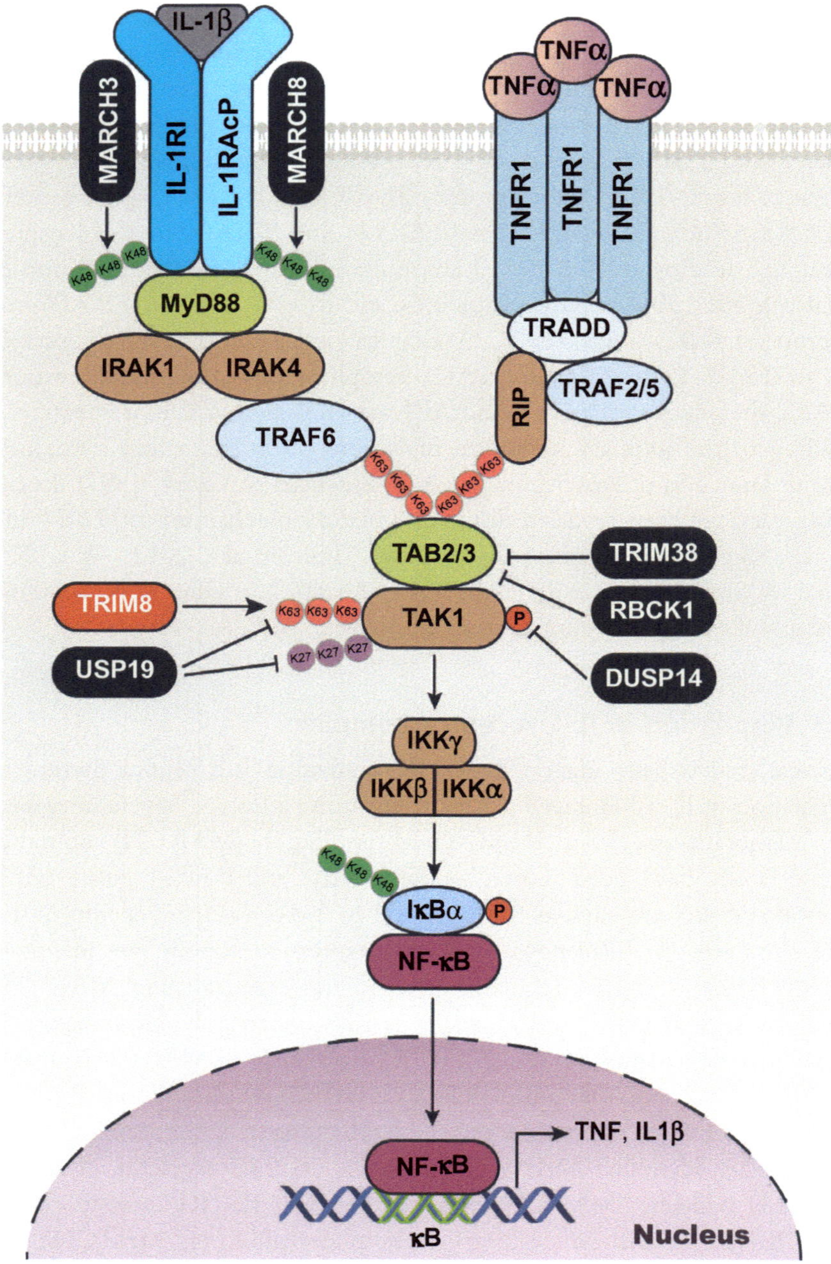

Fig. 6 Molecular mechanisms and regulation of TNF/IL-1β-triggered signaling. After binding of TNF or IL-1β to their respective receptor complexes, RIP1 and TRAF6 undergo polyubiquitination, followed by recruitment of the TAK1-TAB1-TAB2/3 complex and activation of NF-κB and AP1 via IKK and MAPK, respectively, leading to the ultimate

inflammatory death triggered by IL-1β injection and *Listeria monocytogenes* infection (Lin et al., 2018). Our findings suggest that two components of the IL-1 receptor complex are regulated by two distinct MARCH proteins, ensuring the control of excessive inflammatory response upon pathogen infection.

6.2 Regulation of TAK1-TAB1-TAB2/3 complex

The TAK1-TAB1-TAB2/3 complex functions downstream of both TNF and IL-1β signaling, which is tightly regulated by several distinct mechanisms. TRIM8, an E3 ubiquitin ligase, promotes TNF- and IL-1β-triggered NF-κB activation by mediating K63-linked polyubiquitination of TAK1, which is critical for its phosphorylation at T187 and activation (Hu et al., 2014; Li et al., 2011). On the opposite, the deubiquitinase USP19 has been reported to mediate deubiquitination of TAK1. TNF or IL-1β stimulation induces interaction of USP19 with TAK1, followed by deconjugation of K63- and K27-linked polyubiquitin chains from TAK1, leading to impairment of TAK1 activity and disruption of the TAK1-TAB2/3 complex. Consistently, Usp19-deficient mice produces higher levels of inflammatory cytokines and are more susceptible to TNF-α- and IL-1β-triggered septicemia death compared with their wild-type littermates (Lei et al., 2019).

In addition, we also identified a member of the dual-specificity phosphatase family, DUSP14, as a negative regulator of TNF- and IL-1β-triggered NF-κB activation by dephosphorylating TAK1 at T187 (Zheng et al., 2013). DUSP14 constitutively interacts with TAK1, and TNF or IL-1β stimulation further enhances their interaction, leading to DUSP14-mediated dephosphorylation of TAK1 at T187, a residue in the activation loop critically involved in TAK1 activation (Zheng et al., 2013).

TAB2/3, two redundant molecules in TAK1-associated complex, have been shown to undergo degradation via both ubiquitin-proteasomal and endo/lysosomal routes. RBCK1 is associated with TAB2/3 and facilitates their degradation through a proteasome-dependent process (Tian et al., 2007), while TRIM38 is constitutively associated with TAB2/3 and

---

induction of proinflammatory cytokines, chemokines and other effector genes. Various regulatory mechanisms of TNF and IL-1β signaling have been employed by host cells to exert proper inflammatory response. For examples, MARCH3 and MARCH8 mediate K48-linked polyubiquitination of IL-1R and IL-1RAP, respectively, leading degradation their degradation and attenuation of IL-1β-triggered inflammation. The TAK1-TAB2/3 complexes are positively and negatively regulated by TRIM8, TRIM38, RBCK1, USP19 and DUSP14, respectively, as indicated. Please see the figure and text for details.

promotes their lysosome-dependent degradation independent of its E3 ubiquitin ligase activity (Hu et al., 2014). Deficiency of either RBCK1 or TRIM38 potentiates TNF- and IL-1β-induced NF-κB activation as well as induction of inflammatory cytokines, suggesting that these proteins are involved in negative regulation of TNF- and IL-1β-triggered inflammation through distinct mechanisms (Hu et al., 2014).

7. Concluding remarks

For near 20 years, our groups have focused on the molecular mechanisms of antiviral innate immune and inflammatory responses. Discoveries from our groups and many other groups in the world have contributed to our understanding of the major modes of viral nucleic acid-sensing, signaling and regulation of innate immune and inflammatory responses. However, there are many outstanding questions that need to be answered for ultimate understanding of the complicated molecular and cellular mechanisms of antiviral innate immunity. For examples, whether do other sensors, signaling and modulatory components exist in a particular PRR-mediated pathway, and how different nucleic acid-sensing pathways in the same cell are coordinated or cross-talk for an optimal response to an invaded virus? How the distinct post-translational modifications as well as cellular trafficking events are temporally and spatially coordinated and regulated for precisely control of innate immune responses to viral nucleic acids? How viral infection reprograms cellular metabolism? Whether and how these reprogramming events affect viral replication as well as cellular and systemic antiviral immune response? Answering these and other outstanding questions would contribute to further advances on our understanding of pathogen-host interactions.

The ability of recognition of self nucleic acids by certain PRRs makes the innate immune system a double-edged sword. Inappropriate recognition of self nucleic acids and dys-regulated signaling triggered by PRRs are linked with not only autoimmune and inflammatory diseases, but also metabolic disorders and cancers. Therefore, the nucleic acid-sensing pathways would be important targets for development of drugs, adjuvants and immunotherapies for serious human diseases, including infectious and autoimmune diseases and cancers. More research in this area will certainly contribute to our mission to decipher the complicated pathogen-host interactions and to develop therapeutics for the related prevalent human diseases.

Acknowledgments

We thank Ru Zang for assistance with the illustrations, Ming-Ming Hu for critical reading of the manuscript. Work in the authors' laboratory is supported by grants from the State Key R&D Program of China (2017YFA0505800, 2016YFA0502102), and the National Natural Science Foundation of China (31830024, 31630045, 31870870, 31800728).

References

Ablasser, A., Goldeck, M., Cavlar, T., Deimling, T., Witte, G., Rohl, I., et al. (2013). cGAS produces a 2'-5'-linked cyclic dinucleotide second messenger that activates STING. *Nature*, *498*, 380.

Aguirre, S., Maestre, A. M., Pagni, S., Patel, J. R., Savage, T., Gutman, D., et al. (2012). DENV inhibits type I IFN production in infected cells by cleaving human STING. *PLoS Pathogens*, *8*, e1002934.

Akira, S. (2006). TLR signaling. *Current Topics in Microbiology and Immunology*, *311*, 1.

Akira, S., Uematsu, S., & Takeuchi, O. (2006). Pathogen recognition and innate immunity. *Cell*, *124*, 783.

An, T., Li, S., Pan, W., Tien, P., Zhong, B., Shu, H. B., et al. (2015). DYRK2 negatively regulates type I interferon induction by promoting TBK1 degradation via Ser527 phosphorylation. *PLoS Pathogens*, *11*, e1005179.

Andrade, W. A., Firon, A., Schmidt, T., Hornung, V., Fitzgerald, K. A., Kurt-Jones, E. A., et al. (2016). Group B streptococcus degrades cyclic-di-AMP to modulate STING-dependent type I interferon production. *Cell Host & Microbe*, *20*, 49.

Bianchi, K., & Meier, P. (2009). A tangled web of ubiquitin chains: Breaking news in TNF-R1 signaling. *Molecular Cell*, *36*, 736.

Burdette, D. L., Monroe, K. M., Sotelo-Troha, K., Iwig, J. S., Eckert, B., Hyodo, M., et al. (2011). STING is a direct innate immune sensor of cyclic di-GMP. *Nature*, *478*, 515.

Chen, L. T., Hu, M. M., Xu, Z. S., Liu, Y., & Shu, H. B. (2016). MSX1 modulates RLR-mediated innate antiviral signaling by facilitating assembly of TBK1-associated complexes. *Journal of Immunology*, *197*, 199.

Chen, H., Li, Y., Zhang, J., Ran, Y., Wei, J., Yang, Y., et al. (2013). RAVER1 is a coactivator of MDA5-mediated cellular antiviral response. *Journal of Molecular Cell Biology*, *5*, 111.

Chen, R., Li, M., Zhang, Y., Zhou, Q., & Shu, H. B. (2012). The E3 ubiquitin ligase MARCH8 negatively regulates IL-1beta-induced NF-kappaB activation by targeting the IL1RAP coreceptor for ubiquitination and degradation. *Proceedings of the National Academy of Sciences of the United States of America*, *109*, 14128.

Chen, R., Zhang, L., Zhong, B., Tan, B., Liu, Y., & Shu, H. B. (2010). The ubiquitin-specific protease 17 is involved in virus-triggered type I IFN signaling. *Cell Research*, *20*, 802.

Civril, F., Deimling, T., de Oliveira Mann, C. C., Ablasser, A., Moldt, M., Witte, G., et al. (2013). Structural mechanism of cytosolic DNA sensing by cGAS. *Nature*, *498*, 332.

Diao, F., Li, S., Tian, Y., Zhang, M., Xu, L. G., Zhang, Y., et al. (2007). Negative regulation of MDA5- but not RIG-I-mediated innate antiviral signaling by the dihydroxyacetone kinase. *Proceedings of the National Academy of Sciences of the United States of America*, *104*, 11706.

Dobbs, N., Burnaevskiy, N., Chen, D., Gonugunta, V. K., Alto, N. M., & Yan, N. (2015). STING activation by translocation from the ER is associated with infection and autoinflammatory disease. *Cell Host & Microbe*, *18*, 157.

Du, M., & Chen, Z. J. (2018). DNA-induced liquid phase condensation of cGAS activates innate immune signaling. *Science*, *361*, 704.

Ergun, S. L., Fernandez, D., Weiss, T. M., & Li, L. (2019). STING polymer structure reveals mechanisms for activation, hyperactivation, and inhibition. *Cell*, *178*, 290.

Fu, Y. Z., Guo, Y., Zou, H. M., Su, S., Wang, S. Y., Yang, Q., et al. (2019). Human cytomegalovirus protein UL42 antagonizes cGAS/MITA-mediated innate antiviral response. *PLoS Pathogens*, *15*, e1007691.

Fu, Y. Z., Su, S., Gao, Y. Q., Wang, P. P., Huang, Z. F., Hu, M. M., et al. (2017). Human cytomegalovirus tegument protein UL82 inhibits STING-mediated signaling to evade antiviral immunity. *Cell Host & Microbe*, *21*, 231.

Fu, Y. Z., Su, S., Zou, H. M., Guo, Y., Wang, S. Y., Li, S., et al. (2019). Human cytomegalovirus DNA polymerase subunit UL44 antagonizes antiviral immune responses by suppressing IRF3- and NF-kappaB-mediated transcription. *Journal of Virology*, *93*, e00181-19.

Gack, M. U., Shin, Y. C., Joo, C. H., Urano, T., Liang, C., Sun, L., et al. (2007). TRIM25 RING-finger E3 ubiquitin ligase is essential for RIG-I-mediated antiviral activity. *Nature*, *446*, 916.

Ganeshan, K., & Chawla, A. (2014). Metabolic regulation of immune responses. *Annual Review of Immunology*, *32*, 609.

Gao, P., Ascano, M., Wu, Y., Barchet, W., Gaffney, B. L., Zillinger, T., et al. (2013). Cyclic [G(2′,5′)pA(3′,5′)p] is the metazoan second messenger produced by DNA-activated cyclic GMP-AMP synthase. *Cell*, *153*, 1094.

Gao, P., Ascano, M., Zillinger, T., Wang, W., Dai, P., Serganov, A. A., et al. (2013). Structure-function analysis of STING activation by c[G(2',5')pA(3',5')p] and targeting by antiviral DMXAA. *Cell*, *154*, 748.

Gitlin, L., Barchet, W., Gilfillan, S., Cella, M., Beutler, B., Flavell, R. A., et al. (2006). Essential role of mda-5 in type I IFN responses to polyriboinosinic:Polyribocytidylic acid and encephalomyocarditis picornavirus. *Proceedings of the National Academy of Sciences of the United States of America*, *103*, 8459.

Guo, W., Wei, J., Shu, H. B., & Yang, Q. (2019). SNX8 modulates innate immune response to RNA virus by regulating the aggregation of VISA. *Cellular & Molecular Immunology*. https://doi.org/10.1038/s41423-019-0285-2.

Hiscott, J., Grandvaux, N., Sharma, S., Tenoever, B. R., Servant, M. J., & Lin, R. (2003). Convergence of the NF-kappaB and interferon signaling pathways in the regulation of antiviral defense and apoptosis. *Annals of the New York Academy of Sciences*, *1010*, 237.

Holm, C. K., Jensen, S. B., Jakobsen, M. R., Cheshenko, N., Horan, K. A., Moeller, H. B., et al. (2012). Virus-cell fusion as a trigger of innate immunity dependent on the adaptor STING. *Nature Immunology*, *13*, 737.

Hornung, V., Ellegast, J., Kim, S., Brzozka, K., Jung, A., Kato, H., et al. (2006). 5'-Triphosphate RNA is the ligand for RIG-I. *Science*, *314*, 994.

Hou, F., Sun, L., Zheng, H., Skaug, B., Jiang, Q. X., & Chen, Z. J. (2011). MAVS forms functional prion-like aggregates to activate and propagate antiviral innate immune response. *Cell*, *146*, 448.

Hu, M. M., He, W. R., Gao, P., Yang, Q., He, K., Cao, L. B., et al. (2019). Virus-induced accumulation of intracellular bile acids activates the TGR5-beta-arrestin-SRC axis to enable innate antiviral immunity. *Cell Research*, *29*, 193.

Hu, M. M., Liao, C. Y., Yang, Q., Xie, X. Q., & Shu, H. B. (2017). Innate immunity to RNA virus is regulated by temporal and reversible sumoylation of RIG-I and MDA5. *The Journal of Experimental Medicine*, *214*, 973.

Hu, M. M., & Shu, H. B. (2017). Multifaceted roles of TRIM38 in innate immune and inflammatory responses. *Cellular & Molecular Immunology*, *14*, 331.

Hu, M. M., & Shu, H. B. (2018). Cytoplasmic mechanisms of recognition and defense of microbial nucleic acids. *Annual Review of Cell and Developmental Biology*, *34*, 357.

Hu, M. M., & Shu, H. B. (2019). Innate immune response to cytoplasmic DNA: Mechanisms and diseases. *Annual Review of Immunology* in press.
Hu, M. M., Xie, X. Q., Yang, Q., Liao, C. Y., Ye, W., Lin, H., et al. (2015). TRIM38 negatively regulates TLR3/4-mediated innate immune and inflammatory responses by two sequential and distinct mechanisms. *Journal of Immunology*, *195*, 4415.
Hu, M. M., Yang, Q., Xie, X. Q., Liao, C. Y., Lin, H., Liu, T. T., et al. (2016). Sumoylation promotes the stability of the DNA sensor cGAS and the adaptor STING to regulate the kinetics of response to DNA virus. *Immunity*, *45*, 555.
Hu, M. M., Yang, Q., Zhang, J., Liu, S. M., Zhang, Y., Lin, H., et al. (2014). TRIM38 inhibits TNFalpha- and IL-1beta-triggered NF-kappaB activation by mediating lysosome-dependent degradation of TAB2/3. *Proceedings of the National Academy of Sciences of the United States of America*, *111*, 1509.
Hu, Y. H., Zhang, Y., Jiang, L. Q., Wang, S., Lei, C. Q., Sun, M. S., et al. (2015). WDFY1 mediates TLR3/4 signaling by recruiting TRIF. *EMBO Reports*, *16*, 447.
Huang, J., Liu, T., Xu, L. G., Chen, D., Zhai, Z., & Shu, H. B. (2005). SIKE is an IKK epsilon/TBK1-associated suppressor of TLR3- and virus-triggered IRF-3 activation pathways. *The EMBO Journal*, *24*, 4018.
Huang, Z. F., Zou, H. M., Liao, B. W., Zhang, H. Y., Yang, Y., Fu, Y. Z., et al. (2018). Human cytomegalovirus protein UL31 inhibits DNA sensing of cGAS to mediate immune evasion. *Cell Host & Microbe*, *24*, 69.
Ishikawa, H., & Barber, G. N. (2008). STING is an endoplasmic reticulum adaptor that facilitates innate immune signalling. *Nature*, *455*, 674.
Ishikawa, H., Ma, Z., & Barber, G. N. (2009). STING regulates intracellular DNA-mediated, type I interferon-dependent innate immunity. *Nature*, *461*, 788.
Janeway, C. A., Jr. (1989). Introduction: T-cell:B-cell interaction. *Seminars in Immunology*, *1*, 1.
Jiang, L. Q., Xia, T., Hu, Y. H., Sun, M. S., Yan, S., Lei, C. Q., et al. (2018). IFITM3 inhibits virus-triggered induction of type I interferon by mediating autophagosome-dependent degradation of IRF3. *Cellular & Molecular Immunology*, *15*, 858.
Jope, R. S., & Johnson, G. V. (2004). The glamour and gloom of glycogen synthase kinase-3. *Trends in Biochemical Sciences*, *29*, 95.
Kato, H., Takeuchi, O., Sato, S., Yoneyama, M., Yamamoto, M., Matsui, K., et al. (2006). Differential roles of MDA5 and RIG-I helicases in the recognition of RNA viruses. *Nature*, *441*, 101.
Kawai, T., & Akira, S. (2006). TLR signaling. *Cell Death and Differentiation*, *13*, 816.
Konno, H., Konno, K., & Barber, G. N. (2013). Cyclic dinucleotides trigger ULK1 (ATG1) phosphorylation of STING to prevent sustained innate immune signaling. *Cell*, *155*, 688.
Kubota, T., Matsuoka, M., Chang, T. H., Tailor, P., Sasaki, T., Tashiro, M., et al. (2008). Virus infection triggers SUMOylation of IRF3 and IRF7, leading to the negative regulation of type I interferon gene expression. *The Journal of Biological Chemistry*, *283*, 25660.
Kuno, K., & Matsushima, K. (1994). The IL-1 receptor signaling pathway. *Journal of Leukocyte Biology*, *56*, 542.
Lang, X., Tang, T., Jin, T., Ding, C., Zhou, R., & Jiang, W. (2017). TRIM65-catalized ubiquitination is essential for MDA5-mediated antiviral innate immunity. *The Journal of Experimental Medicine*, *214*, 459.
Lei, C. Q., Wu, X., Zhong, X., Jiang, L., Zhong, B., & Shu, H. B. (2019). USP19 inhibits TNF-alpha- and IL-1beta-triggered NF-kappaB activation by deubiquitinating TAK1. *Journal of Immunology*, *203*, 259.
Lei, C. Q., Zhang, Y., Li, M., Jiang, L. Q., Zhong, B., Kim, Y. H., et al. (2015). ECSIT bridges RIG-I-like receptors to VISA in signaling events of innate antiviral responses. *Journal of Innate Immunity*, *7*, 153.

Lei, C. Q., Zhang, Y., Xia, T., Jiang, L. Q., Zhong, B., & Shu, H. B. (2013). FoxO1 negatively regulates cellular antiviral response by promoting degradation of IRF3. *The Journal of Biological Chemistry, 288,* 12596.

Lei, C. Q., Zhong, B., Zhang, Y., Zhang, J., Wang, S., & Shu, H. B. (2010). Glycogen synthase kinase 3beta regulates IRF3 transcription factor-mediated antiviral response via activation of the kinase TBK1. *Immunity, 33,* 878.

Li, Y., Chen, R., Zhou, Q., Xu, Z., Li, C., Wang, S., et al. (2012). LSm14A is a processing body-associated sensor of viral nucleic acids that initiates cellular antiviral response in the early phase of viral infection. *Proceedings of the National Academy of Sciences of the United States of America, 109,* 11770.

Li, Z., Liu, G., Sun, L., Teng, Y., Guo, X., Jia, J., et al. (2015). PPM1A regulates antiviral signaling by antagonizing TBK1-mediated STING phosphorylation and aggregation. *PLoS Pathogens, 11,* e1004783.

Li, X., Shu, C., Yi, G., Chaton, C. T., Shelton, C. L., Diao, J., et al. (2013). Cyclic GMP-AMP synthase is activated by double-stranded DNA-induced oligomerization. *Immunity, 39,* 1019.

Li, Q., Yan, J., Mao, A. P., Li, C., Ran, Y., Shu, H. B., et al. (2011). Tripartite motif 8 (TRIM8) modulates TNFalpha- and IL-1beta-triggered NF-kappaB activation by targeting TAK1 for K63-linked polyubiquitination. *Proceedings of the National Academy of Sciences of the United States of America, 108,* 19341.

Li, S., Zheng, H., Mao, A. P., Zhong, B., Li, Y., Liu, Y., et al. (2010). Regulation of virus-triggered signaling by OTUB1- and OTUB2-mediated deubiquitination of TRAF3 and TRAF6. *The Journal of Biological Chemistry, 285,* 4291.

Li, S., Zhu, M., Pan, R., Fang, T., Cao, Y. Y., Chen, S., et al. (2016). The tumor suppressor PTEN has a critical role in antiviral innate immunity. *Nature Immunology, 17,* 241.

Lian, H., Wei, J., Zang, R., Ye, W., Yang, Q., Zhang, X. N., et al. (2018). ZCCHC3 is a co-sensor of cGAS for dsDNA recognition in innate immune response. *Nature Communications, 9,* 3349.

Lian, H., Zang, R., Wei, J., Ye, W., Hu, M. M., Chen, Y. D., et al. (2018). The zinc-finger protein ZCCHC3 binds RNA and facilitates viral RNA sensing and activation of the RIG-I-like receptors. *Immunity, 49,* 438.

Lin, H., Gao, D., Hu, M. M., Zhang, M., Wu, X. X., Feng, L., et al. (2018). MARCH3 attenuates IL-1beta-triggered inflammation by mediating K48-linked polyubiquitination and degradation of IL-1RI. *Proceedings of the National Academy of Sciences of the United States of America, 115,* 12483.

Lin, H., Li, S., & Shu, H. B. (2019). The membrane-associated MARCH E3 Ligase family: Emerging roles in immune regulation. *Frontiers in Immunology, 10,* 1751.

Lin, D., Zhang, M., Zhang, M. X., Ren, Y., Jin, J., Zhao, Q., et al. (2015). Induction of USP25 by viral infection promotes innate antiviral responses by mediating the stabilization of TRAF3 and TRAF6. *Proceedings of the National Academy of Sciences of the United States of America, 112,* 11324.

Liu, S., Cai, X., Wu, J., Cong, Q., Chen, X., Li, T., et al. (2015). Phosphorylation of innate immune adaptor proteins MAVS, STING, and TRIF induces IRF3 activation. *Science, 347,* aaa2630.

Liu, L. J., Liu, T. T., Ran, Y., Li, Y., Zhang, X. D., Shu, H. B., et al. (2012). The E3 ubiquitin ligase MIB1 negatively regulates basal IkappaBalpha level and modulates NF-kappaB activation. *Cell Research, 22,* 603.

Liu, H., Mintern, J. D., & Villadangos, J. A. (2019). MARCH ligases in immunity. *Current Opinion in Immunology, 58,* 38.

Liu, J., Qian, C., & Cao, X. (2016). Post-translational modification control of innate immunity. *Immunity, 45,* 15.

Liu, Z., Wu, S. W., Lei, C. Q., Zhou, Q., Li, S., Shu, H. B., et al. (2013). Heat shock cognate 71 (HSC71) regulates cellular antiviral response by impairing formation of VISA aggregates. *Protein & Cell, 4*, 373.

Liu, T. T., Yang, Q., Li, M., Zhong, B., Ran, Y., Liu, L. L., et al. (2016). LSm14A plays a critical role in antiviral immune responses by regulating MITA level in a cell-specific manner. *Journal of Immunology, 196*, 5101.

Loo, Y. M., Fornek, J., Crochet, N., Bajwa, G., Perwitasari, O., Martinez-Sobrido, L., et al. (2008). Distinct RIG-I and MDA5 signaling by RNA viruses in innate immunity. *Journal of Virology, 82*, 335.

Luo, W. W., Li, S., Li, C., Lian, H., Yang, Q., Zhong, B., et al. (2016). iRhom2 is essential for innate immunity to DNA viruses by mediating trafficking and stability of the adaptor STING. *Nature Immunology, 17*, 1057.

Luo, W. W., Li, S., Li, C., Zheng, Z. Q., Cao, P., Tong, Z., et al. (2017). iRhom2 is essential for innate immunity to RNA virus by antagonizing ER- and mitochondria-associated degradation of VISA. *PLoS Pathogens, 13*, e1006693.

Luo, W. W., Lian, H., Zhong, B., Shu, H. B., & Li, S. (2016). Kruppel-like factor 4 negatively regulates cellular antiviral immune response. *Cellular & Molecular Immunology, 13*, 65.

Luo, W. W., & Shu, H. B. (2018). Delicate regulation of the cGAS-MITA-mediated innate immune response. *Cellular & Molecular Immunology, 15*, 666.

Ma, Z., & Damania, B. (2016). The cGAS-STING defense pathway and its counteraction by viruses. *Cell Host & Microbe, 19*, 150.

Mao, A. P., Li, S., Zhong, B., Li, Y., Yan, J., Li, Q., et al. (2010). Virus-triggered ubiquitination of TRAF3/6 by cIAP1/2 is essential for induction of interferon-beta (IFN-beta) and cellular antiviral response. *The Journal of Biological Chemistry, 285*, 9470.

Moretti, J., Roy, S., Bozec, D., Martinez, J., Chapman, J. R., Ueberheide, B., et al. (2017). STING senses microbial viability to orchestrate stress-mediated autophagy of the endoplasmic reticulum. *Cell, 171*, 809.

Nazmi, A., Mukhopadhyay, R., Dutta, K., & Basu, A. (2012). STING mediates neuronal innate immune response following Japanese encephalitis virus infection. *Scientific Reports, 2*, 347.

Ni, G., Ma, Z., & Damania, B. (2018). cGAS and STING: At the intersection of DNA and RNA virus-sensing networks. *PLoS Pathogens, 14*, e1007148.

Nie, Y., Ran, Y., Zhang, H. Y., Huang, Z. F., Pan, Z. Y., Wang, S. Y., et al. (2017). GPATCH3 negatively regulates RLR-mediated innate antiviral responses by disrupting the assembly of VISA signalosome. *PLoS Pathogens, 13*, e1006328.

Oshiumi, H., Miyashita, M., Inoue, N., Okabe, M., Matsumoto, M., & Seya, T. (2010). The ubiquitin ligase Riplet is essential for RIG-I-dependent innate immune responses to RNA virus infection. *Cell Host & Microbe, 8*, 496.

Osorio, F., & Reis e Sousa, C. (2011). Myeloid C-type lectin receptors in pathogen recognition and host defense. *Immunity, 34*, 651.

Park, H. H. (2018). Structure of TRAF family: Current understanding of receptor recognition. *Frontiers in Immunology, 9*, 1999.

Pichlmair, A., Schulz, O., Tan, C. P., Naslund, T. I., Liljestrom, P., Weber, F., et al. (2006). RIG-I-mediated antiviral responses to single-stranded RNA bearing 5'-phosphates. *Science, 314*, 997.

Prantner, D., Perkins, D. J., Lai, W., Williams, M. S., Sharma, S., Fitzgerald, K. A., et al. (2012). 5,6-Dimethylxanthenone-4-acetic acid (DMXAA) activates stimulator of interferon gene (STING)-dependent innate immune pathways and is regulated by mitochondrial membrane potential. *The Journal of Biological Chemistry, 287*, 39776.

Qin, Y., Zhou, M. T., Hu, M. M., Hu, Y. H., Zhang, J., Guo, L., et al. (2014). RNF26 temporally regulates virus-triggered type I interferon induction by two distinct mechanisms. *PLoS Pathogens*, *10*, e1004358.

Ran, Y., Liu, T. T., Zhou, Q., Li, S., Mao, A. P., Li, Y., et al. (2011). SENP2 negatively regulates cellular antiviral response by deSUMOylating IRF3 and conditioning it for ubiquitination and degradation. *Journal of Molecular Cell Biology*, *3*, 283.

Ran, Y., Shu, H. B., & Wang, Y. Y. (2014). MITA/STING: A central and multifaceted mediator in innate immune response. *Cytokine & Growth Factor Reviews*, *25*, 631.

Ran, Y., Zhang, J., Liu, L. L., Pan, Z. Y., Nie, Y., Zhang, H. Y., et al. (2016). Autoubiquitination of TRIM26 links TBK1 to NEMO in RLR-mediated innate antiviral immune response. *Journal of Molecular Cell Biology*, *8*, 31.

Schoggins, J. W., MacDuff, D. A., Imanaka, N., Gainey, M. D., Shrestha, B., Eitson, J. L., et al. (2014). Pan-viral specificity of IFN-induced genes reveals new roles for cGAS in innate immunity. *Nature*, *505*, 691.

Schoggins, J. W., Wilson, S. J., Panis, M., Murphy, M. Y., Jones, C. T., Bieniasz, P., et al. (2011). A diverse range of gene products are effectors of the type I interferon antiviral response. *Nature*, *472*, 481.

Shu, H. B., & Wang, Y. Y. (2014). Adding to the STING. *Immunity*, *41*, 871.

Srikanth, S., Woo, J. S., Wu, B., El-Sherbiny, Y. M., Leung, J., Chupradit, K., et al. (2019). The Ca(2+) sensor STIM1 regulates the type I interferon response by retaining the signaling adaptor STING at the endoplasmic reticulum. *Nature Immunology*, *20*, 152.

Sun, W., Li, Y., Chen, L., Chen, H., You, F., Zhou, X., et al. (2009). ERIS, an endoplasmic reticulum IFN stimulator, activates innate immune signaling through dimerization. *Proceedings of the National Academy of Sciences of the United States of America*, *106*, 8653.

Sun, B., Sundstrom, K. B., Chew, J. J., Bist, P., Gan, E. S., Tan, H. C., et al. (2017). Dengue virus activates cGAS through the release of mitochondrial DNA. *Scientific Reports*, *7*, 3594.

Sun, L., Wu, J., Du, F., Chen, X., & Chen, Z. J. (2013). Cyclic GMP-AMP synthase is a cytosolic DNA sensor that activates the type I interferon pathway. *Science*, *339*, 786.

Sun, H., Zhang, Q., Jing, Y. Y., Zhang, M., Wang, H. Y., Cai, Z., et al. (2017). USP13 negatively regulates antiviral responses by deubiquitinating STING. *Nature Communications*, *8*, 15534.

Takaoka, A., Wang, Z., Choi, M. K., Yanai, H., Negishi, H., Ban, T., et al. (2007). DAI (DLM-1/ZBP1) is a cytosolic DNA sensor and an activator of innate immune response. *Nature*, *448*, 501.

Takeuchi, O., & Akira, S. (2010). Pattern recognition receptors and inflammation. *Cell*, *140*, 805.

Taniguchi, T., Ogasawara, K., Takaoka, A., & Tanaka, N. (2001). IRF family of transcription factors as regulators of host defense. *Annual Review of Immunology*, *19*, 623.

Taniguchi, T., & Takaoka, A. (2002). The interferon-alpha/beta system in antiviral responses: A multimodal machinery of gene regulation by the IRF family of transcription factors. *Current Opinion in Immunology*, *14*, 111.

Tao, J., Zhang, X. W., Jin, J., Du, X. X., Lian, T., Yang, J., et al. (2017). Nonspecific DNA binding of cGAS N terminus promotes cGAS activation. *Journal of Immunology*, *198*, 3627.

Tian, Y., Zhang, Y., Zhong, B., Wang, Y. Y., Diao, F. C., Wang, R. P., et al. (2007). RBCK1 negatively regulates tumor necrosis factor- and interleukin-1-triggered NF-kappaB activation by targeting TAB2/3 for degradation. *The Journal of Biological Chemistry*, *282*, 16776.

Unterholzner, L., Keating, S. E., Baran, M., Horan, K. A., Jensen, S. B., Sharma, S., et al. (2010). IFI16 is an innate immune sensor for intracellular DNA. *Nature Immunology*, *11*, 997.

Wang, Q., Liu, X., Cui, Y., Tang, Y., Chen, W., Li, S., et al. (2014). The E3 ubiquitin ligase AMFR and INSIG1 bridge the activation of TBK1 kinase by modifying the adaptor STING. *Immunity*, *41*, 919.

Wang, Y. Y., Liu, L. J., Zhong, B., Liu, T. T., Li, Y., Yang, Y., et al. (2010). WDR5 is essential for assembly of the VISA-associated signaling complex and virus-triggered IRF3 and NF-kappaB activation. *Proceedings of the National Academy of Sciences of the United States of America*, *107*, 815.

Wei, J., Lian, H., Guo, W., Chen, Y. D., Zhang, X. N., Zang, R., et al. (2018). SNX8 modulates innate immune response to DNA virus by mediating trafficking and activation of MITA. *PLoS Pathogens*, *14*, e1007336.

Wisniewski, H. G., & Vilcek, J. (1997). TSG-6: An IL-1/TNF-inducible protein with anti-inflammatory activity. *Cytokine & Growth Factor Reviews*, *8*, 143.

Wu, X., Lei, C. Q., Xia, T., Zhong, X., Yang, Q., & Shu, H. B. (2019). Regulation of TRIF-mediated innate immune response by K27-linked polyubiquitination and deubiquitination. *Nature Communications*, *10*, 1–14.

Wu, M., Xu, L. G., Zhai, Z., & Shu, H. B. (2003). SINK is a p65-interacting negative regulator of NF-kappaB-dependent transcription. *The Journal of Biological Chemistry*, *278*, 27072.

Xia, P., Wang, S., Ye, B., Du, Y., Huang, G., Zhu, P., et al. (2015). Sox2 functions as a sequence-specific DNA sensor in neutrophils to initiate innate immunity against microbial infection. *Nature Immunology*, *16*, 366.

Xia, T., Yi, X., Wu, X., Shang, J., & Shu, H. B. (2019). PTPN1/2-mediated dephosphorylation of MITA/STING promotes its 20S proteasomal degradation and attenuates innate antiviral response. *Proceedings of the National Academy of Sciences of the United States of America*, *116*, 20063–20069.

Xu, L. G., Wang, Y. Y., Han, K. J., Li, L. Y., Zhai, Z., & Shu, H. B. (2005). VISA is an adapter protein required for virus-triggered IFN-beta signaling. *Molecular Cell*, *19*, 727.

Yan, J., Li, Q., Mao, A. P., Hu, M. M., & Shu, H. B. (2014). TRIM4 modulates type I interferon induction and cellular antiviral response by targeting RIG-I for K63-linked ubiquitination. *Journal of Molecular Cell Biology*, *6*, 154.

Yan, B. R., Zhou, L., Hu, M. M., Li, M., Lin, H., Yang, Y., et al. (2017). PKACs attenuate innate antiviral response by phosphorylating VISA and priming it for MARCH5-mediated degradation. *PLoS Pathogens*, *13*, e1006648.

Yang, Y., Liao, B., Wang, S., Yan, B., Jin, Y., Shu, H. B., et al. (2013). E3 ligase WWP2 negatively regulates TLR3-mediated innate immune response by targeting TRIF for ubiquitination and degradation. *Proceedings of the National Academy of Sciences of the United States of America*, *110*, 5115.

Yang, Q., Liu, T. T., Lin, H., Zhang, M., Wei, J., Luo, W. W., et al. (2017). TRIM32-TAX1BP1-dependent selective autophagic degradation of TRIF negatively regulates TLR3/4-mediated innate immune responses. *PLoS Pathogens*, *13*, e1006600.

Yang, Y., Wang, S. Y., Huang, Z. F., Zou, H. M., Yan, B. R., Luo, W. W., et al. (2016). The RNA-binding protein Mex3B is a coreceptor of toll-like receptor 3 in innate antiviral response. *Cell Research*, *26*, 288.

Ye, W., Hu, M. M., Lei, C. Q., Zhou, Q., Lin, H., Sun, M. S., et al. (2017). TRIM8 negatively regulates TLR3/4-mediated innate immune response by blocking TRIF-TBK1 interaction. *Journal of Immunology*, *199*, 1856.

Yin, Q., Tian, Y., Kabaleeswaran, V., Jiang, X., Tu, D., Eck, M. J., et al. (2012). Cyclic di-GMP sensing via the innate immune signaling protein STING. *Molecular Cell*, *46*, 735.

Yoo, Y. S., Park, Y. Y., Kim, J. H., Cho, H., Kim, S. H., Lee, H. S., et al. (2015). The mitochondrial ubiquitin ligase MARCH5 resolves MAVS aggregates during antiviral signalling. *Nature Communications*, *6*, 7910.

You, F., Sun, H., Zhou, X., Sun, W., Liang, S., Zhai, Z., et al. (2009). PCBP2 mediates degradation of the adaptor MAVS via the HECT ubiquitin ligase AIP4. *Nature Immunology*, *10*, 1300.
You, F., Wang, P., Yang, L., Yang, G., Zhao, Y. O., Qian, F., et al. (2013). ELF4 is critical for induction of type I interferon and the host antiviral response. *Nature Immunology*, *14*, 1237.
Zhang, J., Hu, M. M., Wang, Y. Y., & Shu, H. B. (2012). TRIM32 protein modulates type I interferon induction and cellular antiviral response by targeting MITA/STING protein for K63-linked ubiquitination. *The Journal of Biological Chemistry*, *287*, 28646.
Zhang, Y., Lei, C. Q., Hu, Y. H., Xia, T., Li, M., Zhong, B., et al. (2014). Kruppel-like factor 6 is a co-activator of NF-kappaB that mediates p65-dependent transcription of selected downstream genes. *The Journal of Biological Chemistry*, *289*, 12876.
Zhang, C., Shang, G., Gui, X., Zhang, X., Bai, X. C., & Chen, Z. J. (2019). Structural basis of STING binding with and phosphorylation by TBK1. *Nature*, *567*, 394.
Zhang, M., Tian, Y., Wang, R. P., Gao, D., Zhang, Y., Diao, F. C., et al. (2008). Negative feedback regulation of cellular antiviral signaling by RBCK1-mediated degradation of IRF3. *Cell Research*, *18*, 1096.
Zhang, X., Wu, J., Du, F., Xu, H., Sun, L., Chen, Z., et al. (2014). The cytosolic DNA sensor cGAS forms an oligomeric complex with DNA and undergoes switch-like conformational changes in the activation loop. *Cell Reports*, *6*, 421.
Zhang, J., Xu, L. G., Han, K. J., & Shu, H. B. (2004). Identification of a ZU5 and death domain-containing inhibitor of NF-kappaB. *The Journal of Biological Chemistry*, *279*, 17819.
Zhang, Z., Yuan, B., Bao, M., Lu, N., Kim, T., & Liu, Y. J. (2011). The helicase DDX41 senses intracellular DNA mediated by the adaptor STING in dendritic cells. *Nature Immunology*, *12*, 959.
Zhang, M., Zhang, M. X., Zhang, Q., Zhu, G. F., Yuan, L., Zhang, D. E., et al. (2016). USP18 recruits USP20 to promote innate antiviral response through deubiquitinating STING/MITA. *Cell Research*, *26*, 1302.
Zheng, H., Li, Q., Chen, R., Zhang, J., Ran, Y., He, X., et al. (2013). The dual-specificity phosphatase DUSP14 negatively regulates tumor necrosis factor- and interleukin-1-induced nuclear factor-kappaB activation by dephosphorylating the protein kinase TAK1. *The Journal of Biological Chemistry*, *288*, 819.
Zhong, X., Feng, L., Xu, W. H., Wu, X., Ding, Y. D., Zhou, Y., et al. (2019). The zinc-finger protein ZFYVE1 modulates TLR3-mediated signaling by facilitating TLR3 ligand binding. *Cellular & Molecular Immunology*. https://doi.org/10.1038/s41423-019-0265-6.
Zhong, B., Yang, Y., Li, S., Wang, Y. Y., Li, Y., Diao, F., et al. (2008). The adaptor protein MITA links virus-sensing receptors to IRF3 transcription factor activation. *Immunity*, *29*, 538.
Zhong, B., Zhang, L., Lei, C., Li, Y., Mao, A. P., Yang, Y., et al. (2009). The ubiquitin ligase RNF5 regulates antiviral responses by mediating degradation of the adaptor protein MITA. *Immunity*, *30*, 397.
Zhong, B., Zhang, Y., Tan, B., Liu, T. T., Wang, Y. Y., & Shu, H. B. (2010). The E3 ubiquitin ligase RNF5 targets virus-induced signaling adaptor for ubiquitination and degradation. *Journal of Immunology*, *184*, 6249.
Zhou, Q., Lin, H., Wang, S., Wang, S., Ran, Y., Liu, Y., et al. (2014). The ER-associated protein ZDHHC1 is a positive regulator of DNA virus-triggered, MITA/STING-dependent innate immune signaling. *Cell Host & Microbe*, *16*, 450.
Zhou, X., You, F., Chen, H., & Jiang, Z. (2012). Poly(C)-binding protein 1 (PCBP1) mediates housekeeping degradation of mitochondrial antiviral signaling (MAVS). *Cell Research*, *22*, 717.

CHAPTER TWO

Tissue-resident NK cells and other innate lymphoid cells

Jing Zhou[a,b], Zhigang Tian[a,b,*], Hui Peng[a,b,*]
[a]Division of Molecular Medicine, Hefei National Laboratory for Physical Sciences at Microscale, The CAS Key Laboratory of Innate Immunity and Chronic Disease, School of Life Sciences, University of Science and Technology of China, Hefei, Anhui, China
[b]Institute of Immunology, University of Science and Technology of China, Hefei, Anhui, China
*Corresponding authors: e-mail address: tzg@ustc.edu.cn; huipeng@mail.ustc.edu.cn

Contents

Abstract

Natural killer (NK) cells are important innate effectors for their defense against pathogens and tumors without the need of prior sensitization. Along with the growing understanding of basic NK cell biology, it has been widely accepted that NK cells are a heterogeneous population of innate lymphoid cell (ILC) family. Apart from the conventional NK cell (cNK) subset that circulates throughout the body, some non-lymphoid tissues contain tissue-resident NK (trNK) cell subsets, and the composition of NK cell subsets varies greatly with different locations. Except for cNK cells, other ILCs are known as tissue-resident cells. In this review, we summarize the unique properties of trNK cells, discuss their lineage relationship with other ILCs, and highlight recent advances in our understanding of the functions of trNK cells and other ILCs.

Advances in Immunology, Volume 145
ISSN 0065-2776
https://doi.org/10.1016/bs.ai.2019.11.002

1. Introduction

As a component of innate immune system, NK cells lack recombination activating gene (RAG)-dependent rearranged antigen receptors, and express the NK cell surface markers NK1.1, NKp46 or CD49b (DX5) in mice, or CD56 and CD16 in humans (Guillerey, Huntington, & Smyth, 2016). NK cells can quickly respond to stressed cells, and their activation is determined by a complex integration of signals from an array of cell surface activating and inhibitory receptors (Sivori et al., 2019).

Apart from their direct cytotoxicity against infected cells or tumor cells via secretion of granzymes and perforin or expression of ligands for death receptors (Guillerey et al., 2016; Voskoboinik, Smyth, & Trapani, 2006), NK cells are also major producers of various cytokines and chemokines, such as interferon-γ (IFN-γ), tumor necrosis factor-α (TNF-α), granulocyte-macrophage colony-stimulating factor (GM-CSF) and chemokine (C–C motif) ligand 5 (CCL5), thereby contributing to shaping innate and adaptive immune responses (Lam & Lanier, 2017; Schuster, Coudert, Andoniou, & Degli-Esposti, 2016). Therefore, NK cells not only act as killers but also have immunoregulatory functions (Sungur et al., 2013). Furthermore, increasing evidence has revealed that NK cells can mediate antigen-specific immunological memory, challenging the conventional distinction between innate and adaptive immunity (Marcus & Raulet, 2013; Peng & Tian, 2017).

Early studies show that NK cells from different tissues exhibit distinct phenotypic characteristics (Di Santo, 2008; Takeda et al., 2005), and it has been considered to be related to unequal tissue distribution of NK cell subsets at different maturation stages. Recent findings of tissue-resident NK (trNK) cells have greatly improved our understanding of NK cell diversity. Unlike conventional NK (cNK) cells that are circulating and widely distributed, trNK cells are unevenly distributed at different sites with an enrichment in the liver and mucosal barrier (Fu et al., 2017; Peng et al., 2013; Sojka, Plougastel-Douglas, et al., 2014). trNK cells are distinct from cNK cells in expression of cell surface molecules and transcription factors. Different tissue-derived trNK cells share common markers and also have unique tissue-specific features, which may be shaped by local microenvironment factors.

Along with the expanding knowledge of NK cell heterogeneity, new innate cell types that belong to the lymphoid lineage have been sequentially discovered over the past decade. These newly identified populations, together with NK cells and lymphoid tissue-inducer (LTi) cells, constitute the innate lymphoid cell (ILC) family (Vivier et al., 2018). Except for cNK cells, most ILC members are tissue-resident (Gasteiger, Fan, Dikiy, Lee, & Rudensky, 2015), and contribute to multiple physiological and pathological processes, such as tissue remodeling, fetal growth, host defense and inflammation. Moreover, tissue-resident ILCs (trILCs) develop from a common progenitor cell, but require different transcriptional factors for their lineage fate decision. Here, we summarize recent findings of trNK cell subsets with tissue-specific features, discuss lineage relationship between trNK cells and other ILCs, and highlight recent advances in our understanding of the functions of trNK cells and other ILCs.

2. Discovery of liver-resident NK cells: A historical perspective

Liver NK cells were initially defined as "pit cells" in the rat liver with highly characteristic cytoplasmic granules, situating in the liver sinusoids and resembling fruit pits under an electron microscope (Wisse, van't Noordende, van der Meulen, & Daems, 1976). The percentage of NK cells among total hepatic lymphocytes (~50% in humans) is higher than that in many peripheral tissues (Mikulak, Bruni, Oriolo, Di Vito, & Mavilio, 2019). Furthermore, bulk NK cells in murine and human liver display phenotypic and functional properties differing from their counterparts in the spleen and or peripheral blood (Peng & Tian, 2018). Since liver NK cells express relatively low levels of NK cell maturation-associated makers such as CD11b, CD49b (DX5) and Ly49 receptors (Gordon et al., 2012; Kim et al., 2002; Ochi et al., 2004; Takeda et al., 2001, 2005), the peculiarity of liver NK cells was once ascribed to an abundant presence of immature NK cells in the liver.

Consistently, we also noticed that $CD11b^{-}CD27^{-}$ NK cells, which were considered immature, accounted for a large fraction of total liver NK cells in adult mice (Wu, Chen, Wei, Sun, & Tian, 2012). Furthermore, liver and spleen NK cells display different expression patterns of stimulatory receptors and adhesion molecules during ontogeny (Wu, Chen, Wei, et al., 2012). Interestingly, while NK cells in other tissues are scarcely influenced by IFN-γ, liver NK cells were reduced and functionally impaired in IFN-γ-deficient mice (Wu, Chen, Sun, et al., 2012). These findings suggest that there might be a specific developmental pathway for liver NK cells, and the local microenvironment may play important roles in remolding their development. Our further research indicates that murine liver NK cells consist of two distinct subsets, the $CD49a^-CD49b^+$ cNK cell subset and a unique $CD49a^+CD49b^-$ cell subset (Peng et al., 2013). The latter accounts for nearly half of total liver NK cells and takes up residence in the hepatic sinusoids without circulating in the blood, therefore termed liver-resident NK (LrNK) cells (Peng et al., 2013; Sojka, Plougastel-Douglas, et al., 2014). LrNK cells highly express the chemokine receptor CXCR6, and possess memory potential as evidenced by their ability of conferring hapten-specific contact hypersensitivity (CHS) responses (Peng et al., 2013), in accordance with previous finding of liver bulk NK cell-mediated CHS in a CXCR6-dependent manner (O'Leary, Goodarzi, Drayton, & von Andrian, 2006; Paust et al., 2010). The enrichment of this subset in the liver provides an explanation for the early recognition of the unique characteristics of liver bulk NK cells.

Although LrNK cells exhibit an immature phenotype, they maintain their phenotype without further differentiation into $CD49a^-CD49b^+$ cNK cells, suggesting that they are a stable subset rather than developmental intermediates (Peng et al., 2013). Furthermore, murine LrNK cell development is independent on Eomes, which is strictly required for murine cNK cells; the transcription factors T-bet, Hobit, PLZF and AhR are more important for LrNK cell development than for cNK cells (Constantinides, McDonald, Verhoef, & Bendelac, 2014; Mackay et al., 2016; Sojka, Plougastel-Douglas, et al., 2014; Zhang, Shin, Haggadone, & Sunwoo, 2016). Dependence on different transcription factors provide additional evidence that LrNK cells represent a unique cell lineage distinct from cNK cells.

Unique NK cell subsets resembling murine LrNK cells have also been found in human livers, although the identification of human LrNK cells remains controversial. Human $CD49a^+CD56^{bright}$ NK cells could be detected in liver but were rare in peripheral blood and, similar to murine LrNK cells, they had high expression of T-bet but low expression of Eomes (Marquardt et al., 2015). However, the presence and frequency of expression of $CD49a^+$ NK cells in human liver vary significantly among individuals (Marquardt et al., 2015). Further studies by other groups suggested that $CXCR6^+$ or $CD49e^-$ NK cells, which were specifically enriched in the liver, may represent human LrNK cells (Aw Yeang et al., 2017; Cuff et al., 2016; Stegmann et al., 2016). However, in contrast to the expression pattern of T-bet and Eomes in murine NK cells, these cells are $Eomes^{hi}T\text{-}bet^{low}$, while circulating NK cells are $Eomes^{low}T\text{-}bet^{hi}$ (Aw Yeang et al., 2017; Harmon et al., 2016), suggesting species differences in defining mouse and human NK cell subsets.

3. trNK cells in other tissues

The finding of LrNK cells provides an example for research into trNK cells in other tissues. Besides the liver, trNK cells are also found in the uterus, skin, kidney, salivary gland and adipose tissue (Cortez et al., 2016; O'Sullivan et al., 2016; Sojka, Plougastel-Douglas, et al., 2014; Victorino et al., 2015). trNK cells across different tissues share similarities and also display distinctive features.

NK cells are abundantly present in the uterus during early pregnancy, constituting approximately 70% of uterine lymphocytes (Fu & Wei, 2016). Compelling evidence highlighting a beneficial role of uterine NK cells in protecting fetus and promoting fetal development has been provided (Sojka, Yang, & Yokoyama, 2018). For instance, human $CD56^{bright}CD27^{+}$ decidual NK cells can inhibit Th17 cell differentiation through secreting IFN-γ, thereby contributing to maintaining maternal-fetal tolerance (Fu et al., 2013). Regarding subset composition of uterine NK cells, recent studies revealed that $CD49a^{+}$ trNK cells represent the predominant population in the uterus of virgin mice (Sojka, Plougastel-Douglas, et al., 2014). During pregnancy, although both trNK and cNK cell numbers increase in the mouse uterus, only trNK cells actively proliferate and represent the source of the expanding pool of uterine NK cells (Sojka, Yang, Plougastel-Douglas, et al., 2018). In contrast to LrNK cells that express low levels of Eomes and strictly rely on T-bet, $CD49a^{+}$ trNK cells in the uterus have high expression of Eomes, and their number is not significantly changed in T-bet-deficient mice. Transcription factors specifying the fate of uterus-resident NK cells are still unclear. Uterine trNK cells in mice and humans can secret several types of growth-promoting factors, and play a vital role in promoting early fetal growth (Fu et al., 2017). Among $CD49a^{+}$ uterine NK cells, a minor fraction is Eomes negative. These $CD49b^{+}Eomes^{-}$ cells, termed ILC1s, are analogous to LrNK cells and express high levels of the memory marker CXCR6 (Filipovic et al., 2018), raising a possibility of their memory potential.

The kidney also contains $CD49a^{+}CD49b^{-}$ trNK cells, which account for 15–20% of kidney NK cells (Victorino et al., 2015). Kidney-resident NK cells were moderately reduced in T-bet-deficient mice but increased in NFIL3-deficient mice (Victorino et al., 2015). In salivary glands, $CD49a^{+}CD49b^{+}$ NK cells with tissue-resident properties represent the predominant population (Cortez et al., 2016), and neither T-bet nor NFIL3 is required for their development (Cortez et al., 2016; Cortez, Fuchs, Cella, Gilfillan, & Colonna, 2014). The composition of NK cell subsets is more complicated for those in the adipose tissue, which comprises three distinct subsets (Boulenouar et al., 2017; O'Sullivan et al., 2016). In addition to the $CD49a^+CD49b^+Eomes^-$ trNK cell and $CD49a^-CD49b^+Eomes^+$ cNK cell subsets, $CD49a^-CD49b^-Eomes^+$ NK cells occupy a substantial fraction of adipose NK cells, and they are regarded as an immature stage of cNK cells for their ability of generating $CD49a^-CD49b^+Eomes^+$ cNK cells (O'Sullivan et al., 2016). This finding suggests that a local development pathway may exist for adipose NK cells.

Differences in NK cell subset composition and trNK cell diversity across different tissues might be related to tissue-specific microenvironment factors. For example, TGF-β is abundant in the salivary gland, and it also plays a vital role in shaping the characteristics of salivary gland trNK cells (Cortez et al., 2016). However, it remains largely unknown about which tissue-specific factors impact trNK cells in other tissues and how these factors coordinate with cellular intrinsic factors. An in vitro method for induction of $CD49a^+Eomes^{-/+}$ NK cells resembling trNK cells from bone marrow progenitors has been established (Ni et al., 2018). By using this method, IL-15 was found to be critical for the development and maintenance of $CD49a^+Eomes^-$ NK cells, while adding IL-4 could promote the expression of Eomes and convert $CD49a^+Eomes^-$ NK cells into $CD49a^+Eomes^+$ NK cells. These findings further hints at a role of environmental factors in shaping trNK cells and also provide a tool for studying trNK cell development.

4. Lineage relationship between trNK and other ILCs

With the discovery of newly identified ILC subsets, the ILC family has been expanding over the past decade (Vivier et al., 2018). Based on their cytokine secretion profiles, developmental requirements and functions, a nomenclature for ILCs proposed in 2013 categorized ILC subsets into three groups: group 1, 2 and 3 ILCs (Spits et al., 2013). Recently, a new classification model has been proposed based on the developmental pathways, in which ILCs are divided into five populations, including NK cells, ILC1s, ILC2s, ILC3s and LTi cells (Vivier et al., 2018).

According to the earlier proposed nomenclature for ILCs, NK cells and ILC1s belong to group 1 ILCs (Spits et al., 2013), as they share many similarities. For example, both of NK cells and ILC1s express NK cell-related markers such as NK1.1, NKp46 and the transcription factor T-bet.

A common functional property for them is the ability to produce IFN-γ during pathogen infections and tumor development (Gao et al., 2017; Klose et al., 2014), and this is also an important characteristic to distinguish them from other ILC subsets. While NK cells and ILC1s are IL-15-dependent, ILC2s, ILC3s and LTi cells rely on IL-7 for their maintenance (Kang & Coles, 2012; Moro et al., 2010; Yang et al., 2018). Despite such similarities, ILC1s are regarded as a lineage that develops separately from NK cells. Based on recent studies of ILC development, it has been increasingly accepted that all ILCs originate from a common innate lymphoid progenitor (CILPs), which further differentiate into NK cell precursors (NKPs) or into common helper innate lymphoid progenitors (CHILPs) (Klose et al., 2014; Yu et al., 2016). While NKPs only generate cNK cells, CHILPs give rise to lymphoid tissue inducer progenitors (LTiPs) and innate lymphoid cell precursors (ILCPs) that finally differentiate into ILC1s, ILC2s, or ILC3s (Vivier et al., 2018; Yu et al., 2016). Thus, regarding the developmental relationship, ILC1s seem to be more closely related to ILC2s and ILC3s rather than NK cells.

However, the phenotypic distinction between NK cells and ILC1s still blurs. Given that ILC1s express the cell surface molecules such as CD49a and CD69, which are initially used to characterize trNK cells, and they also exhibit tissue-resident properties (Tang et al., 2016), it is particularly difficult to discriminate trNK cells from ILC1s. This leads to a phenomenon for a cell population with two titles, called the "trNK cell" or "ILC1". Considering that the cell surface phenotype is hardly to discriminate these two populations, cell surface markers combined with transcription factors may better identify trNK cells and ILC1s. For example, in the murine uterus, trNK cells and ILC1s are identified using the expression patterns of CD49a and Eomes. The $CD49a^{+}Eomes^{-}$ subset is called uterine ILC1s, and the $CD49a^{+}Eomes^{+}$ subset is regarded as trNK cells (Filipovic et al., 2018; Fu et al., 2017). Whether this nomenclature also applies to other tissues needs further investigation. Moreover, since ILC1s are functionally defined as non-cytotoxic cells (Spits et al., 2013; Vivier et al., 2018), the effector functions should also be taken into account.

5. Functions of trNK cells and other ILCs

5.1 Functions of trNK cells/ILC1s

While our knowledge about NK cell functions are majorly obtained from previous studies on cNK cells or bulk NK cells (a mixture of both cNK and trNK cells), researchers are beginning to investigate the functions of different NK cell subsets and their relevance to diseases. It is now known that trNK cells/ILC1s are actively involved in multiple processes, such as antimicrobial defense, regulation of adaptive immunity, tumor immunoevasion and fetal growth.

LrNK cells are initially functionally featured by their ability to remember haptens in CHS models. Our recent study further indicated that the IL-7Rα$^+$CD49a$^+$ subset, which originated from draining lymph nodes and chose the liver for their long-term maintenance in an IL-7R signaling-dependent manner, possessed memory potential after hapten sensitization (Wang et al., 2018; Wang, Peng, & Tian, 2019). In addition to remembering haptens, LrNK cells can also remember encountered antigen from influenza virus after primary infection, and are more protective during secondary infection (Li et al., 2017). However, the mechanisms underlying how LrNK cells recognize different haptens and antigens and how they migrate to the sites of effector function, remain unclear.

NK cells play a critical role in viral clearance during murine cytomegalovirus (MCMV) infection, and accumulating evidence has highlighted the importance of Ly49H$^+$ cNK cells in this process (Arase, Mocarski, Campbell, Hill, & Lanier, 2002; Brown et al., 2001; Dokun et al., 2001; Sun, Beilke, & Lanier, 2009). However, recent studies demonstrate that trNK cells/ILC1s produce IFN-γ at local sites of MCMV infection and their responses are more rapidly than cNK cells, thus providing the major source of IFN-γ at the early infection stage and conferring host protection (Weizman et al., 2017). Moreover, similar to Ly49H$^+$ cNK cells, LrNK cells can also acquire MCMV-specific memory through recognition of the MCMV-encoded glycoprotein m12 (Weizman et al., 2019).

Beyond being innate immune effectors, NK cells can also act as modulators of adaptive immune responses through multiple mechanisms. Our group found that LrNK cells were enriched with genes associated with negative regulation and immune tolerance, and expressed an array of inhibitory molecules (Zhou et al., 2019). By using LrNK cells-deficient mice and cell transfer strategy, we demonstrated that LrNK cells negatively regulated the antiviral activity of hepatic T Cells via the PD-1/PD-L1 interaction during viral infection (Zhou et al., 2019). A more recent study also reported the negative regulatory role of LrNK cells in suppressing CD4$^+$ T cells proliferation in autoimmune cholangitis (Zhao et al., 2019). In humans, CD49a$^+$ LrNK cells accumulated in the liver of in hepatocellular carcinoma patient, which was correlated with poor prognosis (Sun et al., 2019), suggesting a probable role for them in tumor development.

trNK cells/ILC1s in other tissues also display diverse functions. In chronic MCMV infection, salivary gland trNK cells can eliminate $CD4^+$ T cells in a TRAIL-dependent manner and inhibit infection-induced autoimmunity (Schuster et al., 2014). In the kidney, trNK cells play a key role in mediating ischemic-reperfusion injury (Victorino et al., 2015). Additionally, ILC1s in adipose enable local macrophage toward M1 polarization, leading to adipose tissue inflammation and insulin resistance (Lee et al., 2016; O'Sullivan et al., 2016; Wensveen et al., 2015). Intriguingly, trNK cell in the uterus not only promote immune tolerance at the maternal-fetal interface, but also act as a "nurse," to promote fetal development by producing growth-promoting factors (Andreotti et al., 2018; Fu et al., 2013, 2017). Tumor-infiltrating ILC1s exhibit potent cytotoxic activities against tumor cells (Dadi et al., 2016); however, they may also help tumors escape from immune surveillance (Gao et al., 2017). Mucosal ILC1s participate in host defense against *T. gondii* and *Clostridium* infection (Abt et al., 2015; Klose et al., 2014) , and contribute to colitis through IFN-γ secretion (Buonocore et al., 2010).

5.2 Functions of ILC2s

ILC2s are considered the innate counterparts of Th2 cells. They can secrete type 2 cytokines such as IL-5, IL-9, IL-13, and amphiregulin in response to thymic stromal lymphopoietin (TSLP), IL-25, and IL-33 (Gurram & Zhu, 2019; Panda & Colonna, 2019), and rely on GATA3 for their development and functionality (Furusawa et al., 2013; Hoyler et al., 2012; Klein Wolterink et al., 2013; Yagi et al., 2014). ILC2s are tissue-resident cells (Gasteiger et al., 2015; Moro et al., 2010), with distribution in the lung (Beale et al., 2014; Oliphant et al., 2014), intestine (von Moltke, Ji, Liang, & Locksley, 2016), adipose tissue (Brestoff et al., 2015; Moro et al., 2010), skin (Kim et al., 2013; Roediger et al., 2013), islet (Dalmas et al., 2017) and liver (Li et al., 2014; McHedlidze et al., 2013).

Regarding ILC2 functions, it has been increasingly appreciated that ILC2s are important for the initiation of type 2 immune responses, thereby contributing to protective immunity against helminth infection and tissue repair (Bernink, Germar, & Spits, 2014). For example, ILC2-derived IL-4 drives Th2 cell differentiation following helminth infection (Pelly et al., 2016). ILC2s promote IL-13 production by Th2 cells dependently on MHC-II and PD-L1, leading to enhanced expulsion of gastrointestinal helminth (Oliphant et al., 2014; Schwartz et al., 2017). Furthermore, adipose-resident ILC2s regulate inflammation via interaction with local immune cells or adipocytes, and prevent diet-induced obesity (Brestoff et al., 2015; Hams, Locksley, McKenzie, & Fallon, 2013; Moro et al., 2010). In the islet, IL-33-activated ILC2s can promote macrophages and dendritic cells to produce retinoic acid, which in turn enhances insulin secretion (Dalmas et al., 2017). In the liver, ILC2-derived IL-13 is required for hepatic stellate cell activation, and contributes to hepatic fibrosis (McHedlidze et al., 2013). ILC2s also play a role in inducing cholangiocyte hyperplasia and cholangiocarcinoma (Li et al., 2014). However, they can protect the liver injury upon virus challenge via limiting the inflammatory response of neutrophils, macrophages and T cells (Liang et al., 2013, 2019). ILC2 functions can be regulated by local environmental stimuli. For instance, type I and type II interferons and IL-27 can restrain ILC2 cell-mediated immunopathology (Duerr et al., 2016). In rhinovirus-induced asthma exacerbation, IL-25 production from asthmatic epithelial cells upon viral infection could enhance the ability of ILC2s in driving type 2 immunity and allergic pulmonary inflammation (Beale et al., 2014).

5.3 Functions of ILC3s and LTi cells

ILC3s and LTi cells constitute the group 3 ILCs, and they are featured by their dependence on the transcription factor RORγt and ability of producing IL-17 and/or IL-22 (Eberl et al., 2004; Sanos et al., 2009). They exhibit tissue-resident properties and are preferentially distributed in the small intestine lamina propria, mesenteric lymph node, salivary gland and lung (Gasteiger et al., 2015).

ILC3s and LTi cells are important in lymphoid organogenesis, tissue remodeling, inflammation as well as host protective immunity against infections (Ebbo, Crinier, Vely, & Vivier, 2017; Gasteiger & Rudensky, 2014; Ignacio, Breda, & Camara, 2017; Lam & Lanier, 2017; Spits, Bernink, & Lanier, 2016; Walker, Barlow, & McKenzie, 2013). ILC3s were initially recognized as a unique subset of NK cells and named NK-22 cells, as they express NK cell markers and provide an innate source of IL-22 for mucosal immunity in humans and mice (Cella et al., 2009). IL-22 produced by ILC3s can enhance the proliferation of intestinal stem cells and maintain intestinal homeostasis (Guo et al., 2014; Vivier et al., 2018). Moreover, IL-22-producing NKp46$^+$ ILC3s provide innate mucosal immune defense against intestinal pathogen *Citrobacter rodentium* (Satoh-Takayama et al., 2008). Similarly, LTi cells can also secrete IL-22 and promote the production of antimicrobial molecules (Sanos et al., 2009). However, it has also been reported that ILC3s can directly limit commensal bacteria-specific $CD4^+$ T cell responses through MHC II-dependent induction of cell death, and this process is independent on IL-17A, IL-22 or IL-23 (Hepworth et al., 2013, 2015).

6. Conclusion

The discovery of trNK cells and other trILC subsets has greatly improved our understanding of innate immunity, leading to a redefined map for hematopoietic lineages. Recent advances have highlighted the importance of trILCs in shaping adaptive immunity, suggesting a coordination between local and systemic immune system. Although our knowledge of these newly identified cells is increasing, many questions remain to be addressed in this field: (1) What factors are involved in determining the diversity of trNK cells across different tissues? (2) How do trNK cells and other trILCs originate during ontogeney? Since they are maintained locally during adult life without external supplement, are they maintained by self-proliferation or by local hematopoietic progenitors? (3) How can we precisely discriminate trNK cells from ILC1s? Although LrNK cells have been found in mice and humans, do trNK cells exist in other human tissues? If so, how is their relevance to human diseases? Answering these questions would enable a better understanding of regional immunity, and provide insights into therapeutic strategy for human diseases.

Acknowledgments

This work was supported by the National Natural Science Foundation of China (Grant Nos. 81788101, 91642105, 81821001 and 91542000).

References

Abt, M. C., Lewis, B. B., Caballero, S., Xiong, H., Carter, R. A., Susac, B., et al. (2015). Innate immune defenses mediated by two ILC subsets are critical for protection against acute clostridium difficile infection. *Cell Host & Microbe, 18*, 27–37.

Andreotti, J. P., Paiva, A. E., Prazeres, P., Guerra, D. A. P., Silva, W. N., Vaz, R. S., et al. (2018). The role of natural killer cells in the uterine microenvironment during pregnancy. *Cellular & Molecular Immunology, 15*, 941–943.

Arase, H., Mocarski, E. S., Campbell, A. E., Hill, A. B., & Lanier, L. L. (2002). Direct recognition of cytomegalovirus by activating and inhibitory NK cell receptors. *Science, 296*, 1323–1326.

Aw Yeang, H. X., Piersma, S. J., Lin, Y., Yang, L., Malkova, O. N., Miner, C., et al. (2017). Cutting edge: Human CD49e- NK cells are tissue resident in the liver. *Journal of Immunology, 198*, 1417–1422.

Beale, J., Jayaraman, A., Jackson, D. J., Macintyre, J. D., Edwards, M. R., Walton, R. P., et al. (2014). Rhinovirus-induced IL-25 in asthma exacerbation drives type 2 immunity and allergic pulmonary inflammation. *Science Translational Medicine*, *6*, 256ra134.

Bernink, J. H., Germar, K., & Spits, H. (2014). The role of ILC2 in pathology of type 2 inflammatory diseases. *Current Opinion in Immunology*, *31*, 115–120.

Boulenouar, S., Michelet, X., Duquette, D., Alvarez, D., Hogan, A. E., Dold, C., et al. (2017). Adipose type one innate lymphoid cells regulate macrophage homeostasis through targeted cytotoxicity. *Immunity*, *46*, 273–286.

Brestoff, J. R., Kim, B. S., Saenz, S. A., Stine, R. R., Monticelli, L. A., Sonnenberg, G. F., et al. (2015). Group 2 innate lymphoid cells promote beiging of white adipose tissue and limit obesity. *Nature*, *519*, 242–246.

Brown, M. G., Dokun, A. O., Heusel, J. W., Smith, H. R., Beckman, D. L., Blattenberger, E. A., et al. (2001). Vital involvement of a natural killer cell activation receptor in resistance to viral infection. *Science*, *292*, 934–937.

Buonocore, S., Ahern, P. P., Uhlig, H. H., Ivanov, I. I., Littman, D. R., Maloy, K. J., et al. (2010). Innate lymphoid cells drive interleukin-23-dependent innate intestinal pathology. *Nature*, *464*, 1371–1375.

Cella, M., Fuchs, A., Vermi, W., Facchetti, F., Otero, K., Lennerz, J. K., et al. (2009). A human natural killer cell subset provides an innate source of IL-22 for mucosal immunity. *Nature*, *457*, 722–725.

Constantinides, M. G., McDonald, B. D., Verhoef, P. A., & Bendelac, A. (2014). A committed precursor to innate lymphoid cells. *Nature*, *508*, 397–401.

Cortez, V. S., Cervantes-Barragan, L., Robinette, M. L., Bando, J. K., Wang, Y., Geiger, T. L., et al. (2016). Transforming growth factor-beta signaling guides the differentiation of innate lymphoid cells in salivary glands. *Immunity*, *44*, 1127–1139.

Cortez, V. S., Fuchs, A., Cella, M., Gilfillan, S., & Colonna, M. (2014). Cutting edge: Salivary gland NK cells develop independently of Nfil3 in steady-state. *Journal of Immunology*, *192*, 4487–4491.

Cuff, A. O., Robertson, F. P., Stegmann, K. A., Pallett, L. J., Maini, M. K., Davidson, B. R., et al. (2016). Eomeshi NK cells in human liver are long-lived and do not recirculate but can be replenished from the circulation. *Journal of Immunology*, *197*, 4283–4291.

Dadi, S., Chhangawala, S., Whitlock, B. M., Franklin, R. A., Luo, C. T., Oh, S. A., et al. (2016). Cancer immunosurveillance by tissue-resident innate lymphoid cells and innate-like T cells. *Cell*, *164*, 365–377.

Dalmas, E., Lehmann, F. M., Dror, E., Wueest, S., Thienel, C., Borsigova, M., et al. (2017). Interleukin-33-activated islet-resident innate lymphoid cells promote insulin secretion through myeloid cell retinoic acid production. *Immunity*, *47*, 928–942.e927.

Di Santo, J. P. (2008). Functionally distinct NK-cell subsets: Developmental origins and biological implications. *European Journal of Immunology*, *38*, 2948–2951.

Dokun, A. O., Kim, S., Smith, H. R., Kang, H. S., Chu, D. T., & Yokoyama, W. M. (2001). Specific and nonspecific NK cell activation during virus infection. *Nature Immunology*, *2*, 951–956.

Duerr, C. U., McCarthy, C. D., Mindt, B. C., Rubio, M., Meli, A. P., Pothlichet, J., et al. (2016). Type I interferon restricts type 2 immunopathology through the regulation of group 2 innate lymphoid cells. *Nature Immunology*, *17*, 65–75.

Ebbo, M., Crinier, A., Vely, F., & Vivier, E. (2017). Innate lymphoid cells: Major players in inflammatory diseases. *Nature Reviews Immunology*, *17*, 665–678.

Eberl, G., Marmon, S., Sunshine, M. J., Rennert, P. D., Choi, Y., & Littman, D. R. (2004). An essential function for the nuclear receptor RORgamma(t) in the generation of fetal lymphoid tissue inducer cells. *Nature Immunology*, *5*, 64–73.

Filipovic, I., Chiossone, L., Vacca, P., Hamilton, R. S., Ingegnere, T., Doisne, J. M., et al. (2018). Molecular definition of group 1 innate lymphoid cells in the mouse uterus. *Nature Communications*, *9*, 4492.
Fu, B., Li, X., Sun, R., Tong, X., Ling, B., Tian, Z., et al. (2013). Natural killer cells promote immune tolerance by regulating inflammatory TH17 cells at the human maternal-fetal interface. *Proceedings of the National Academy of Sciences of the United States of America*, *110*, E231–E240.
Fu, B., & Wei, H. (2016). Decidual natural killer cells and the immune microenvironment at the maternal-fetal interface. *Science China. Life Sciences*, *59*, 1224–1231.
Fu, B., Zhou, Y., Ni, X., Tong, X., Xu, X., Dong, Z., et al. (2017). Natural killer cells promote fetal development through the secretion of growth-promoting factors. *Immunity*, *47*, 1100–1113 e1106.
Furusawa, J., Moro, K., Motomura, Y., Okamoto, K., Zhu, J., Takayanagi, H., et al. (2013). Critical role of p38 and GATA3 in natural helper cell function. *Journal of Immunology*, *191*, 1818–1826.
Gao, Y., Souza-Fonseca-Guimaraes, F., Bald, T., Ng, S. S., Young, A., Ngiow, S. F., et al. (2017). Tumor immunoevasion by the conversion of effector NK cells into type 1 innate lymphoid cells. *Nature Immunology*, *18*, 1004–1015.
Gasteiger, G., Fan, X., Dikiy, S., Lee, S. Y., & Rudensky, A. Y. (2015). Tissue residency of innate lymphoid cells in lymphoid and nonlymphoid organs. *Science*, *350*, 981–985.
Gasteiger, G., & Rudensky, A. Y. (2014). Interactions between innate and adaptive lymphocytes. *Nature Reviews Immunology*, *14*, 631–639.
Gordon, S. M., Chaix, J., Rupp, L. J., Wu, J., Madera, S., Sun, J. C., et al. (2012). The transcription factors T-bet and Eomes control key checkpoints of natural killer cell maturation. *Immunity*, *36*, 55–67.
Guillerey, C., Huntington, N. D., & Smyth, M. J. (2016). Targeting natural killer cells in cancer immunotherapy. *Nature Immunology*, *17*, 1025–1036.
Guo, X., Qiu, J., Tu, T., Yang, X., Deng, L., Anders, R. A., et al. (2014). Induction of innate lymphoid cell-derived interleukin-22 by the transcription factor STAT3 mediates protection against intestinal infection. *Immunity*, *40*, 25–39.
Gurram, R. K., & Zhu, J. (2019). Orchestration between ILC2s and Th2 cells in shaping type 2 immune responses. *Cellular & Molecular Immunology*, *16*, 225–235.
Hams, E., Locksley, R. M., McKenzie, A. N., & Fallon, P. G. (2013). Cutting edge: IL-25 elicits innate lymphoid type 2 and type II NKT cells that regulate obesity in mice. *Journal of Immunology*, *191*, 5349–5353.
Harmon, C., Robinson, M. W., Fahey, R., Whelan, S., Houlihan, D. D., Geoghegan, J., et al. (2016). Tissue-resident Eomes(hi) T-bet(lo) CD56(bright) NK cells with reduced proinflammatory potential are enriched in the adult human liver. *European Journal of Immunology*, *46*, 2111–2120.
Hepworth, M. R., Fung, T. C., Masur, S. H., Kelsen, J. R., McConnell, F. M., Dubrot, J., et al. (2015). Immune tolerance. Group 3 innate lymphoid cells mediate intestinal selection of commensal bacteria-specific CD4(+) T cells. *Science*, *348*, 1031–1035.
Hepworth, M. R., Monticelli, L. A., Fung, T. C., Ziegler, C. G., Grunberg, S., Sinha, R., et al. (2013). Innate lymphoid cells regulate CD4+ T-cell responses to intestinal commensal bacteria. *Nature*, *498*, 113–117.
Hoyler, T., Klose, C. S., Souabni, A., Turqueti-Neves, A., Pfeifer, D., Rawlins, E. L., et al. (2012). The transcription factor GATA-3 controls cell fate and maintenance of type 2 innate lymphoid cells. *Immunity*, *37*, 634–648.
Ignacio, A., Breda, C. N. S., & Camara, N. O. S. (2017). Innate lymphoid cells in tissue homeostasis and diseases. *World Journal of Hepatology*, *9*, 979–989.
Kang, J., & Coles, M. (2012). IL-7: The global builder of the innate lymphoid network and beyond, one niche at a time. *Seminars in Immunology*, *24*, 190–197.

Kim, S., Iizuka, K., Kang, H. S. P., Dokun, A., French, A. R., Greco, S., et al. (2002). In vivo developmental stages in murine natural killer cell maturation. *Nature Immunology*, *3*, 523–528.

Kim, B. S., Siracusa, M. C., Saenz, S. A., Noti, M., Monticelli, L. A., Sonnenberg, G. F., et al. (2013). TSLP elicits IL-33-independent innate lymphoid cell responses to promote skin inflammation. *Science Translational Medicine*, *5*, 170ra116.

Klein Wolterink, R. G., Serafini, N., van Nimwegen, M., Vosshenrich, C. A., de Bruijn, M. J., Fonseca Pereira, D., et al. (2013). Essential, dose-dependent role for the transcription factor Gata3 in the development of IL-5+ and IL-13+ type 2 innate lymphoid cells. *Proceedings of the National Academy of Sciences of the United States of America*, *110*, 10240–10245.

Klose, C. S. N., Flach, M., Mohle, L., Rogell, L., Hoyler, T., Ebert, K., et al. (2014). Differentiation of type 1 ILCs from a common progenitor to all helper-like innate lymphoid cell lineages. *Cell*, *157*, 340–356.

Lam, V. C., & Lanier, L. L. (2017). NK cells in host responses to viral infections. *Current Opinion in Immunology*, *44*, 43–51.

Lee, B. C., Kim, M. S., Pae, M., Yamamoto, Y., Eberle, D., Shimada, T., et al. (2016). Adipose natural killer cells regulate adipose tissue macrophages to promote insulin resistance in obesity. *Cell Metabolism*, *23*, 685–698.

Li, J., Razumilava, N., Gores, G. J., Walters, S., Mizuochi, T., Mourya, R., et al. (2014). Biliary repair and carcinogenesis are mediated by IL-33-dependent cholangiocyte proliferation. *Journal of Clinical Investigation*, *124*, 3241–3251.

Li, T., Wang, J., Wang, Y., Chen, Y., Wei, H., Sun, R., et al. (2017). Respiratory influenza virus infection induces memory-like liver NK cells in mice. *Journal of Immunology*, *198*, 1242–1252.

Liang, Y., Jie, Z., Hou, L., Aguilar-Valenzuela, R., Vu, D., Soong, L., et al. (2013). IL-33 induces nuocytes and modulates liver injury in viral hepatitis. *Journal of Immunology*, *190*, 5666–5675.

Liang, Y., Yi, P., Yuan, D. M. K., Jie, Z., Kwota, Z., Soong, L., et al. (2019). IL-33 induces immunosuppressive neutrophils via a type 2 innate lymphoid cell/IL-13/STAT6 axis and protects the liver against injury in LCMV infection-induced viral hepatitis. *Cellular & Molecular Immunology*, *16*, 126–137.

Mackay, L. K., Minnich, M., Kragten, N. A., Liao, Y., Nota, B., Seillet, C., et al. (2016). Hobit and Blimp1 instruct a universal transcriptional program of tissue residency in lymphocytes. *Science*, *352*, 459–463.

Marcus, A., & Raulet, D. H. (2013). Evidence for natural killer cell memory. *Current Biology*, *23*, R817–R820.

Marquardt, N., Béziat, V., Nyström, S., Hengst, J., Ivarsson, M. A., Kekäläinen, E., et al. (2015). Cutting edge: Identification and characterization of human intrahepatic CD49a+ NK cells. *Journal of Immunology*, *194*, 2467–2471.

McHedlidze, T., Waldner, M., Zopf, S., Walker, J., Rankin, A. L., Schuchmann, M., et al. (2013). Interleukin-33-dependent innate lymphoid cells mediate hepatic fibrosis. *Immunity*, *39*, 357–371.

Mikulak, J., Bruni, E., Oriolo, F., Di Vito, C., & Mavilio, D. (2019). Hepatic natural killer cells: Organ-specific sentinels of liver immune homeostasis and physiopathology. *Frontiers in Immunology*, *10*, 946.

Moro, K., Yamada, T., Tanabe, M., Takeuchi, T., Ikawa, T., Kawamoto, H., et al. (2010). Innate production of T(H)2 cytokines by adipose tissue-associated c-Kit(+)Sca-1(+) lymphoid cells. *Nature*, *463*, 540–544.

Ni, X., Fu, B., Zhang, J., Sun, R., Tian, Z., & Wei, H. (2018). Cytokine-based generation of CD49a+Eomes-/+ natural killer cell subsets. *Frontiers in Immunology*, *9*, 2126.

Ochi, M., Ohdan, H., Mitsuta, H., Onoe, T., Tokita, D., Hara, H., et al. (2004). Liver NK cells expressing TRAIL are toxic against self hepatocytes in mice. *Hepatology*, *39*, 1321–1331.
O'Leary, J. G., Goodarzi, M., Drayton, D. L., & von Andrian, U. H. (2006). T cell- and B cell-independent adaptive immunity mediated by natural killer cells. *Nature Immunology*, *7*, 507–516.
Oliphant, C. J., Hwang, Y. Y., Walker, J. A., Salimi, M., Wong, S. H., Brewer, J. M., et al. (2014). MHCII-mediated dialog between group 2 innate lymphoid cells and CD4(+) T cells potentiates type 2 immunity and promotes parasitic helminth expulsion. *Immunity*, *41*, 283–295.
O'Sullivan, T. E., Rapp, M., Fan, X., Weizman, O. E., Bhardwaj, P., Adams, N. M., et al. (2016). Adipose-resident group 1 innate lymphoid cells promote obesity-associated insulin resistance. *Immunity*, *45*, 428–441.
Panda, S. K., & Colonna, M. (2019). Innate lymphoid cells in mucosal immunity. *Frontiers in Immunology*, *10*, 861.
Paust, S., Gill, H. S., Wang, B. Z., Flynn, M. P., Moseman, E. A., Senman, B., et al. (2010). Critical role for the chemokine receptor CXCR6 in NK cell-mediated antigen-specific memory of haptens and viruses. *Nature Immunology*, *11*, 1127–1135.
Pelly, V. S., Kannan, Y., Coomes, S. M., Entwistle, L. J., Ruckerl, D., Seddon, B., et al. (2016). IL-4-producing ILC2s are required for the differentiation of TH2 cells following Heligmosomoides polygyrus infection. *Mucosal Immunology*, *9*, 1407–1417.
Peng, H., Jiang, X., Chen, Y., Sojka, D. K., Wei, H., Gao, X., et al. (2013). Liver-resident NK cells confer adaptive immunity in skin-contact inflammation. *Journal of Clinical Investigation*, *123*, 1444–1456.
Peng, H., & Tian, Z. (2017). Natural killer cell memory: Progress and implications. *Frontiers in Immunology*, *8*, 1143.
Peng, H., & Tian, Z. (2018). NK cells in liver homeostasis and viral hepatitis. *Science China. Life Sciences*, *61*, 1477–1485.
Roediger, B., Kyle, R., Yip, K. H., Sumaria, N., Guy, T. V., Kim, B. S., et al. (2013). Cutaneous immunosurveillance and regulation of inflammation by group 2 innate lymphoid cells. *Nature Immunology*, *14*, 564–573.
Sanos, S. L., Bui, V. L., Mortha, A., Oberle, K., Heners, C., Johner, C., et al. (2009). RORgammat and commensal microflora are required for the differentiation of mucosal interleukin 22-producing NKp46+ cells. *Nature Immunology*, *10*, 83–91.
Satoh-Takayama, N., Vosshenrich, C. A., Lesjean-Pottier, S., Sawa, S., Lochner, M., Rattis, F., et al. (2008). Microbial flora drives interleukin 22 production in intestinal NKp46+ cells that provide innate mucosal immune defense. *Immunity*, *29*, 958–970.
Schuster, I. S., Coudert, J. D., Andoniou, C. E., & Degli-Esposti, M. A. (2016). "Natural regulators": NK cells as modulators of T cell immunity. *Frontiers in Immunology*, *7*, 235.
Schuster, I. S., Wikstrom, M. E., Brizard, G., Coudert, J. D., Estcourt, M. J., Manzur, M., et al. (2014). TRAIL+ NK cells control CD4+ T cell responses during chronic viral infection to limit autoimmunity. *Immunity*, *41*, 646–656.
Schwartz, C., Khan, A. R., Floudas, A., Saunders, S. P., Hams, E., Rodewald, H. R., et al. (2017). ILC2s regulate adaptive Th2 cell functions via PD-L1 checkpoint control. *Journal of Experimental Medicine*, *214*, 2507–2521.
Sivori, S., Vacca, P., Del Zotto, G., Munari, E., Mingari, MC., & Moretta, L. (2019). Human NK cells: surface receptors, inhibitory checkpoints, and translational applications. *Cellular & Molecular Immunology*, *16*, 430–441.
Sojka, D. K., Plougastel-Douglas, B., Yang, L., Pak-Wittel, M. A., Artyomov, M. N., Ivanova, Y., et al. (2014). Tissue-resident natural killer (NK) cells are cell lineages distinct from thymic and conventional splenic NK cells. *eLife*, *3*, e01659.

Sojka, D. K., Yang, L., Plougastel-Douglas, B., Higuchi, D. A., Croy, B. A., & Yokoyama, W. M. (2018). Cutting edge: Local proliferation of uterine tissue-resident NK cells during decidualization in mice. *Journal of Immunology*, *201*, 2551–2556.

Sojka, D. K., Yang, L., & Yokoyama, W. M. (2018). Uterine natural killer cells: To protect and to nurture. *Birth Defects Research*, *110*, 1531–1538.

Spits, H., Artis, D., Colonna, M., Diefenbach, A., Di Santo, J. P., Eberl, G., et al. (2013). Innate lymphoid cells—A proposal for uniform nomenclature. *Nature Reviews Immunology*, *13*, 145–149.

Spits, H., Bernink, J. H., & Lanier, L. (2016). NK cells and type 1 innate lymphoid cells: Partners in host defense. *Nature Immunology*, *17*, 758–764.

Stegmann, K. A., Robertson, F., Hansi, N., Gill, U., Pallant, C., Christophides, T., et al. (2016). CXCR6 marks a novel subset of T-bet(lo)Eomes(hi) natural killer cells residing in human liver. *Scientific Reports*, *6*, 26157.

Sun, J. C., Beilke, J. N., & Lanier, L. L. (2009). Adaptive immune features of natural killer cells. *Nature*, *457*, 557–561.

Sun, H., Liu, L., Huang, Q., Liu, H., Huang, M., Wang, J., et al. (2019). Accumulation of tumor-infiltrating CD49a(+) NK cells correlates with poor prognosis for human hepatocellular carcinoma. *Cancer Immunology Research*, *7*, 1535–1546.

Sungur, C. M., Tang-Feldman, Y. J., Ames, E., Alvarez, M., Chen, M., Longo, D. L., et al. (2013). Murine natural killer cell licensing and regulation by T regulatory cells in viral responses. *Proceedings of the National Academy of Sciences of the United States of America*, *110*, 7401–7406.

Takeda, K., Cretney, E., Hayakawa, Y., Ota, T., Akiba, H., Ogasawara, K., et al. (2005). TRAIL identifies immature natural killer cells in newborn mice and adult mouse liver. *Blood*, *105*, 2082–2089.

Takeda, K., Hayakawa, Y., Smyth, M. J., Kayagaki, N., Yamaguchi, N., Kakuta, S., et al. (2001). Involvement of tumor necrosis factor-related apoptosis-inducing ligand in surveillance of tumor metastasis by liver natural killer cells. *Nature Medicine*, *7*, 94–100.

Tang, L., Peng, H., Zhou, J., Chen, Y., Wei, H., Sun, R., et al. (2016). Differential phenotypic and functional properties of liver-resident NK cells and mucosal ILC1s. *Journal of Autoimmunity*, *67*, 29–35.

Victorino, F., Sojka, D. K., Brodsky, K. S., McNamee, E. N., Masterson, J. C., Homann, D., et al. (2015). Tissue-resident NK cells mediate ischemic kidney injury and are not depleted by anti-asialo-GM1 antibody. *Journal of Immunology*, *195*, 4973–4985.

Vivier, E., Artis, D., Colonna, M., Diefenbach, A., Di Santo, J. P., Eberl, G., et al. (2018). Innate lymphoid cells: 10 Years on. *Cell*, *174*, 1054–1066.

von Moltke, J., Ji, M., Liang, H. E., & Locksley, R. M. (2016). Tuft-cell-derived IL-25 regulates an intestinal ILC2-epithelial response circuit. *Nature*, *529*, 221–225.

Voskoboinik, I., Smyth, M. J., & Trapani, J. A. (2006). Perforin-mediated target-cell death and immune homeostasis. *Nature Reviews Immunology*, *6*, 940–952.

Walker, J. A., Barlow, J. L., & McKenzie, A. N. (2013). Innate lymphoid cells—How did we miss them? *Nature Reviews Immunology*, *13*, 75–87.

Wang, X., Peng, H., Cong, J., Lian, Z., Wei, H., Sun, R., et al. (2018). Memory formation and long-term maintenance of IL-7Ralpha(+) ILC1s via a lymph node-liver axis. *Nature Communications*, *9*, 4854.

Wang, X., Peng, H., & Tian, Z. (2019). Innate lymphoid cell memory. *Cellular & Molecular Immunology*, *16*, 423–429.

Weizman, O. E., Adams, N. M., Schuster, I. S., Krishna, C., Pritykin, Y., Lau, C., et al. (2017). ILC1 confer early host protection at initial sites of viral infection. *Cell*, *171*, 795–808 e712.

Weizman, O. E., Song, E., Adams, N. M., Hildreth, A. D., Riggan, L., Krishna, C., et al. (2019). Mouse cytomegalovirus-experienced ILC1s acquire a memory response dependent on the viral glycoprotein m12. *Nature Immunology*, *20*, 1004–1011.
Wensveen, F. M., Jelenčić, V., Valentić, S., Šestan, M., Wensveen, T. T., Theurich, S., et al. (2015). NK cells link obesity-induced adipose stress to inflammation and insulin resistance. *Nature Immunology*, *16*, 376–385.
Wisse, E., van't Noordende, J. M., van der Meulen, J., & Daems, W. T. (1976). The pit cell: Description of a new type of cell occurring in rat liver sinusoids and peripheral blood. *Cell and Tissue Research*, *173*, 423–435.
Wu, X., Chen, Y., Sun, R., Wei, H., & Tian, Z. (2012). Impairment of hepatic NK cell development in IFN-gamma deficient mice. *Cytokine*, *60*, 616–625.
Wu, X., Chen, Y., Wei, H., Sun, R., & Tian, Z. (2012). Development of murine hepatic NK cells during ontogeny: Comparison with spleen NK cells. *Clinical and Developmental Immunology*, *2012*, 2012.
Yagi, R., Zhong, C., Northrup, D. L., Yu, F., Bouladoux, N., Spencer, S., et al. (2014). The transcription factor GATA3 is critical for the development of all IL-7Ralpha-expressing innate lymphoid cells. *Immunity*, *40*, 378–388.
Yang, J., Cornelissen, F., Papazian, N., Reijmers, R. M., Llorian, M., Cupedo, T., et al. (2018). IL-7-dependent maintenance of ILC3s is required for normal entry of lymphocytes into lymph nodes. *Journal of Experimental Medicine*, *215*, 1069–1077.
Yu, Y., Tsang, J. C., Wang, C., Clare, S., Wang, J., Chen, X., et al. (2016). Single-cell RNA-seq identifies a PD-1(hi) ILC progenitor and defines its development pathway. *Nature*, *539*, 102–106.
Zhang, L. H., Shin, J. H., Haggadone, M. D., & Sunwoo, J. B. (2016). The aryl hydrocarbon receptor is required for the maintenance of liver-resident natural killer cells. *Journal of Experimental Medicine*, *213*, 2249–2257.
Zhao, Z., Lu, F., Ma, H., Wang, Y., Yang, W., Long, J., et al. (2019). Liver-resident NK cells suppress autoimmune cholangitis and limit the proliferation of CD4(+) T cells. *Cellular & Molecular Immunology*, https://doi.org/10.1038/s41423-019-0199-z.
Zhou, J., Peng, H., Li, K., Qu, K., Wang, B., Wu, Y., et al. (2019). Liver-resident NK cells control antiviral activity of hepatic T cells via the PD-1-PD-L1 axis. *Immunity*, *50*, 403–417 e404.

CHAPTER THREE

The strategies of targeting the NLRP3 inflammasome to treat inflammatory diseases

Hua Jiang[a], Tao Gong[a,*], Rongbin Zhou[a,b,*]

[a]Hefei National Laboratory for Physical Sciences at Microscale, CAS Key Laboratory of Innate Immunity and Chronic Disease, School of Basic Medical Sciences, Division of Life Science and Medicine, University of Science and Technology of China, Hefei, China
[b]CAS Centre for Excellence in Cell and Molecular Biology, University of Science and Technology of China, Hefei, China
*Corresponding authors: e-mail address: gtao@ustc.edu.cn; zrb1980@ustc.edu.cn

Contents

Advances in Immunology, Volume 145
ISSN 0065-2776
https://doi.org/10.1016/bs.ai.2019.11.003

Abstract

The NLRP3 inflammasome is a cytoplasmic multiprotein complex, the assembly of which can be initiated in response to various exogenous or endogenous danger signals. Excessive activation of the NLRP3 inflammasome has been implicated in the pathogenesis of a wide variety of human inflammatory diseases, suggesting that the NLRP3 inflammasome is a potential target for the treatment of these diseases. However, clinical drugs targeting the NLRP3 inflammasome are still not available. Recent data have elucidated the different signaling pathways or events that can control NLRP3 inflammasome activation and have provided some potential compounds with anti-NLRP3 inflammasome activity. Here, we summarize the molecular mechanisms and diseases involved in NLRP3 inflammasome activation and discuss the potential strategies targeting different aspects of the NLRP3 inflammasome and its implications for the treatment of inflammatory diseases.

1. Introduction

To date, 22 human Nod-like Receptors (NLRs) and 34 mouse NLRs have been identified (Harton, Linhoff, Zhang, & Ting, 2002). All NLRs have a similar tripartite domain organization (Martinon, Mayor, & Tschopp, 2009). A leucine-rich repeat (LRR) domain located in the C-terminal domain of NLRs participates in ligand sensing and auto-regulation. A nucleotide-binding oligomerization domain (NACHT domain) is the central domain responsible for nucleotide binding and self-oligomerization. An effector domain of NLRs usually located in the N-terminus region contains a caspase activation and recruitment domain (CARD) or pyrin domain (PYD), both of which belong to the death domain superfamily and are involved in homotypic protein-protein interactions and signal transduction to other downstream PYD- or CARD-containing proteins (Gross, Thomas, Guarda, & Tschopp, 2011). One of the most important functions of NLRs is to form the multiprotein complex termed the "inflammasome" in sensing and recognizing pathogen-associated molecular patterns (PAMPs) and damage-associated molecular patterns (DAMPs). Different NLRs, such as NLRP1 (NLR family pyrin domain-containing 1), NLRP3, NLRP6 and NLRC4 (NLR family CARD domain-containing protein 4), can recognize various kinds of PAMPs and DAMPs, resulting in local or systemic inflammation reactions by the activation of inflammasomes, with which the hosts hence establish a critical defense line against the infection and other danger signals

(Gong, Jiang, & Zhou, 2018). Numerous studies have indicated that excessive activation of the inflammasome can elicit acute or chronic inflammation and result in various human diseases (Awad et al., 2018). In addition, many studies have indicated that the treatment of these inflammatory diseases needs a balanced and appropriate control of inflammasome-driven inflammation (Awad et al., 2018; Mangan et al., 2018; Voet, Srinivasan, Lamkanfi, & van Loo, 2019).

Unlike other inflammasomes, which usually sense a special kind of stimulus, the NLRP3 inflammasome can be activated not only by the broadest range of PAMPs, such as bacterial toxins, microbial pore-forming toxins and cytoplasmic lipopolysaccharides (LPS), but also by various DAMPs, including the crystalline particles monosodium urate (MSU), alum, silica, asbestos and amyloid-β as well as the endogenous intermediate metabolites ATP and saturated fatty acids (Dostert et al., 2008; Mariathasan et al., 2006; Wang et al., 2014). Given the broadest range of PAMPs and DAMPs recognized by NLRP3, the NLRP3 inflammasome is one of the most important inflammasomes that is broadly implicated in the pathogenesis of various human diseases, such as neurodegenerative diseases, metabolic disorders and autoimmune diseases (Mangan et al., 2018; Strowig, Henao-Mejia, Elinav, & Flavell, 2012). Recent data have elucidated the different molecules or events that can regulate NLRP3 inflammasome activation and have provided several potential compounds with anti-NLRP3 inflammasome activity. In this review, we will discuss the molecular mechanisms and diseases involved in NLRP3 inflammasome activation. Specifically, we will highlight the strategies of targeting the NLRP3 inflammasome and their clinical potential to treat NLRP3-related inflammatory diseases.

2. Molecular mechanisms of NLRP3 inflammasome activation

As generally accepted, a two-signal model, referred to as the "priming" signal and the "activation" signal, has been proposed during the activation of the NLRP3 inflammasome (Gong, Jiang, & Zhou, 2018; Gong, Yang, Jin, Jiang, & Zhou, 2018). Usually, the priming signal provided by microbial or endogenous molecules is transduced through the Toll-like receptor (TLR) signaling pathway, which facilitates the activation of the NF-KB pathway. Then, the basal expression of precursor IL-1β and NLRP3 protein are significantly increased. It is worth noting that the priming signal can also induce the posttranscriptional modification of NLRP3, such as the deubiquitination and phosphorylation of NLRP3, to facilitate subsequent NLRP3 inflammasome activation (Py, Kim, Vakifahmetoglu-Norberg, & Yuan, 2013; Song et al., 2017). Once primed, a wide variety of DAMPs and PAMPs trigger the assembly of NLRP3 in a homotypic interaction manner between its NACHT domain. A cluster of PYD of NLRP3 is formed to interact with the PYD of adaptor protein ASC, which then leads to the formation of ASC speck. Clustered ASC recruits pro-caspase-1 *via* their homotypic CARD domains, eventually leading to the autocleavage and maturation of pro-caspase-1. The activation of caspase-1 leads to the cleavage of precursor IL-1β and IL-18, as well as gasdermin D (GSDMD). The cleavage of GSDMD separates it into an N-terminal "GSDMD-N" domain and a C-terminal "GSDMD-C" domain (Kayagaki et al., 2015; Shi et al., 2015). GSDMD-N itself could be inserted into the lipid bilayer of the plasma membrane, which is necessary and sufficient for cytotoxic pore formation (Aglietti et al., 2016; Ding et al., 2016; Kayagaki et al., 2015; Liu et al., 2016; Sborgi et al., 2016; Shi et al., 2015). The formation of cytotoxic pores induces inflammatory cell death, termed "pyroptosis," and plays a key role in the release of mature IL-1β and IL-18.

Given the broad range of NLRP3 activators, it is impossible for NLRP3 to directly interact or sense all of the activators, suggesting that common cellular molecules or events may be induced by multiple NLRP3 activators to promote the assembly and activation of the NLRP3 inflammasome (Jo, Kim, Shin, & Sasakawa, 2016; Man & Kanneganti, 2015). Indeed, previous studies have proposed multiple cellular events, such as ion fluxes, mitochondrial damage, lysosomal rupture and Golgi dispersal, to explain how the NLRP3 inflammasome is activated (Fig. 1).

Intracellular fluctuations of multiple ions, including K^+, Ca^{2+} and Cl^-, have been reported to promote NLRP3 inflammasome activation (Gong, Jiang, et al., 2018; Gong, Yang, et al., 2018). K^+ efflux is the most accepted mechanism of NLRP3 inflammasome activation. Currently, it is thought that K^+ efflux is induced in response to most NLRP3 agonists (Muñoz-Planillo et al., 2013). In addition, the activation of the NLRP3 inflammasome by various stimuli can be inhibited by a high concentration of extracellular K^+, and K^+-free medium was sufficient to induce NLRP3 inflammasome activation in the absence of any NLRP3 agonist (Muñoz-Planillo et al., 2013; Petrilli et al., 2007). However, it should be noted that the inhibition of K^+ efflux can not only suppress NLRP3 inflammasome activation but also greatly attenuate the activation of the NLRP1b inflammasome, and further research is required to determine whether

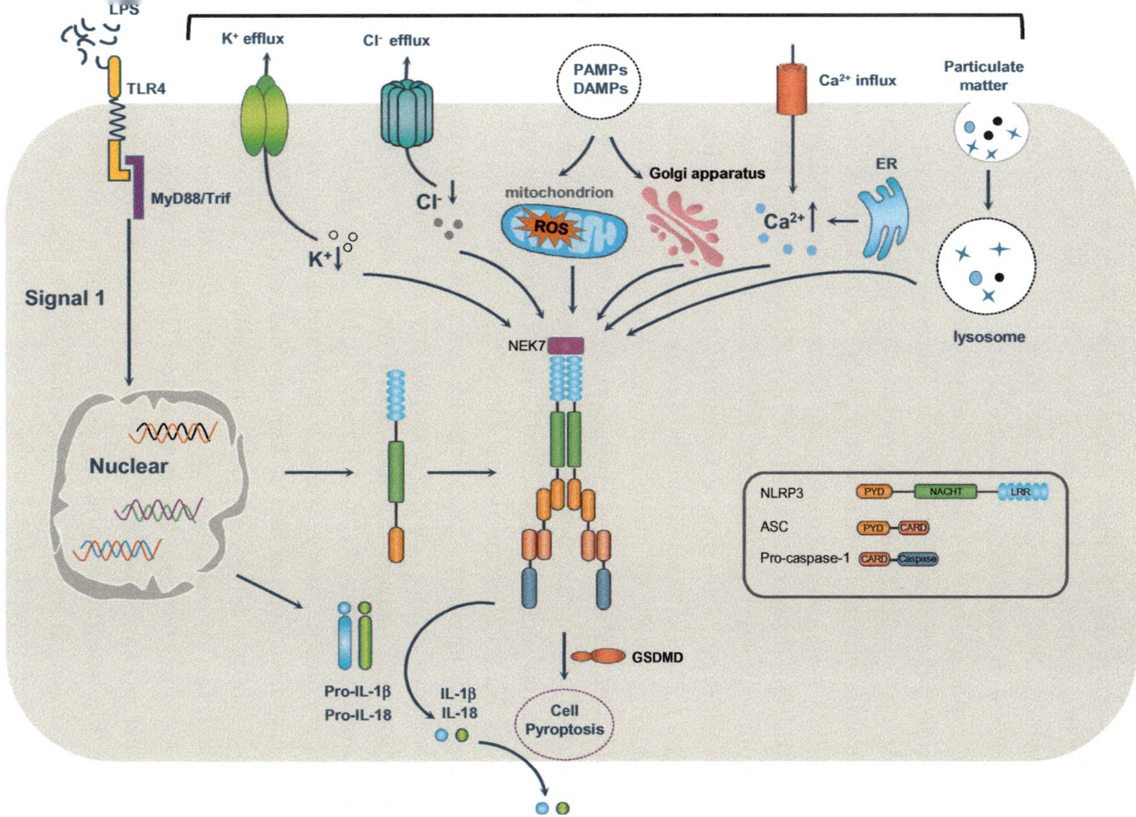

Fig. 1 Two-signal activation model of NLRP3 inflammasome. As generally accepted, a two-signal model has been proposed during the activation of NLRP3 inflammasome. Usually, the signal 1 provided by microbial or endogenous molecules is transduced through the TLR signaling pathway, which facilitates the activation of NF-KB pathway to promote the expression of NLRP3 and pro-IL-1β. Signal 2 provided by a broad range of PAMPs and DAMPs, is suggested to induce multiple cellular events, such as K^+ efflux, Cl^- efflux, Ca^{2+} mobilization, mitochondria damage, lysosomal rupture and Golgi dispersal to promote the assembly and activation of NLRP3 inflammasome. Activated NLRP3 inflammasome processes the cytokine precursor (pro-IL-1β/pro-IL-18) into mature form and induces cell pyroptosis in a caspase-1 dependent manner. Secretion of the IL-1β and IL-18 result in local or systemic inflammation, which further promote the development of various chronic diseases.

K^+ efflux is specifically sensed by the NLRP3 inflammasome (Petrilli et al., 2007). Intracellular Ca^{2+} mobilization can also occur in response to the stimulation of various NLRP3 activators, such as ATP, the bacterial second messengers cyclic-di-GMP and cyclic-di-AMP, the complement membrane attack complex, liposomes and the plant lectins (Abdul-Sater et al., 2013; Gong et al., 2017; Ito, Yanagi, & Ichinohe, 2012; Triantafilou, Hughes, Triantafilou, & Morgan, 2013). Previous studies have suggested that intracellular Ca^{2+} mobilization, caused by extracellular and intracellular stores, may both play an important role in NLRP3 inflammasome activation, at least in some conditions (Murakami et al., 2012). However, several studies have indicated that Ca^{2+} mobilization is necessary but not sufficient for NLRP3 inflammasome activation because many Ca^{2+} flux agonists, such a LPS and the Ca^{2+} ionophore ionomycin, cannot induce NLRP3 inflammasome activation (Murakami et al., 2012; Zanoni et al., 2009). A recent study by our colleagues found that NLRP3 inflammasome agonists, such as ATP and nigericin, can induce significant Cl^- efflux in bone marrow-derived macrophages (BMDMs) (Tang et al., 2017). In addition, the substitution of extracellular Cl^- with gluconate can enhance NLRP3 inflammasome activation. Moreover, Cl^--free medium can lead to Cl^- efflux, spontaneous NLRP3 inflammasome activation and IL-1β release in BMDMs. These results suggest that Cl^- efflux is also necessary and sufficient to activate the NLRP3 inflammasome (Tang et al., 2017).

Mitochondria play an important role in the initiation of the inflammatory response in innate immune cells, and several previous studies have connected mitochondrial damage to the activation of the NLRP3 inflammasome (Gurung, Lukens, & Kanneganti, 2015; Mills, Kelly, & O'Neill, 2017). Mitochondrial damage was initially proposed to be involved in NLRP3 inflammasome activation by Dr. Tschopp and colleagues (Zhou, Yazdi, Menu, & Tschopp, 2011). Mitochondrial damage induced by NLRP3 stimuli allows the generation and accumulation of reactive oxygen species (ROS). In addition, tremendous mitochondrial DNA (mtDNA) will be exposed to the cytoplasm (Nakahira et al., 2011). Zhong and colleagues recently stated that TLR-dependent priming signals trigger the synthesis of novel mtDNA that is critical for the activation of NLRP3 (Zhong et al., 2018). Consistent with previous studies, Zhong and colleagues also observed that NLRP3 activators initiate the production of mitochondrial ROS (mtROS) that convert mtDNA to an oxidized form (Zhong et al., 2018; Zhong, Sanchez-Lopez, & Karin, 2016; Zhong, Umemura, et al., 2016). As a potent inducer of IL-1β production, oxidized mtDNA has been identified to co-localize with NLRP3 and promote the activation of the NLRP3 inflammasome (Shimada et al., 2012; Zhong et al., 2018). Although the exact role of the mitochondria in NLRP3 activation remains to be revealed, we could conclude that mtROS and mtROS-induced mtDNA oxidation occupy a central role in the orchestration of NLRP3 inflammasome activation.

Some nondegradable particulates, such as alum, MSU, or aggregated amyloid-β, have been verified to activate the NLRP3 inflammasome. One of the most common explanations is 'frustrated' phagocytosis. Many nondigestible particles can be taken up into the intracellular phagolysosomes by sensed macrophages, which results in the release of stress substances and lysosomal proteases into the cytoplasm. Cathepsin B is one of the most important lysosomal proteases that has been broadly reported to activate the NLRP3 inflammasome (Halle et al., 2008; Hornung et al., 2008).

The newest research has extremely replenished the activated mechanisms of NLRP3 inflammasome. Chen and colleagues suggested that NLRP3 could be recruited to the disassembled trans-Golgi network (TGN) by the interaction of its conserved polybasic region with negatively charged phosphatidylinositol-4-phosphate (PtdIns4P) in response to various NLRP3 stimuli. Then, the TGN will act as a scaffold for the aggregation and polymerization of NLRP3 and ASC (Chen & Chen, 2018).

In addition to canonical NLRP3 inflammasome activation, a caspase-11-dependent NLRP3 inflammasome can be activated in response to the invasion of gram-negative bacteria, also known as noncanonical NLRP3 inflammasome activation (Kayagaki et al., 2011). Further study revealed that caspase-11 can directly sense intracellular LPS from bacteria independent of the classic LPS membrane receptor TLR4 (Hagar, Powell, Aachoui, Ernst, & Miao, 2013; Kayagaki et al., 2013). Similar to caspase-11 in mice, Shi and colleagues found that caspase-4 and caspase-5 expressed in human monocytes, epithelial cells and keratinocytes could directly bind to intracellular LPS and lipid A with a high specificity and affinity (Shi et al., 2014). Remarkably, activated human caspase-4 can trigger the activation of the noncanonical NLRP3 inflammasome without a need for a signal provided by the canonical NLRP3 activator (Casson et al., 2015; Kajiwara et al., 2014; Shi et al., 2015, 2014). During noncanonical inflammasome activation, caspase-11 (in human caspase-4/5) can cleave GSDMD and pannexin-1, which promote the formation of cytotoxic pores or the opening of nonselective channels in the plasma membrane, respectively, inducing the subsequent NLRP3 activation and pyroptosis (Kayagaki et al., 2015; Yang et al., 2015).

During the past decades, tremendous effort has been made in the investigation of the molecular mechanisms of NLRP3 inflammasome activation; however, there are still many problems to be answered. Future studies still need to focus on mechanistic research on how complicated signals are integrated into a common activated signal to activate the NLRP3 inflammasome.

3. Role of NLRP3 inflammasome in human diseases

Moderate activation of the NLRP3 inflammasome benefits host defenses against bacteria, viruses and parasites; however, excessive activation of the NLRP3 inflammasome is implicated in the pathogenesis of genetic and acquired inflammatory diseases, such as cryopyrin-associated periodic syndromes (CAPS), metabolic syndrome, neurodegenerative disease and inflammatory bowel disease (IBD) (Franchi, Munoz-Planillo, & Nunez, 2012; Strowig et al., 2012).

Gain-of-function mutations of NLRP3 are correlated with a group of rare genetic autoinflammatory disorders termed CAPS, containing familial cold autoinflammatory syndrome (FCAS), Muckle-Wells syndrome (MWS), and chronic infantile neurological, cutaneous, and articular (CINCA) syndrome (Gattorno et al., 2007). These diseases are characterized by recurrent fever, rash and arthropathies as well as various degrees of neurological complications (Aganna et al., 2002; Hoffman, Mueller, Broide, Wanderer, & Kolodner, 2001; Shinkai, McCalmont, & Leslie, 2008).

A group of obesity-related metabolic syndromes, such as T2D and gout, has been confirmed to be related to the sustained activation of the NLRP3 inflammasome (Duewell et al., 2010; Schroder, Zhou, & Tschopp, 2010; So & Martinon, 2017). In particular, sustained activation of the NLRP3 inflammasome in adipose-tissue-infiltrating macrophages results in metabolic inflammation, which further aggravates the inflammation environment in insulin-sensitive tissues (Vandanmagsar et al., 2011). During β-cell failure in T2D, NLRP3 could be activated *via* alternative mechanisms. Primarily, β-cell-derived mitochondrial ROS are continuously produced in response to hyperglycemia, which results in the dissociation of thioredoxin-interacting protein (TXNIP) from thioredoxin and then activation of NLRP3 (Zhou, Tardivel, Thorens, Choi, & Tschopp, 2010). Second, continuous hyperinsulinemia is accompanied by a large quantity deposition of amyloid polypeptide (IAPP, also termed amylin) around the islet cells, which has been confirmed to specifically activate the NLRP3 inflammasome

(Seino, 2001). Consistent with the observation, human *IAPP*-transgenic mice displayed a higher expression of IL-1β in the pancreatic macrophages than wild-type mice (Masters et al., 2010). Gout is a type of inflammatory arthritis in humans caused by the precipitation of monosodium urate (MSU) crystals in joints. The pathological hallmark of a typical gout attack is the large quantity of neutrophil influx into the synovium and joint fluid (Dalbeth, Merriman, & Stamp, 2016). Considerable MSU accumulation within joints was found to interact with resident joint cells and infiltrating neutrophils. Numerous studies have indicated that MSU crystals can act as a "danger" signal to induce the activation of NLRP3 inflammasome and the release of IL-1β, which plays a crucial role in the recruitment of neutrophils and the subsequent activation of the downstream innate immune response (Martinon, Petrilli, Mayor, Tardivel, & Tschopp, 2006; Shi, Evans, & Rock, 2003).

Neurodegenerative diseases such as Parkinson's disease (PD) and Alzheimer's disease (AD) are a group of disorders characterized by progressively impaired memory, decision making, judgment, language and orientation to physical surroundings (Nussbaum & Ellis, 2003). Chronic neuroinflammation, which occurs with an irreversible exhaustion of dopaminergic neurons, mitochondrial dysfunction, and a widespread deposition of misfolded protein aggregates of amyloid-β (Aβ), plays an important role in the pathogenesis of these neurodegenerative diseases. In the failure of neurons during PD and AD, accumulating evidence suggests that persistent accumulation of Aβ, α-synuclein and prions could directly trigger and sustain NLRP3 inflammasome activation and thereby result in central nervous system (CNS) inflammation and neuropathology (Heneka et al., 2013; Voet et al., 2019). Recent findings in human PD brains suggest that activated microglia are the major source of the NLRP3 inflammasome, which may provide new insight into the mechanisms of NLRP3 activation in microglia implicated in PD pathophysiology (Gordon et al., 2018).

Inflammatory bowel diseases (IBD), such as Crohn's disease (CD) and ulcerative colitis (UC), are characterized by chronic and relapsed inflammation in the gastrointestinal tract (Torres, Mehandru, Colombel, & Peyrin-Biroulet, 2017; Ungaro, Mehandru, Allen, Peyrin-Biroulet, & Colombel, 2017). By using an acute or chronic epithelial impaired colitis animal model, several groups have indicated that a deficiency of caspase-1 or NLRP3 could significantly improve colitis (Bauer et al., 2010; Siegmund, Lehr, Fantuzzi, & Dinarello, 2001). However, with the same animal model, some other groups have found that knockout of NLRP3, caspase-1 and ASC in mice resulted in exacerbated disease severity (Allen et al., 2010; Dupaul-Chicoine et al., 2010; Hirota et al., 2011; Yao et al., 2017). Another work has provided an alternative explanation about these opposite results. In this work, the authors claimed that the NLRP6 inflammasome is involved in the steady-state regulation of the gut commensal microbiota (Elinav et al., 2011). The deficiency of the NLRP6 inflammasome contributes to changes in the microbiota communities and the pro-inflammatory activation of some bacteria. Therefore, the opposite results may be explained by discrepancies in microbiota communities in different animal facilities.

Collectively, NLRP3 inflammasome has been implicated to take part in the pathogenesis of various important human diseases, in most of which NLRP3 activation plays a harmful role in the occurrence and progress. Actually, all the NLRP3-related diseases described above have no effective therapy. Treatment of these diseases by targeting of the NLRP3 inflammasome may be able to provide a novel clinical pathway in the future.

4. Targeting the upstream events of the NLRP3 inflammasome

As mentioned above, multiple cellular events, such as ion fluxes, mitochondrial damage and lysosomal rupture, has been proposed to induce the activation of NLRP3 inflammasome. The inhibition of these cellular events may be an alternative strategy to prevent the excessive activation of the NLRP3 inflammasome (Table 1).

4.1 Inhibition of ion fluxes

As mentioned above, many studies have verified that the NLRP3 inflammasome can be activated by disordered ion fluxes, including those of K^+, Ca^{2+}, and Cl^- (Gong, Jiang, et al., 2018; Gong, Yang, et al., 2018). Indeed, several inhibitors have been identified to limit the activation of the NLRP3 inflammasome by inhibiting ion fluxes. Youm and colleagues found that β-hydroxybutyrate blocks K^+ efflux and attenuates caspase-1 activation and IL-1β secretion in primed macrophages (Youm et al., 2015). Several inhibitors of Ca^{2+} mobilization, such as 2-APB, XeC and U73122, have been reported to inhibit the activation of the NLRP3 inflammasome in response to different NLRP3 agonists (Gong, Jiang, et al., 2018; Gong, Yang, et al., 2018). In addition, several studies have indicated that targeting of the Cl^- channel by its blockers, such as 5-nitro-2-(3-phenylpropylamino) benzoic

Table 1 Targeting the upstream signaling of NLRP3 inflammasome.

Target	Inhibitor	Mechanism of action	References
K^+ efflux	β-hydroxybutyrate	K^+ efflux is required for the binding of NEK7 to NLRP3, which is essential for the assembly of NLRP3 inflammasome	He, Zeng, Yang, Motro, and Nunez (2016) and Youm et al. (2015)
Ca^{2+} mobilization	2-APB, XeC and U73122	Mitochondrial Ca^{2+} overload results in mitochondrial damage, mROS production and mtDNA oxidation	Gong, Jiang, et al. (2018) and Gong, Yang, et al. (2018)
Cl^- efflux	NPPB, DIDS, IAA94	Cl^- efflux is necessary for the interaction between NEK7 and NLRP3 and the formation of NLRP3-ASC complex	Compan et al. (2012), Daniels et al. (2016), and Tang et al. (2017)
ROS	NAC, APDC, DPI	Oxidized mtDNA can be directly sensed by NLRP3, which results in the assemble of NLRP3	Dostert et al. (2008), Zhong et al. (2018), and Zhou et al. (2011)
Cathepsin B	CA-074-Me	Some nondegradable particulates can induce lysosomal rupture and cathepsin B release to activate the NLRP3 inflammasome	Halle et al. (2008) and Hornung et al. (2008)

acid (NPPB), 4,4′-diisothiocyano-2,2′-stilbenedisulfonic acid (DIDS), flufenamic acid, mefenamic acid and IAA94, can specifically inhibit NLRP3 inflammasome activation rather than the AIM2 or NLRC4 inflammasomes (Compan et al., 2012; Daniels et al., 2016; Tang et al., 2017). Although the inhibition of ion fluxes can be effective for the limitation of NLRP3 activation, it may also lead to side effects. For example, some important calmodulins that are distributed on the membrane of mitochondria and endoplasmic reticulum are the direct targets of Ca^{2+} flux inhibitors. The modification of these calmodulins to limit the activation of the NLRP3 inflammasome will inevitably elicit potent off-target effects (Murakami et al., 2012). Thus, the blocker's specificity or its side effect must be fully considered to inhibit ion fluxes, and the inhibition of ion fluxes may not be a potential strategy to treat NLRP3 inflammasome-driven diseases in the clinic.

4.2 Inhibition of mitochondrial ROS

Previous research and the latest data both have clearly indicated that accumulated mtROS and mtROS-induced mitochondrial damage are critical and necessary for the activation of the NLRP3 inflammasome (Zhong et al., 2018; Zhou et al., 2011). Since the oxidized mtDNA derived from the damaged mitochondria could be directly sensed by NLRP3, the blockade of mtROS production by using ROS scavengers such as *N*-acetyl-L-cysteine (NAC) or (2*R*, 4*R*)-4-aminopyrro lidine-2,4-dicarboxylate (APDC) can largely mitigate the ability of asbestos, MSU, ATP and nigericin to activate the NLRP3 inflammasome (Dostert et al., 2008). Additionally, the phagocytosis of particles results in the accumulation of ROS in a NADPH oxidase-dependent manner, and the inhibition of NADPH oxidase with its specific inhibitors diphenylene iodonium (DPI) and apocynin or the knockdown of the NADPH oxidase subunit p22phox extremely diminish the activation of the NLRP3 inflammasome and the production of IL-1β (Dostert et al., 2008). However, some clinical studies suggest that patients with defective NADPH oxidase subunits display normal or even increased caspase-1 activity, and some well-known ROS inhibitors actually promote the activation of NLRP3 (Bauernfeind et al., 2011; Meissner et al., 2010; van de Veerdonk et al., 2010). In addition, as ROS are widely involved in multiple signaling pathways, the inhibition of NLRP3 inflammasome activation by ROS inhibitors is inevitable to provoke off-target effects. We could conclude that targeting the cellular ROS accumulated in the macrophages at least in part contributes to the control of NLRP3 activation, and more specific ROS inhibitors that selectively target the mitochondria should be developed and verified in the future.

4.3 Inhibition of cathepsin B

As mentioned above, cathepsin B is one of the most important lysosomal proteases that have been reported to activate the NLRP3 inflammasome (Halle et al., 2008; Hornung et al., 2008). Targeting cathepsin B by using its specific inhibitor CA-074-Me or knocking out cathepsin B through genetic engineering methods can only partially diminish particle agonist-induced activation of the NLRP3 inflammasome, which may mean that other unclear NLRP3 activating factors may also participate in particle agonist-induced NLRP3 activation (Hornung et al., 2008). Interestingly, Bruchard and colleagues have indicated that antitumor chemotherapeutic agents, gemcitabine (Gem) and 5-fluorouracil (5FU) activate the NLRP3 inflammasome in myeloid-derived suppressor cells (MDSCs) in a cathepsin B-dependent manner (Bruchard et al., 2013). Thus, targeting cathepsin B may be feasible to inhibit only particle agonist-induced NLRP3 inflammasome.

5. Targeting the components of the NLRP3 inflammasome

In addition to NLRP3, adaptor protein ASC, caspase-1 and nima-related kinase 7 (NEK7) are now all known as core components of the NLRP3 complex. The inhibition of NLRP3 inflammasome activation by targeting these core components can be sufficient and necessary to alleviate NLRP3-related inflammatory diseases.

5.1 Inhibition of NEK7, ASC or caspase-1

NEK7 was recently identified and characterized as a key component of the NLRP3 complex, and its deletion nearly abolishes the activation of the NLRP3 inflammasome in response to various NLRP3 agonists. Upstream signaling, including K^+ efflux and mtROS, has been proposed to trigger the interaction between NEK7 and NLRP3, facilitating the formation of the NLRP3 inflammasome complex (He et al., 2016; Shi et al., 2016). However, it should be noted that the mechanisms by which ionic changes or ROS production engage the interaction between NEK7 and NLRP3 are still not clear. In addition, due to the wide expression and pivotal role of NEK7 in mitosis, it is difficult to develop a highly selective NEK7 inhibitor to inhibit NLRP3 inflammasome activation without disturbing other cellular physiological processes (Salem et al., 2010).

Several chemicals have also been reported to inhibit the NLRP3 inflammasome by targeting the ASC adaptor. For example, Lee showed that caffeic acid phenethyl ester (CAPE) suppressed MSU-induced caspase-1 activation and IL-1β production by directly targeting ASC and blocking the formation of ASC dimers and NLRP3-ASC assembly, which substantially contributes to the alleviation of pathological symptoms of gouty arthritis in mice (Lee et al., 2016).

Scientists have made considerable effort to develop specific caspase-1 inhibitors, among which the chemical VX-765 is one of the best studied. Wannamaker and colleagues showed that the oral administration of VX-765 specifically inhibited the release of IL-1β and IL-18 and ameliorated the severity of diseases in mouse models of rheumatoid arthritis and skin inflammation (Wannamaker et al., 2007). Another study recently indicated that an intravenous bolus of VX-765, combined with a platelet inhibitor, can protect against myocardial infarction in rats (Yang et al., 2017). In addition, the capase-1 inhibitor pralnacasan also inhibits the secretion of IL-1β and contributes to the improvement of diseases in mouse models, such as streptococcal cell wall (SCW)-induced arthritis and ventilator-induced lung injury (Joosten et al., 2009; Timmermans et al., 2013). In addition, it has also been shown that the inhibition of caspase-1 with pralnacasan can significantly decrease the IL-1β content in adipose tissue and robustly attenuate insulin resistance during obesity (Stienstra et al., 2010).

Taken together, these results indicate that although targeting NEK7 is special for the limitation of NLRP3 inflammasome activation, there is presently no direct way to target NEK7, and the inhibition of NEK7 will also inevitably produce undesired effects. As the core complements of the inflammasome complex, ASC and caspase-1 are involved in the formation of multiple inflammasome complexes, such as NLRP3, NLRP1b, AIM2, NLRC4, NLRP6 and the Pyrin inflammasome, and the inhibition of either ASC or caspase-1 is bound to inhibit the activation of other inflammasomes at the same time. Some undesirable effects *in vivo* inevitably result, and the immune balance of the host can be disturbed. Therefore, the inhibition of the NLRP3 inflammasome by targeting NEK7, ASC or caspase-1 may not be an advisable research direction in the future.

5.2 Inhibition of NLRP3 self

In light of the fact that the inhibition of NLRP3 activation by targeting both the upstream activating signaling and the other components of the NLRP3 complex, including NEK7, ASC and caspase-1, will inevitably result in an unexpected cascade reaction *in vivo*, several scientists have now turned their efforts toward the control of NLRP3 inflammasome activation by directly targeting the NLRP3 protein itself. Indeed, the NLRP3 protein is the most important component of the NLRP3 complex, the targeting of which is

Table 2 Targeting site, mechanism and improved diseases of NLRP3-targeting inhibitors.

Inhibitor	Targeting site	Inhibitory mechanism	Disease model	References
MCC950	Within or close to Walker B motif	Inhibits ATP hydrolysis of NLRP3	CAPS, stroke, EAE, atherosclerosis, AD, asthma, NAFLD	Coll et al. (2015), Dempsey et al. (2017), Kim et al. (2017), Mridha et al. (2017), Ren et al. (2018), and van der Heijden et al. (2017)
CY-09	ATP-binding site	Inhibits ATPase activity of NLRP3	Gouty arthritis, CAPS, T2D	Jiang et al. (2017)
Oridonin	Cys279	Inhibits NEK7-NLRP3 interaction	Peritonitis, gouty arthritis, T2D	He et al. (2018)
Tranilast	–	Inhibits NLRP3 self-oligomerization	Gouty arthritis, CAPS, T2D	Huang et al. (2018)

attractive and practicable. Several compounds have displayed specific inhibitory effects on the NLRP3 inflammasome *via* direct targeting of NLRP3 (Table 2).

Coll and colleagues found that MCC950 is a specific and potent inhibitor of the NLRP3 inflammasome at an extremely low dose (Coll et al., 2015). It can inhibit ATP-induced NLRP3 activation and IL-1β secretion with a half-maximal inhibitory concentration (IC50) of 8.1 nM in human monocytes. MCC950 has shown excellent anti-inflammatory function in several NLRP3-dependent disease models, such as murine models of CAPS, multiple sclerosis (MS), stroke, atherosclerosis, AD, asthma, non-alcoholic fatty liver disease (NAFLD) (Coll et al., 2015; Dempsey et al., 2017; Kim et al., 2017; Mridha et al., 2017; Ren et al., 2018; van der Heijden et al., 2017). In addition, MCC950 could improve neuroinflammation-related neurodegeneration by disrupting the activation of NLRP3 in microglia and astrocytes (Gordon et al., 2018). Interestingly, previous data have indicated that MCC950 could dose-dependently inhibit nigericin-induced chloride efflux in *Nlrp3*$^{-/-}$ BMDMs, which correlated with its inhibitory activity for NLRP3 activation, suggesting that MCC950 might suppress inflammasome activation by targeting chloride efflux (Tang et al., 2017). Two recent studies have indicated that MCC950 could directly target the NLRP3 protein at a site within or close to the Walker B motif. Binding of MCC950 to NLRP3 inhibits its ATP hydrolysis and blocks NLRP3 assemble (Coll & Hill, 2019; Tapia-Abellan et al., 2019). Indeed, MCC950 has been tested in phase II clinical trials for rheumatoid arthritis. However, the clinical trials were not continued further, as MCC950 was found to induce liver injury in some cases (Mangan et al., 2018). Both the inhibitory mechanism of the NLRP3 inflammasome and the cause of this liver toxicity signal need to be further investigated.

CY-09, a novel small molecule, has recently been identified to highly and specifically inhibit the activation of the NLRP3 inflammasome (Jiang et al., 2017). A mechanistic study indicated that CY-09 disrupts the assembly of the NLRP3 complex by suppressing the ATPase activity of NLRP3, which is achieved through competitive binding to the ATP-binding site on the NACHT domain of NLRP3. *In vivo* data indicated that the chronic administration of CY-09 reverses NLRP3-dependent inflammation in a mouse model of T2D. In addition, *in vivo* data also confirmed that CY-09 treatment increased survival in a mouse model of Muckle-Wells syndrome (MWS) and suppressed MSU-induced IL-1β production and neutrophil influx, both of which suggest that CY-09 is active *in vivo*. Furthermore, *ex vivo* data also indicated that CY-09 can inhibit the preactivated NLRP3 inflammasome in synovial fluid cells (SFCs) from patients with gout, suggesting the clinical potential of CY-09 in the treatment of rheumatic diseases (Jiang et al., 2017).

Some natural ingredients of traditional Chinese herbs also displayed significant and specific inhibitory effects on NLRP3 inflammasome activation. A work from our laboratory recently identified oridonin, a bioactive ent-kaurane diterpenoid, which specifically inhibits the activation of the NLRP3 inflammasome at a very low dose (He et al., 2018). Oridonin is the major active constituent of *Rabdosia rubescens*, which is often used in traditional Chinese medicine. Mechanistic research indicated that oridonin could covalently bind to the cysteine 279 site on the NACHT domain of NLRP3 and then inhibit NEK7-NLRP3 interaction and prevent NLRP3 complex assembly and NLRP3 activation (He et al., 2018). *In vivo* data also provided evidence showing that oridonin could suppress NLRP3 activation and that it had remarkable preventive or therapeutic effects on the mouse models of NLRP3-driven diseases, including peritonitis, gouty arthritis and T2D.

In addition, tranilast, an old clinical drug, is an analog of the tryptophan metabolite and has been used to treat various inflammatory diseases in clinics, including bronchial asthma, atypical dermatitis, allergic conjunctivitis, and hypertrophic scars (Darakhshan & Pour, 2015). Most recently, we identified that tranilast could directly target the NACHT domain of NLRP3 and disturb the assembly of the NLRP3 complex, which substantially inhibits the activation of the NLRP3 inflammasome *in vitro* (Huang et al., 2018). Additionally, tranilast could prevent or treat NLRP3-dependent inflammatory diseases in mouse models of gouty arthritis, CAPS, and T2D. More importantly, tranilast can also inhibit the preactivated NLRP3 inflammasome in SFCs from patients with gout. As a relatively safe and well-tolerated drug, the clinical therapeutic effect of tranilast on NLRP3-related diseases needs to be further tested in the future.

Taken together, these works listed above not only evidence that targeting the NLRP3 inflammasome is feasible for the treatment of inflammatory diseases but also suggest that NLRP3 itself could be targeted with its specific antagonists.

6. Targeting the positive regulators of NLRP3 inflammasome

Previous studies have revealed several molecular regulators that are involved in the activation of the NLRP3 inflammasome. The inhibition of these proteins may be an alternative strategy to prevent the excessive activation of the NLRP3 inflammasome (Table 3).

6.1 Inhibition of NLRP3-interacting proteins

Previous studies have shown that several proteins can bind to NLRP3 and induce the posttranscriptional modification of NLRP3, facilitating NLRP3 inflammasome activation. It was reported that deubiquitinated modification of NLRP3 by deubiquitinase BRCC3 is critical for the activation of NLRP3, inhibition of which by isopeptidase inhibitor G5 will induce polyubiquitination of both the NACHT domain and the LRR domain of NLRP3 and inhibit the activation of the NLRP3 inflammasome (Py et al., 2013). Consistent with this, posttranslational ubiquitination modification of NLRP3 by E3 ligase ariadne homolog 2 (ARIH2) was also shown to negatively regulate the activation of the NLRP3 inflammasome in macrophages by directly interacting with the NACHT domain of

Table 3 Targeting the regulators of NLRP3 inflammasome.

Targeting the positive regulators of NLRP3 inflammasome

Target	Inhibitor	Mechanism of action	References
BRCC3	G5	Promotes NLRP3 activation by facilitating deubiquitination of NLRP3	Py et al. (2013)
JNK1	SP600125	Promotes NLRP3 activation by facilitating phosphorylation of NLRP3	Song et al. (2017)
PTPN22	–	Promotes NLRP3 activation by facilitating dephosphorization of NLRP3	Spalinger et al. (2016)
GBP5	–	Interacts with NLRP3 and facilitates NLRP3 inflammasome assembly	Shenoy et al. (2012)
HSP90	Geldanamycin	Interacts with NLRP3 and facilitates NLRP3 inflammasome assembly	Mayor, Martinon, De Smedt, Petrilli, and Tschopp (2007)
Syk	R406, BAY 61-3606	Promotes NLRP3 activation by facilitating phosphorylation of ASC	Hara et al. (2013)
JNK	SP600125, TAT-TI-JIP$_{153–163}$		
IKKα	–	Promotes NLRP3 activation by interacting with ASC	Martin et al. (2014)
LUBAC	–	Promotes NLRP3 activation by facilitating linear ubiquitination of ASC	Rodgers et al. (2014)

Targeting the negative regulators of NLRP3 inflammasome

Target	Activator	Mechanism of action	References
AhR	TCDD, FICZ	Inhibits NLRP3 transcription	Huai et al. (2014)
BCL6	–		Chen et al. (2017)
A20	–	Inhibits NLRP3 and pro-IL-1β expression	Walle et al. (2014)
TTP	–		Haneklaus et al. (2017)
miR-7/9/115/223	–	Inhibits NLRP3 expression	Chen et al. (2015), Feng et al. (2017), Neudecker et al. (2017), Wang et al. (2017), and Zhou et al. (2016)
SHP	Fenofibrate, AICAR	Interacts with NLRP3 and inhibits NLRP3 inflammasome assembly	Bochner and Ames (1982), Yang, He, et al. (2015), and Zambon and Cusi (2007)
GPSM3	–		Giguere et al. (2014)
NO or others	IFNs	Inhibits NLRP3 activation by inducing the nitrosylation of NLRP3	Guarda et al. (2011), Mayer-Barber et al. (2011), and Mishra et al. (2013)
EP2/4	PGE2	Inhibits NLRP3 activation by facilitating phosphorylation of NLRP3	Mortimer et al. (2016)
TGR5	Bile acids	Inhibits NLRP3 activation by facilitating phosphorylation of NLRP3	Guo et al. (2016)

Continued

Table 3 Targeting the regulators of NLRP3 inflammasome.—cont'd

Targeting the negative regulators of NLRP3 inflammasome

Target	Activator	Mechanism of action	References
DRD1	Dopamine, A-68930	Inhibits NLRP3 activation by facilitating NLRP3 ubiquitination and degradation	Yan et al. (2015)
ATG16L1	–	Inhibits NLRP3 activation by eliminating active inflammasome or facilitating mitophagy	Saitoh et al. (2008) and Zhong, Sanchez-Lopez, et al. (2016)
FBXL2	–	Inhibits NLRP3 activation by facilitating NLRP3 ubiquitination and degradation	Han et al. (2015)
HSF1-β-catenin axis	–	Inhibits NLRP3 activation through XBP1 inhibition	Yue et al. (2016)
SIRT3	Honokiol	Inhibits NLRP3 activation by inhibiting ROS production	Zhao, Zhang, Sui, Zhu, and Zeng (2016)
PPAR-γ	Rosiglitazone	Inhibits NLRP3 activation through regulating mitochondrial function	Miao et al. (2014)
TRIM30	–	Inhibits NLRP3 activation via decreasing the generation of ROS	Hu et al. (2010)

NLRP3 (Kawashima et al., 2017). Recently, Song and colleagues revealed that c-Jun N-terminal kinase 1 (JNK1)-dependent NLRP3 phosphorylation at the S194 residue in the priming stage is critical for NLRP3 deubiquitination and accelerates its self-oligomerization and subsequent inflammasome activation, blocking the activation of JNK1 with the JNK inhibitor SP600125 can markedly disrupt the activation of the NLRP3 inflammasome (Song et al., 2017). Additionally, dephosphorization of NLRP3 at the Tyr861 residue by protein tyrosine phosphatase nonreceptor 22 (PTPN22) was also found to contribute to the regulation of NLRP3 inflammasome-related diseases. Knockdown of PTPN22 will reduce the secretion of IL-1β *in vitro,* and loss of PTPN22 in murine models results in reduced peritonitis (Spalinger et al., 2016). Further study indicated that PTPN22-mediated NLRP3 activation and IL-1β secretion occurred in an autophagy-dependent manner. Treatment with the autophagy inhibitor 3-MA and bafilomycin A_1 or the PI3K inhibitor wortmannin abrogates the inhibitory effect on NLRP3 activation observed upon loss of PTPN22 (Spalinger et al., 2017).

In addition to inducing the posttranscriptional modification of NLRP3, several proteins can interact with NLRP3 and facilitate NLRP3 inflammasome assembly. For example, guanylate-binding protein 5 (GBP5) has been shown to promote NLRP3 activation in response to ATP, nigericin, and bacteria but not MSU or other particulate matter (Shenoy et al., 2012). Genetic deficiency or specific inhibition of GBP5 should effectively limit the activation of NLRP3 (Shenoy et al., 2012). In addition, the SGT1-HSP90 complex has been reported to interact with NLRP3 and promote the activation of the NLRP3 inflammasome, inhibition of HSP90 with its specific inhibitor geldanamycin has been shown to abrogate the activation of NLRP3 *in vitro* and improve NLRP3-dependent gout *in vivo* (Mayor et al., 2007).

6.2 Inhibition of ASC-interacting proteins

Similar to NLRP3, previous studies have shown that several proteins can also bind to ASC and facilitate the activation of multiple inflammasomes, including the NLRP3 inflammasome. Originally, Hara and colleagues found that ASC was phosphorylated by Syk and JNK during NLRP3 and AIM2 inflammasome activation, inhibition of ASC phosphorylation with Syk-specific inhibitors R406 (1 μM) and BAY 61-3606 (10 μM) as well as JNK inhibitors SP600125 (40 μM) and TAT-TI-$JIP_{153-163}$ (40 μM) could significantly decrease the production of IL-18 in response to the activation of NLRP3 and AIM2 inflammasome (Hara et al., 2013). Further study indicated that phosphorylation of Tyr144 in mouse ASC plays a crucial role in ASC speck formation and inflammasome assembly. However, it should also be noted that how Syk and JNK mediate the activation of NLRP3 and AIM2 inflammasomes has not been answered (Hara et al., 2013). Another recent study has shown that basal IκB kinase α (IKKα) plays a critical regulatory role in ASC-dependent inflammasome activation (Martin et al., 2014). Further mechanistic research indicated that IKKα regulates ATP-induced NLRP3 inflammasome activation by directly interacting with ASC, which is dependent on the dephosphorization of Ser193 and Ser16 residues at ASC by serine/threonine phosphatase PP2A (Martin et al., 2014). Rodgers and colleagues found that HOIL-1L, the subunit of the linear ubiquitination assembly complex (LUBAC), plays an important role in the linear ubiquitination of ASC and the formation of the NLRP3-ASC complex independent of its role in NF-κB-mediated transcription activity (Rodgers et al., 2014).

7. Targeting the negative regulators of NLRP3 inflammasome

Recent studies have also revealed several molecular regulators and physiological processes that decrease the expression of NLRP3 protein or inhibit NLRP3 inflammasome assembly. The activation of these proteins or processes may be an alternative strategy to prevent the excessive activation of the NLRP3 inflammasome (Table 3).

7.1 Targeting the molecules that decrease NLRP3 expression

As generally accepted, increased expression of NLRP3 protein and the precursor of IL-1β during the priming stage is necessary for the substantial activation of the NLRP3 inflammasome, and inhibition of the expression of NLRP3 can surely decrease the activation of the NLRP3 inflammasome. Previous studies have indicated that the expression of NLRP3 protein can be inhibited both at the transcriptional and posttranslational levels. It has been reported that activated aryl hydrocarbon receptor (AhR) inhibits NLRP3 transcription by directly binding to the xenobiotic response element (XRE) motif of the NLRP3 promoter and decreasing the expression of NLRP3, which substantially contributes to the limitation of caspase-1 activation and IL-1β secretion in peritoneal macrophages (Huai et al., 2014). The activation of AhR by its specific agonists, such as 2,3,7,8-tetrachlorodibenzo-*p*-dioxin (TCDD, a common dioxin) or its endogenous ligand tryptophan photoproduct 6-formylindolo-[3,2-*b*]-carbazole (FICZ), could significantly decrease the expression levels of both NLRP3 and the precursor of IL-1β. In addition, a recent study indicated that B-cell lymphoma 6 (BCL6) could suppress renal NLRP3 activation by directly targeting its promoter region (Chen et al., 2017). The upregulation of BCL6 by its specific agonists may indicate a potential pathway in treating NLRP3-related inflammatory diseases. However, no such inhibitors have been developed so far. Similar to this, Lamcanfi and colleagues recently found that the deficiency of A20 in macrophages will increase the basal and LPS-induced expression of NLRP3 and the precursor of IL-1β, and the deficiency of A20 in macrophages significantly strengthens NLRP3-dependent caspase-1 activation, pyroptosis and IL-1β secretion in response to particle stimuli *in vivo* (Walle et al., 2014). The upregulation of A20 or decreasing its degradation by genetic engineering or pharmacological methods should be a potential strategy for the treatment of arthritis. Moreover, the RNA-binding protein tristetraprolin (TTP) was recently identified as a negative regulator of the NLRP3 inflammasome *via* directly targeting AU-rich elements in the NLRP3 3′-untranslated region (UTR) and decreasing both NLRP3 and IL-1β expression (Haneklaus, O'Neil, Clark, Masters, & O'Neill, 2017).

Several miRNAs were found to inhibit the expression of NLRP3 by directly targeting the NLRP3 gene. For example, miR-223 has been shown to exhibit an inhibitory effect on the NLRP3 inflammasome by directly binding to the 3′ untranslated region of NLRP3, contributing to the attenuation of experimental colitis (Neudecker et al., 2017). Feng and colleagues found that $Ly6G^+$ neutrophil-derived miR-223 contributes to the alleviation of mitochondrial damage-associated molecular pattern (DAMP)-induced acute lung injury/acute respiratory distress syndrome (ALI/ARDS) by inhibiting NLRP3 expression and IL-1β release (Feng et al., 2017). Interestingly, miR-7 was also found to directly target the 3′ untranslated region of the NLRP3 gene and abrogate its expression in microglia, which substantially contributes to the improvement of NLRP3-mediated neuroinflammation (Zhou et al., 2016). In addition, miR-9 and miR-155 have inhibitory effects on the NLRP3 inflammasome *in vivo* by targeting the JAK1/STAT pathway and ERK signaling pathway, respectively (Chen et al., 2015; Wang et al., 2017). Given the excellent inhibitory effect of the above miRNAs on NLRP3 activation, a novel gene therapy pathway may be worthy of an attempt to treat NLRP3-related inflammatory diseases by developing the related antisense RNA.

7.2 Targeting NLRP3-interacting proteins

The orphan nuclear receptor small heterodimer partner (SHP) has been shown to negatively regulate the activation of the NLRP3 inflammasome by directly targeting NLRP3, a deficiency of which will enhance the activation of the NLRP3 inflammasome and significantly strengthen the pathological responses in mouse models of kidney tubular necrosis and peritoneal gout (Yang, He, Munoz-Planillo, Liu, & Nunez, 2015). Increasing SHP expression by the SHP-inducing drugs fenofibrate (a fibrate class drug for the treatment of hypercholesterolemia) and AICAR (5-amino-1-β-D-ribofuranosyl-imidazole-4-carboxamide (also known as ZMP), an analog of AMP14), could significantly attenuate the activation of NLRP3 (Bochner & Ames, 1982; Yang, He, et al., 2015; Zambon & Cusi, 2007). In addition, it is worth noting that G protein signaling modulator-3 (GPSM3) has been identified as a direct NLRP3-interacting protein and a negative regulator of IL-1β production (Giguere et al., 2014). The induction of GPSM3 expression by some chemicals or genetic engineering pathways may be an attractive way to restrict NLRP3 inflammasome activation.

7.3 Targeting interferons (IFNs) signaling

A previous study has indicated that type I IFN suppresses the activation of the NLRP3 and NLRP1 inflammasome in a STAT1-dependent manner (Guarda et al., 2011). Interestingly, a later study indicated that not only the type I IFN but also the $CD4^+$ T cell-derived IFN-γ could inhibit the production of IL-1α and IL-1β in response to the infection by *Mycobacterium tuberculosis* (Mayer-Barber et al., 2011). Indeed, as one of the most important adaptive immune cytokines, IFN-γ has recently been shown to inhibit the assembly of the NLRP3 complex by generating nitric oxide and inducing the nitrosylation of NLRP3 (Mishra et al., 2013). The inhibition of NLRP3 activation with IFNs may be a feasible pathway for the treatment of NLRP3-driven diseases upon infection, but the treatment of other NLRP3-driven chronic diseases, such as T2D and atherosclerosis, in this way seems impossible.

7.4 Targeting cyclic adenosine monophosphate (cAMP)

Cyclic adenosine monophosphate (cAMP) was the original "second messenger" to be identified. Recent studies have revealed that several GPCR agonists, such as prostaglandin E2 (PGE2), bile acids and the neurotransmitter dopamine, can inhibit the activation of the NLRP3 inflammasome in a cAMP-dependent manner (Guo et al., 2016; Mortimer, Moreau, MacDonald, & Chadee, 2016; Sokolowska et al., 2015; Yan et al., 2015). It has been indicated that the PGE2-cAMP-protein kinase A (PKA) axis induces the phosphorylation of NLRP3 at Ser295 located in its NACHT domain, which attenuates the ATPase activity of NLRP3 and restrains the rapid activation of the NLRP3 inflammasome (Mortimer et al., 2016). The mutation of Ser295 of NLRP3 abrogates the PKA-induced phosphorylation of NLRP3 and has been linked to the autoimmune disease cryopyrin-associated periodic syndrome (CAPS) (Mortimer et al., 2016). Similar to this study, a study carried out by Wang and colleagues indicated that bile acids could specifically inhibit the activation of NLRP3 by binding to its cell membrane receptor TGR5 (transmembrane G protein-coupled receptor-5; also known as GPR131) and then elevate the cellular content of cyclic AMP (cAMP) and trigger the activation of protein kinase A (PKA), which subsequently facilitates the phosphorylation and ubiquitination of NLRP3 (Guo et al., 2016). However, Hao and coworkers most recently found that bile acids could not inhibit but rather activate the NLRP3 inflammasome by activating both the priming signal and the activation signal through farnesoid X receptor (FXR) *in vitro* (Hao et al., 2017). It is of interest to note that FXR, as a master regulator of bile acid homeostasis, is sharply reduced in the liver in a mouse model of LPS-induced endotoxemia. The conflicting results of the two groups may be due to their different experimental systems; on the other hand, bile acids themselves can function as immune balancers by activating different receptors. In addition to promoting PKA-dependent NLRP3 phosphorylation, it has also been reported that the neurotransmitter dopamine activates dopamine receptor 1 (DRD1) and increases the intracellular level of cAMP, which facilitates NLRP3 K48-ubiquitination and degradation *via* the E3 ubiquitin ligase MARCH7 (Yan et al., 2015). The activation of DRD1 by dopamine or DRD1 agonist A-68930 inhibited NLRP3 inflammasome activation in microglia and astrocytes and prevented neurotoxin 1-methyl-4-phenyl-1,2,3,6-tetrahydropyridine (MPTP)-induced neuroinflammation (Yan et al., 2015). As indicated by these studies, cAMP signaling has been shown to involve the inhibition of the NLRP3 inflammasome. However, cAMP has been verified as one of the most important intracellular second messengers, and it takes part in various critical cellular metabolism pathways, the content of which should be maintained at the homeostasis level. Therefore, all efforts to increase the intracellular content of cAMP and inhibit NLRP3 activation may inevitably elicit other undesired responses.

7.5 Targeting autophagy and ubiquitination

Autophagy is one of the most important cell physiological processes in tumorigenesis, ontogenesis, aging and inflammation (Fernandez et al., 2018; Ghislat & Lawrence, 2018; Rosenfeldt et al., 2013). Several studies have shown that a deficiency of autophagy-related protein 16-like 1 (ATG16L1) facilitates IL-1β release in response to the stimulation of NLRP3 agonists, which means that autophagy takes part in the negative regulation of the NLRP3 inflammasome (Saitoh et al., 2008; Zhong, Sanchez-Lopez, et al., 2016). In addition, ubiquitination, another important intracellular event, has been reported to control both the degradation rate of NLRP3 and its ability to self-oligomerize (Han et al., 2015; Song et al., 2016; Yan et al., 2015). For example, the E3 ubiquitin ligase F-boxO3 (FBXO3) induced by TLR activation is critical and necessary for the ubiquitination and degradation of another F-box protein, F-box L2 (FBXL2), which could directly target the amino acid site of Lys689 on NLRP3 and initiate the K48-linked ubiquitination and degradation of NLRP3 (Han et al., 2015). The inhibition of FBXO3 with the small-molecule inhibitor benzathine (BC-1215) restores the expression of FBXL2, which substantially decreases the expression of NLRP3 protein and the production of IL-1β and IL-18 in macrophages during NLRP3 activation (Mallampalli et al., 2013). Inducing autophagy and ubiquitination with some special chemicals may contribute to the restriction of NLRP3 activation to some extent, however, other physiological processes involved in autophagy or ubiquitination will be unavoidably disturbed. Therefore, it is not be recommended to develop a NLRP3 inhibitor based on autophagy and ubiquitination inducers.

7.6 Targeting other regulators

The myeloid heat shock transcription factor 1 (HSF1)-β-catenin axis has been found to negatively regulate the activation of the NLRP3 inflammasome through X-box-binding protein (XBP1) inhibition in a mouse model of liver ischemia/reperfusion injury (Yue et al., 2016). Notably, the inhibition of XBP1 activity could significantly reduce NLRP3 activation, leading to reduced caspase-1 activation and IL-1β secretion in this liver injury model. It may be worthwhile to try to inhibit NLRP3 activation by targeting XBP1 with its specific inhibitors, such as STF-08030, trierixin and tunicamycin (Futamura et al., 2007; Jiang, Niwa, & Koong, 2015; Tanabe et al., 2018).

Sirtuin-3 (SIRT3), an NAD (+)-dependent deacetylase, was shown to be necessary for the limitation of NLRP3 activation and IL-1β and IL-18 production, which substantially contributes to the amelioration of kidney dysfunction in a mouse model of acute kidney injury (Zhao et al., 2016). Interestingly, Honokiol (a polyphenolic lignan from *Magnolia grandiflora*) is a specific activator of SIRT3 and has excellent antioxidant activity in several experimental models. It is possible that the beneficial function of Honokiol may be contributed at least in part by its NLRP3-inhibitory effect (Lu et al., 2017; Ramesh et al., 2018).

Previous studies have indicated that a high-fat diet could induce the activation of NLRP3 *in vivo* in a mouse obesity model (Yan et al., 2013; Zhou et al., 2010). An interesting study demonstrated that CGI-58 (comparative gene identification-58), an important cofactor for adipose triglyceride lipase, is critical for the negative regulation of high-fat diet-induced NLRP3 activation by maintaining PPAR-γ signaling and mitochondrial homeostasis in macrophages (Miao et al., 2014). Thus, some groups quickly realized that the activation of PPAR-γ may contribute to the inhibition of the NLRP3 inflammasome. Indeed, rosiglitazone, the agonist of PPAR-γ, has been indicated to ameliorate airway inflammation and neuroinflammation *in vivo*, which may be closely related to the activation of the NLRP3 inflammasome (Cheng, Li, Wang, Cheng, & Liu, 2018; Dempsey et al., 2017; Meng et al., 2019). The control of the excessive activation of NLRP3 in astrocytes and microglia may represent a potential idea in treating inflammation-driven neurodegeneration, such as that in AD, PD and amyotrophic lateral sclerosis (ALS) (Gordon et al., 2018).

It has been reported that tripartite-motif protein 30 (TRIM30) inhibits the activation of NLRP3 by decreasing the generation of ROS in response to the specific agonists of NLRP3 (Hu et al., 2010). The overexpression of TRIM30 *in vivo* has been confirmed to attenuate reactive oxygen species production and NLRP3 activation (Hu et al., 2010).

8. Targeting the IL-1/IL-1R interaction

Upon activation of the NLRP3 inflammasome, the pro-inflammatory cytokine IL-1β will be produced and released outside the inflammatory cells. IL-1β is one of the most common cytokines involved in NLRP3-driven diseases (Mantovani, Dinarello, Molgora, & Garlanda, 2019). Therefore, IL-1β represents the primary target in restricting NLRP3-driven inflammation. Naturally, several agents that target the IL-1/IL-1 receptor (IL-1R) axis have been subjected to clinical trials (Table 4). To date, three IL-1/IL-1R-targeted agents have been certified: the IL-1 receptor antagonist anakinra, the soluble decoy receptor rilonacept and the neutralizing monoclonal anti-IL-1β antibody canakinumab (Dinarello, Simon, & van der Meer, 2012), among which canakinumab and anakinra are presently available for clinical use (So & Martinon, 2017). Additionally, a monoclonal antibody targeting IL-1R and a neutralizing anti-IL-1α antibody are now in clinical trials (Dinarello et al., 2012). Canakinumab directly targets IL-1β due to its specific immune recognition, while anakinra inhibits the signaling of IL-1/IL-1R *via* its blocking of the interaction between IL-1α/β and IL-1R. Naturally, different mechanisms of action will lead to different clinical efficacies. Anakinra was primarily developed to treat NLRP3-driven disorders such as CAPS and rheumatoid arthritis. However, the advantage of anakinra in clinical practice is limited due to its short plasma half-life (4–6 h) and the inconvenience for patients to maintain the treatment (Granowitz et al., 1992). In contrast, canakinumab has a much longer half-life (26 days), which makes it convenient for patients to maintain the

Table 4 Existing IL-1/IL-1 receptor inhibitors.

Inhibitor	Mode of target	Half-life (h)	Administration	References
Anakinra	IL-1 receptor antagonist	4–6	Subcutaneous	Granowitz et al. (1992) and So and Martinon (2017)
Canakinumab	Anti-IL-1β antibody	624–672	Subcutaneous	Chakraborty et al. (2012) and So and Martinon (2017)
Rilonacept	Soluble IL-1 decoy receptor	192-216	Subcutaneous	Dinarello et al. (2012)

treatment (Chakraborty et al., 2012). Indeed, pharmacological inhibition of IL-1 could significantly ameliorate the severity of gout in patients who have no response to conventional treatments or in whom NSAIDs, colchicine or glucocorticoid steroids are forbidden. Most recently, a research group has shown that continuous treatment with canakinumab could significantly reduce the incidence of atherosclerotic plaques in patients with high C-reactive protein (CRP) levels (Aday & Ridker, 2018). Moreover, with canakinumab treatment, the incidence of arthritis and gout in patients was also significantly decreased (Ridker et al., 2017). Taken together, these results show that therapies based on the targeting of the IL-1/IL-1R axis represent an attractive option in the treatment of NLRP3-driven diseases. However, there are still some inevitable problems. First, all three therapeutic agents need to be administered by injection, therefore the treatment can be inconvenient and painful (Moran et al., 2013). Second, regardless of the source, the blocking of all IL-1β signaling will increase the risk of infection. Additionally, strategies that only block the IL-1/IL-1R axis will have decreased efficacy in the treatment of NLRP3-driven diseases, which are also driven by other pro-inflammatory cytokines, such as IL-18 and HMGB1 (Keyel, 2014).

In summary, although targeting of the IL-1/IL-1R axis has shown clinical potential under some conditions, the identification of selective and direct NLRP3 inhibitors to treat NLRP3-related disorders remains an exciting goal. Future inhibitors have the potential to increase specificity and decrease the side effects.

9. Concluding remarks (opportunities and challenges)

During the past two decades, one of the most important achievements in the field of innate immunity is the discovery of "inflammasomes," which function as a critical protein platform and control the processing of IL-1β and IL-18 as well as the initiation of pyroptosis. Despite many critical problems that have not yet been resolved, excessive activation of inflammasomes *in vivo* has been confirmed to result in multiple inflammatory diseases in humans (Mangan et al., 2018). NLRP3 could recognize the broadest range of PAMPs and DAMPs, the result of which is that the NLRP3 inflammasome occupies a central position for immune sensing in the innate immune system. Therapies targeting the NLRP3 inflammasome have attractive potential. However, several studies have confirmed that unspecific effects will be elicited *in vivo* if the therapeutic strategies are designed by targeting the upstream or downstream signaling events of the NLRP3 inflammasome rather than the NLRP3 protein itself. To avoid potential side effects, the right chemicals should directly target the NLRP3 protein itself, rather than other signaling events. Great effort has been made to screen chemical libraries, and several compounds have been identified, including MCC950, CY-09, tranilast and oridonin, all of which have shown strong inhibitory activity for the NLRP3 inflammasome and beneficial effects in experimental mouse models of NLRP3 activation-related diseases (Coll et al., 2015; Dempsey et al., 2017; He et al., 2018; Huang et al., 2018; Jiang et al., 2017; Kim et al., 2017; Mridha et al., 2017; Ren et al., 2018; van der Heijden et al., 2017). In addition, all four compounds suppress the activation of the NLRP3 inflammasome by directly targeting the NACHT domain of NLRP3. These works not only confirmed that targeting NLRP3 is feasible in inhibiting the NLRP3 inflammasome but also showed that compounds directly targeting NLRP3 could demonstrate druggability in the treatment of NLRP3 inflammasome-related diseases. We believe that more selective NLRP3 inhibitors will be identified in the future with the rapidly growing advances in high-throughput screening platforms. Moreover, in contrast to the inhibition of the NLRP3 inflammasome, the activation of the NLRP3 inflammasome may also represent a novel strategy in the treatment of some inflammation-related diseases. For example, the activation of the NLRP3 inflammasome in the tumor microenvironment may help to re-arouse dormant tumor killer cells, which will facilitate anti-tumor immunity and contribute to the control of tumorigenesis and metastasis (Moossavi, Parsamanesh, Bahrami, Atkin, & Sahebkar, 2018).

Acknowledgments

This work was supported by the National Key R&D program of China (2019YFA0508503), the Strategic Priority Research Program of the Chinese Academy of Sciences (XDB29030102), NSFC (31770991, 91742202, 81525013, 81722022, 81788101, 81821001) and the Young Talent Support Program and the Fundamental Research Funds for the Central Universities.

References

Abdul-Sater, A. A., Tattoli, I., Jin, L., Grajkowski, A., Levi, A., Koller, B. H., et al. (2013). Cyclic-di-GMP and cyclic-di-AMP activate the NLRP3 inflammasome. *EMBO Reports*, *14*, 900.

Aday, A. W., & Ridker, P. M. (2018). Antiinflammatory therapy in clinical care: The CANTOS trial and beyond. *Frontiers in cardiovascular medicine*, *5*, 62.

Aganna, E., Martinon, F., Hawkins, P. N., Ross, J. B., Swan, D. C., Booth, D. R., et al. (2002). Association of mutations in the NALP3/CIAS1/PYPAF1 gene with a broad phenotype including recurrent fever, cold sensitivity, sensorineural deafness, and AA amyloidosis. *Arthritis and Rheumatism*, *46*, 2445.

Aglietti, R. A., Estevez, A., Gupta, A., Ramirez, M. G., Liu, P. S., Kayagaki, N., et al. (2016). GsdmD p30 elicited by caspase-11 during pyroptosis forms pores in membranes. *Proceedings of the National Academy of Sciences of the United States of America*, *113*, 7858.

Allen, I. C., TeKippe, E. M., Woodford, R. M., Uronis, J. M., Holl, E. K., Rogers, A. B., et al. (2010). The NLRP3 inflammasome functions as a negative regulator of tumorigenesis during colitis-associated cancer. *The Journal of Experimental Medicine*, *207*, 1045.

Awad, F., Assrawi, E., Louvrier, C., Jumeau, C., Georgin-Lavialle, S., Grateau, G., et al. (2018). Inflammasome biology, molecular pathology and therapeutic implications. *Pharmacology & Therapeutics*, *187*, 133.

Bauer, C., Duewell, P., Mayer, C., Lehr, H. A., Fitzgerald, K. A., Dauer, M., et al. (2010). Colitis induced in mice with dextran sulfate sodium (DSS) is mediated by the NLRP3 inflammasome. *Gut*, *59*, 1192.

Bauernfeind, F., Bartok, E., Rieger, A., Franchi, L., Nunez, G., & Hornung, V. (2011). Cutting edge: Reactive oxygen species inhibitors block priming, but not activation, of the NLRP3 inflammasome. *Journal of Immunology*, *187*, 613.

Bochner, B. R., & Ames, B. N. (1982). ZTP (5-amino 4-imidazole carboxamide riboside 5'-triphosphate): A proposed alarmone for 10-formyl-tetrahydrofolate deficiency. *Cell*, *29*, 929.

Bruchard, M., Mignot, G., Derangere, V., Chalmin, F., Chevriaux, A., Vegran, F., et al. (2013). Chemotherapy-triggered cathepsin B release in myeloid-derived suppressor cells activates the Nlrp3 inflammasome and promotes tumor growth. *Nature Medicine*, *19*, 57.

Casson, C. N., Yu, J., Reyes, V. M., Taschuk, F. O., Yadav, A., Copenhaver, A. M., et al. (2015). Human caspase-4 mediates noncanonical inflammasome activation against gram-negative bacterial pathogens. *Proceedings of the National Academy of Sciences of the United States of America*, *112*, 6688.

Chakraborty, A., Tannenbaum, S., Rordorf, C., Lowe, P. J., Floch, D., Gram, H., et al. (2012). Pharmacokinetic and pharmacodynamic properties of canakinumab, a human anti-interleukin-1beta monoclonal antibody. *Clinical Pharmacokinetics*, *51*, e1.

Chen, J., & Chen, Z. J. (2018). PtdIns4P on dispersed trans-Golgi network mediates NLRP3 inflammasome activation. *Nature*, *564*, 71.

Chen, S., Smith, B. A., Iype, J., Prestipino, A., Pfeifer, D., Grundmann, S., et al. (2015). MicroRNA-155-deficient dendritic cells cause less severe GVHD through reduced migration and defective inflammasome activation. *Blood*, *126*, 103.

Chen, D., Xiong, X. Q., Zang, Y. H., Tong, Y., Zhou, B., Chen, Q., et al. (2017). BCL6 attenuates renal inflammation via negative regulation of NLRP3 transcription. *Cell Death & Disease*, *8*, e3156.

Cheng, Y., Li, S., Wang, M., Cheng, C., & Liu, R. (2018). Peroxisome proliferator activated receptor gamma (PPARgamma) agonist rosiglitazone ameliorate airway inflammation by inhibiting toll-like receptor 2 (TLR2)/nod-like receptor with pyrin domain containing 3 (NLRP3) inflammatory corpuscle activation in asthmatic mice. *Medical Science Monitor*, *24*, 9045.

Coll, R. C., & Hill, J. R. (2019). MCC950 directly targets the NLRP3 ATP-hydrolysis motif for inflammasome inhibition. *Nature Chemical Biology*, *15*, 556.

Coll, R. C., Robertson, A. A., Chae, J. J., Higgins, S. C., Munoz-Planillo, R., Inserra, M. C., et al. (2015). A small-molecule inhibitor of the NLRP3 inflammasome for the treatment of inflammatory diseases. *Nature Medicine*, *21*, 248.

Compan, V., Baroja-Mazo, A., Lopez-Castejon, G., Gomez, A. I., Martinez, C. M., Angosto, D., et al. (2012). Cell volume regulation modulates NLRP3 inflammasome activation. *Immunity*, *37*, 487.

Dalbeth, N., Merriman, T. R., & Stamp, L. K. (2016). Gout. *Lancet*, *388*, 2039.

Daniels, M. J., Rivers-Auty, J., Schilling, T., Spencer, N. G., Watremez, W., Fasolino, V., et al. (2016). Fenamate NSAIDs inhibit the NLRP3 inflammasome and protect against Alzheimer's disease in rodent models. *Nature Communications*, *7*, 12504.

Darakhshan, S., & Pour, A. B. (2015). Tranilast: A review of its therapeutic applications. *Pharmacological Research*, *91*, 15.

Dempsey, C., Rubio Araiz, A., Bryson, K. J., Finucane, O., Larkin, C., Mills, E. L., et al. (2017). Inhibiting the NLRP3 inflammasome with MCC950 promotes non-phlogistic clearance of amyloid-beta and cognitive function in APP/PS1 mice. *Brain, Behavior, and Immunity*, *61*, 306.

Dinarello, C. A., Simon, A., & van der Meer, J. W. (2012). Treating inflammation by blocking interleukin-1 in a broad spectrum of diseases. *Nature Reviews. Drug Discovery*, *11*, 633.

Ding, J., Wang, K., Liu, W., She, Y., Sun, Q., Shi, J., et al. (2016). Pore-forming activity and structural autoinhibition of the gasdermin family. *Nature*, *535*, 111.

Dostert, C., Petrilli, V., Van Bruggen, R., Steele, C., Mossman, B. T., & Tschopp, J. (2008). Innate immune activation through Nalp3 inflammasome sensing of asbestos and silica. *Science*, *320*, 674.

Duewell, P., Kono, H., Rayner, K. J., Sirois, C. M., Vladimer, G., Bauernfeind, F. G., et al. (2010). NLRP3 inflammasomes are required for atherogenesis and activated by cholesterol crystals. *Nature*, *464*, 1357.

Dupaul-Chicoine, J., Yeretssian, G., Doiron, K., Bergstrom, K. S., McIntire, C. R., LeBlanc, P. M., et al. (2010). Control of intestinal homeostasis, colitis, and colitis-associated colorectal cancer by the inflammatory caspases. *Immunity*, *32*, 367.

Elinav, E., Strowig, T., Kau, A. L., Henao-Mejia, J., Thaiss, C. A., Booth, C. J., et al. (2011). NLRP6 inflammasome regulates colonic microbial ecology and risk for colitis. *Cell*, *145*, 745.

Feng, Z., Qi, S., Zhang, Y., Qi, Z., Yan, L., Zhou, J., et al. (2017). Ly6G+ neutrophil-derived miR-223 inhibits the NLRP3 inflammasome in mitochondrial DAMP-induced acute lung injury. *Cell Death & Disease*, *8*, e3170.

Fernandez, A. F., Sebti, S., Wei, Y., Zou, Z., Shi, M., McMillan, K. L., et al. (2018). Disruption of the beclin 1-BCL2 autophagy regulatory complex promotes longevity in mice. *Nature*, *558*, 136.

Franchi, L., Munoz-Planillo, R., & Nunez, G. (2012). Sensing and reacting to microbes through the inflammasomes. *Nature Immunology*, *13*, 325.

Futamura, Y., Tashiro, E., Hironiwa, N., Kohno, J., Nishio, M., Shindo, K., et al. (2007). Trierixin, a novel Inhibitor of ER stress-induced XBP1 activation from Streptomyces sp. II. structure elucidation. *Journal of Antibiotics (Tokyo)*, *60*, 582.

Gattorno, M., Tassi, S., Carta, S., Delfino, L., Ferlito, F., Pelagatti, M. A., et al. (2007). Pattern of interleukin-1beta secretion in response to lipopolysaccharide and ATP before and after interleukin-1 blockade in patients with CIAS1 mutations. *Arthritis and Rheumatism*, *56*, 3138.

Ghislat, G., & Lawrence, T. (2018). Autophagy in dendritic cells. *Cellular & Molecular Immunology*, *15*, 944.

Giguere, P. M., Gall, B. J., Ezekwe, E. A., Jr., Laroche, G., Buckley, B. K., Kebaier, C., et al. (2014). G Protein signaling modulator-3 inhibits the inflammasome activity of NLRP3. *The Journal of Biological Chemistry*, *289*, 33245.

Gong, T., Jiang, W., & Zhou, R. (2018). Control of Inflammasome Activation by Phosphorylation. *Trends in Biochemical Sciences*, *43*, 685.

Gong, T., Wang, X., Yang, Y., Yan, Y., Yu, C., Zhou, R., et al. (2017). Plant lectins activate the NLRP3 inflammasome to promote inflammatory disorders. *Journal of Immunology*, *198*, 2082.

Gong, T., Yang, Y., Jin, T., Jiang, W., & Zhou, R. (2018). Orchestration of NLRP3 inflammasome activation by ion fluxes. *Trends in Immunology*, *39*, 393.

Gordon, R., Albornoz, E. A., Christie, D. C., Langley, M. R., Kumar, V., Mantovani, S., et al. (2018). Inflammasome inhibition prevents alpha-synuclein pathology and dopaminergic neurodegeneration in mice. *Science Translational Medicine*, *10*, eaah4066.

Granowitz, E. V., Porat, R., Mier, J. W., Pribble, J. P., Stiles, D. M., Bloedow, D. C., et al. (1992). Pharmacokinetics, safety and immunomodulatory effects of human recombinant interleukin-1 receptor antagonist in healthy humans. *Cytokine*, *4*, 353.

Gross, O., Thomas, C. J., Guarda, G., & Tschopp, J. (2011). The inflammasome: An integrated view. *Immunological Reviews*, *243*, 136.

Guarda, G., Braun, M., Staehli, F., Tardivel, A., Mattmann, C., Forster, I., et al. (2011). Type I interferon inhibits interleukin-1 production and inflammasome activation. *Immunity*, *34*, 213.

Guo, C., Xie, S., Chi, Z., Zhang, J., Liu, Y., Zhang, L., et al. (2016). Bile acids control inflammation and metabolic disorder through inhibition of NLRP3 inflammasome. *Immunity*, *45*, 802.

Gurung, P., Lukens, J. R., & Kanneganti, T. D. (2015). Mitochondria: Diversity in the regulation of the NLRP3 inflammasome. *Trends in Molecular Medicine*, *21*, 193.

Hagar, J. A., Powell, D. A., Aachoui, Y., Ernst, R. K., & Miao, E. A. (2013). Cytoplasmic LPS activates caspase-11: Implications in TLR4-independent endotoxic shock. *Science*, *341*, 1250.

Halle, A., Hornung, V., Petzold, G. C., Stewart, C. R., Monks, B. G., Reinheckel, T., et al. (2008). The NALP3 inflammasome is involved in the innate immune response to amyloid-beta. *Nature Immunology*, *9*, 857.

Han, S., Lear, T. B., Jerome, J. A., Rajbhandari, S., Snavely, C. A., Gulick, D. L., et al. (2015). Lipopolysaccharide primes the NALP3 inflammasome by inhibiting its ubiquitination and degradation mediated by the SCFFBXL2 E3 ligase. *The Journal of Biological Chemistry*, *290*, 18124.

Haneklaus, M., O'Neil, J. D., Clark, A. R., Masters, S. L., & O'Neill, L. A. J. (2017). The RNA-binding protein Tristetraprolin (TTP) is a critical negative regulator of the NLRP3 inflammasome. *The Journal of Biological Chemistry*, *292*, 6869.

Hao, H., Cao, L., Jiang, C., Che, Y., Zhang, S., Takahashi, S., et al. (2017). Farnesoid X receptor regulation of the NLRP3 inflammasome underlies cholestasis-associated sepsis. *Cell Metabolism*, *25*, 856.

Hara, H., Tsuchiya, K., Kawamura, I., Fang, R., Hernandez-Cuellar, E., Shen, Y., et al. (2013). Phosphorylation of the adaptor ASC acts as a molecular switch that controls the formation of speck-like aggregates and inflammasome activity. *Nature Immunology*, *14*, 1247.

Harton, J. A., Linhoff, M. W., Zhang, J., & Ting, J. P. (2002). Cutting edge: CATERPILLER: A large family of mammalian genes containing CARD, pyrin, nucleotide-binding, and leucine-rich repeat domains. *Journal of Immunology*, *169*, 4088.

He, H., Jiang, H., Chen, Y., Ye, J., Wang, A., Wang, C., et al. (2018). Oridonin is a covalent NLRP3 inhibitor with strong anti-inflammasome activity. *Nature Communications*, *9*, 2550.

He, Y., Zeng, M. Y., Yang, D., Motro, B., & Nunez, G. (2016). NEK7 is an essential mediator of NLRP3 activation downstream of potassium efflux. *Nature*, *530*, 354.

Heneka, M. T., Kummer, M. P., Stutz, A., Delekate, A., Schwartz, S., Vieira-Saecker, A., et al. (2013). NLRP3 is activated in Alzheimer's disease and contributes to pathology in APP/PS1 mice. *Nature*, *493*, 674.

Hirota, S. A., Ng, J., Lueng, A., Khajah, M., Parhar, K., Li, Y., et al. (2011). NLRP3 inflammasome plays a key role in the regulation of intestinal homeostasis. *Inflammatory Bowel Diseases*, *17*, 1359.

Hoffman, H. M., Mueller, J. L., Broide, D. H., Wanderer, A. A., & Kolodner, R. D. (2001). Mutation of a new gene encoding a putative pyrin-like protein causes familial cold autoinflammatory syndrome and Muckle-Wells syndrome. *Nature Genetics*, *29*, 301.

Hornung, V., Bauernfeind, F., Halle, A., Samstad, E. O., Kono, H., Rock, K. L., et al. (2008). Silica crystals and aluminum salts activate the NALP3 inflammasome through phagosomal destabilization. *Nature Immunology*, *9*, 847.

Hu, Y., Mao, K., Zeng, Y., Chen, S., Tao, Z., Yang, C., et al. (2010). Tripartite-motif protein 30 negatively regulates NLRP3 inflammasome activation by modulating reactive oxygen species production. *Journal of Immunology*, *185*, 7699.

Huai, W., Zhao, R., Song, H., Zhao, J., Zhang, L., Gao, C., et al. (2014). Aryl hydrocarbon receptor negatively regulates NLRP3 inflammasome activity by inhibiting NLRP3 transcription. *Nature Communications*, *5*, 4738.

Huang, Y., Jiang, H., Chen, Y., Wang, X., Yang, Y., Tao, J., et al. (2018). Tranilast directly targets NLRP3 to treat inflammasome-driven diseases. *EMBO Molecular Medicine*, *10*, e8689.

Ito, M., Yanagi, Y., & Ichinohe, T. (2012). Encephalomyocarditis virus viroporin 2B activates NLRP3 inflammasome. *PLoS Pathogens*, *8*, e1002857.

Jiang, H., He, H., Chen, Y., Huang, W., Cheng, J., Ye, J., et al. (2017). Identification of a selective and direct NLRP3 inhibitor to treat inflammatory disorders. *The Journal of Experimental Medicine*, *214*, 3219.

Jiang, D., Niwa, M., & Koong, A. C. (2015). Targeting the IRE1alpha-XBP1 branch of the unfolded protein response in human diseases. *Seminars in Cancer Biology*, *33*, 48.

Jo, E. K., Kim, J. K., Shin, D. M., & Sasakawa, C. (2016). Molecular mechanisms regulating NLRP3 inflammasome activation. *Cellular & Molecular Immunology*, *13*, 148.

Joosten, L. A., Netea, M. G., Fantuzzi, G., Koenders, M. I., Helsen, M. M., Sparrer, H., et al. (2009). Inflammatory arthritis in caspase 1 gene-deficient mice: Contribution of proteinase 3 to caspase 1-independent production of bioactive interleukin-1beta. *Arthritis and Rheumatism*, *60*, 3651.

Kajiwara, Y., Schiff, T., Voloudakis, G., Gama Sosa, M. A., Elder, G., Bozdagi, O., et al. (2014). A critical role for human caspase-4 in endotoxin sensitivity. *Journal of Immunology*, *193*, 335.

Kawashima, A., Karasawa, T., Tago, K., Kimura, H., Kamata, R., Usui-Kawanishi, F., et al. (2017). ARIH2 ubiquitinates NLRP3 and negatively regulates NLRP3 inflammasome activation in macrophages. *Journal of Immunology*, *199*, 3614.

Kayagaki, N., Stowe, I. B., Lee, B. L., O'Rourke, K., Anderson, K., Warming, S., et al. (2015). Caspase-11 cleaves gasdermin D for non-canonical inflammasome signalling. *Nature*, *526*, 666.

Kayagaki, N., Warming, S., Lamkanfi, M., Vande Walle, L., Louie, S., Dong, J., et al. (2011). Non-canonical inflammasome activation targets caspase-11. *Nature*, *479*, 117.

Kayagaki, N., Wong, M. T., Stowe, I. B., Ramani, S. R., Gonzalez, L. C., Akashi-Takamura, S., et al. (2013). Noncanonical inflammasome activation by intracellular LPS independent of TLR4. *Science*, *341*, 1246.

Keyel, P. A. (2014). How is inflammation initiated? individual influences of IL-1, IL-18 and HMGB1. *Cytokine*, *69*, 136.

Kim, R. Y., Pinkerton, J. W., Essilfie, A. T., Robertson, A. A. B., Baines, K. J., Brown, A. C., et al. (2017). Role for NLRP3 inflammasome-mediated, IL-1beta-dependent responses in severe, steroid-resistant asthma. *American Journal of Respiratory and Critical Care Medicine*, *196*, 283.

Lee, H. E., Yang, G., Kim, N. D., Jeong, S., Jung, Y., Choi, J. Y., et al. (2016). Targeting ASC in NLRP3 inflammasome by caffeic acid phenethyl ester: A novel strategy to treat acute gout. *Scientific Reports*, *6*, 38622.

Liu, X., Zhang, Z., Ruan, J., Pan, Y., Magupalli, V. G., Wu, H., et al. (2016). Inflammasome-activated gasdermin D causes pyroptosis by forming membrane pores. *Nature*, *535*, 153.

Lu, J., Zhang, H., Chen, X., Zou, Y., Li, J., Wang, L., et al. (2017). A small molecule activator of SIRT3 promotes deacetylation and activation of manganese superoxide dismutase. *Free Radical Biology & Medicine*, *112*, 287.

Mallampalli, R. K., Coon, T. A., Glasser, J. R., Wang, C., Dunn, S. R., Weathington, N. M., et al. (2013). Targeting F box protein Fbxo3 to control cytokine-driven inflammation. *Journal of Immunology*, *191*, 5247.

Man, S. M., & Kanneganti, T. D. (2015). Regulation of inflammasome activation. *Immunological Reviews*, *265*, 6.

Mangan, M. S. J., Olhava, E. J., Roush, W. R., Seidel, H. M., Glick, G. D., & Latz, E. (2018). Targeting the NLRP3 inflammasome in inflammatory diseases. *Nature Reviews. Drug Discovery*, *17*, 588.

Mantovani, A., Dinarello, C. A., Molgora, M., & Garlanda, C. (2019). Interleukin-1 and related cytokines in the regulation of inflammation and immunity. *Immunity*, *50*, 778.

Mariathasan, S., Weiss, D. S., Newton, K., McBride, J., O'Rourke, K., Roose-Girma, M., et al. (2006). Cryopyrin activates the inflammasome in response to toxins and ATP. *Nature*, *440*, 228.

Martin, B. N., Wang, C., Willette-Brown, J., Herjan, T., Gulen, M. F., Zhou, H., et al. (2014). IKKalpha negatively regulates ASC-dependent inflammasome activation. *Nature Communications*, *5*, 4977.

Martinon, F., Mayor, A., & Tschopp, J. (2009). The inflammasomes: Guardians of the body. *Annual Review of Immunology*, *27*, 229.

Martinon, F., Petrilli, V., Mayor, A., Tardivel, A., & Tschopp, J. (2006). Gout-associated uric acid crystals activate the NALP3 inflammasome. *Nature*, *440*, 237.

Masters, S. L., Dunne, A., Subramanian, S. L., Hull, R. L., Tannahill, G. M., Sharp, F. A., et al. (2010). Activation of the NLRP3 inflammasome by islet amyloid polypeptide provides a mechanism for enhanced IL-1beta in type 2 diabetes. *Nature Immunology*, *11*, 897.

Mayer-Barber, K. D., Andrade, B. B., Barber, D. L., Hieny, S., Feng, C. G., Caspar, P., et al. (2011). Innate and adaptive interferons suppress IL-1alpha and IL-1beta production by distinct pulmonary myeloid subsets during Mycobacterium tuberculosis infection. *Immunity*, *35*, 1023.

Mayor, A., Martinon, F., De Smedt, T., Petrilli, V., & Tschopp, J. (2007). A crucial function of SGT1 and HSP90 in inflammasome activity links mammalian and plant innate immune responses. *Nature Immunology*, *8*, 497.

Meissner, F., Seger, R. A., Moshous, D., Fischer, A., Reichenbach, J., & Zychlinsky, A. (2010). Inflammasome activation in NADPH oxidase defective mononuclear phagocytes from patients with chronic granulomatous disease. *Blood*, *116*, 1570.

Meng, Q. Q., Feng, Z. C., Zhang, X. L., Hu, L. Q., Wang, M., Zhang, H. F., et al. (2019). PPAR-gamma activation exerts an anti-inflammatory effect by suppressing the NLRP3 inflammasome in spinal cord-derived neurons. *Mediators of Inflammation*, *2019*, 6386729.

Miao, H., Ou, J., Ma, Y., Guo, F., Yang, Z., Wiggins, M., et al. (2014). Macrophage CGI-58 deficiency activates ROS-inflammasome pathway to promote insulin resistance in mice. *Cell Reports*, *7*, 223.

Mills, E. L., Kelly, B., & O'Neill, L. A. J. (2017). Mitochondria are the powerhouses of immunity. *Nature Immunology*, *18*, 488.

Mishra, B. B., Rathinam, V. A., Martens, G. W., Martinot, A. J., Kornfeld, H., Fitzgerald, K. A., et al. (2013). Nitric oxide controls the immunopathology of tuberculosis by inhibiting NLRP3 inflammasome-dependent processing of IL-1beta. *Nature Immunology*, *14*, 52.

Moossavi, M., Parsamanesh, N., Bahrami, A., Atkin, S. L., & Sahebkar, A. (2018). Role of the NLRP3 inflammasome in cancer. *Molecular Cancer*, *17*, 13.

Moran, A., Bundy, B., Becker, D. J., DiMeglio, L. A., Gitelman, S. E., Goland, R., et al. (2013). Interleukin-1 antagonism in type 1 diabetes of recent onset: Two multicentre, randomised, double-blind, placebo-controlled trials. *Lancet, 381*, 1905.

Mortimer, L., Moreau, F., MacDonald, J. A., & Chadee, K. (2016). NLRP3 inflammasome inhibition is disrupted in a group of auto-inflammatory disease CAPS mutations. *Nature Immunology, 17*, 1176.

Mridha, A. R., Wree, A., Robertson, A. A. B., Yeh, M. M., Johnson, C. D., Van Rooyen, D. M., et al. (2017). NLRP3 inflammasome blockade reduces liver inflammation and fibrosis in experimental NASH in mice. *Journal of Hepatology, 66*, 1037.

Muñoz-Planillo, R., Kuffa, P., Martínez-Colón, G., Smith, B. L., Rajendiran, T. M., & Núñez, G. (2013). K+ efflux is the common trigger of NLRP3 inflammasome activation by bacterial toxins and particulate matter. *Immunity, 38*, 1142.

Murakami, T., Ockinger, J., Yu, J., Byles, V., McColl, A., Hofer, A. M., et al. (2012). Critical role for calcium mobilization in activation of the NLRP3 inflammasome. *Proceedings of the National Academy of Sciences of the United States of America, 109*, 11282.

Nakahira, K., Haspel, J. A., Rathinam, V. A., Lee, S. J., Dolinay, T., Lam, H. C., et al. (2011). Autophagy proteins regulate innate immune responses by inhibiting the release of mitochondrial DNA mediated by the NALP3 inflammasome. *Nature Immunology, 12*, 222.

Neudecker, V., Haneklaus, M., Jensen, O., Khailova, L., Masterson, J. C., Tye, H., et al. (2017). Myeloid-derived miR-223 regulates intestinal inflammation via repression of the NLRP3 inflammasome. *The Journal of Experimental Medicine, 214*, 1737.

Nussbaum, R. L., & Ellis, C. E. (2003). Alzheimer's disease and Parkinson's disease. *The New England Journal of Medicine, 348*, 1356.

Petrilli, V., Papin, S., Dostert, C., Mayor, A., Martinon, F., & Tschopp, J. (2007). Activation of the NALP3 inflammasome is triggered by low intracellular potassium concentration. *Cell Death and Differentiation, 14*, 1583.

Py, B. F., Kim, M. S., Vakifahmetoglu-Norberg, H., & Yuan, J. (2013). Deubiquitination of NLRP3 by BRCC3 critically regulates inflammasome activity. *Molecular Cell, 49*, 331.

Ramesh, S., Govindarajulu, M., Lynd, T., Briggs, G., Adamek, D., Jones, E., et al. (2018). SIRT3 activator Honokiol attenuates beta-Amyloid by modulating amyloidogenic pathway. *PLoS One, 13* e0190350.

Ren, H., Kong, Y., Liu, Z., Zang, D., Yang, X., Wood, K., et al. (2018). Selective NLRP3 (pyrin domain-containing protein 3) inflammasome inhibitor reduces brain injury after intracerebral hemorrhage. *Stroke, 49*, 184.

Ridker, P. M., Everett, B. M., Thuren, T., MacFadyen, J. G., Chang, W. H., Ballantyne, C., et al. (2017). Antiinflammatory therapy with canakinumab for atherosclerotic disease. *The New England Journal of Medicine, 377*, 1119.

Rodgers, M. A., Bowman, J. W., Fujita, H., Orazio, N., Shi, M., Liang, Q., et al. (2014). The linear ubiquitin assembly complex (LUBAC) is essential for NLRP3 inflammasome activation. *The Journal of Experimental Medicine, 211*, 1333.

Rosenfeldt, M. T., O'Prey, J., Morton, J. P., Nixon, C., MacKay, G., Mrowinska, A., et al. (2013). p53 status determines the role of autophagy in pancreatic tumour development. *Nature, 504*, 296.

Saitoh, T., Fujita, N., Jang, M. H., Uematsu, S., Yang, B. G., Satoh, T., et al. (2008). Loss of the autophagy protein Atg16L1 enhances endotoxin-induced IL-1beta production. *Nature, 456*, 264.

Salem, H., Rachmin, I., Yissachar, N., Cohen, S., Amiel, A., Haffner, R., et al. (2010). Nek7 kinase targeting leads to early mortality, cytokinesis disturbance and polyploidy. *Oncogene, 29*, 4046.

Sborgi, L., Ruhl, S., Mulvihill, E., Pipercevic, J., Heilig, R., Stahlberg, H., et al. (2016). GSDMD membrane pore formation constitutes the mechanism of pyroptotic cell death. *The EMBO Journal*, *35*, 1766.

Schroder, K., Zhou, R., & Tschopp, J. (2010). The NLRP3 inflammasome: A sensor for metabolic danger? *Science*, *327*, 296.

Seino, S. (2001). S20G mutation of the amylin gene is associated with Type II diabetes in Japanese. Study Group of Comprehensive Analysis of Genetic Factors in Diabetes Mellitus. *Diabetologia*, *44*, 906.

Shenoy, A. R., Wellington, D. A., Kumar, P., Kassa, H., Booth, C. J., Cresswell, P., et al. (2012). GBP5 promotes NLRP3 inflammasome assembly and immunity in mammals. *Science*, *336*, 481.

Shi, Y., Evans, J. E., & Rock, K. L. (2003). Molecular identification of a danger signal that alerts the immune system to dying cells. *Nature*, *425*, 516.

Shi, H., Wang, Y., Li, X., Zhan, X., Tang, M., Fina, M., et al. (2016). NLRP3 activation and mitosis are mutually exclusive events coordinated by NEK7, a new inflammasome component. *Nature Immunology*, *17*, 250.

Shi, J., Zhao, Y., Wang, Y., Gao, W., Ding, J., Li, P., et al. (2014). Inflammatory caspases are innate immune receptors for intracellular LPS. *Nature*, *514*, 187.

Shi, J., Zhao, Y., Wang, K., Shi, X., Wang, Y., Huang, H., et al. (2015). Cleavage of GSDMD by inflammatory caspases determines pyroptotic cell death. *Nature*, *526*, 660.

Shimada, K., Crother, T. R., Karlin, J., Dagvadorj, J., Chiba, N., Chen, S., et al. (2012). Oxidized mitochondrial DNA activates the NLRP3 inflammasome during apoptosis. *Immunity*, *36*, 401.

Shinkai, K., McCalmont, T. H., & Leslie, K. S. (2008). Cryopyrin-associated periodic syndromes and autoinflammation. *Clinical and Experimental Dermatology*, *33*, 1.

Siegmund, B., Lehr, H. A., Fantuzzi, G., & Dinarello, C. A. (2001). IL-1 beta -converting enzyme (caspase-1) in intestinal inflammation. *Proceedings of the National Academy of Sciences of the United States of America*, *98*, 13249.

So, A. K., & Martinon, F. (2017). Inflammation in gout: Mechanisms and therapeutic targets. *Nature Reviews Rheumatology*, *13*, 639.

Sokolowska, M., Chen, L. Y., Liu, Y., Martinez-Anton, A., Qi, H. Y., Logun, C., et al. (2015). Prostaglandin E2 inhibits NLRP3 inflammasome activation through EP4 receptor and intracellular cyclic AMP in human macrophages. *Journal of Immunology*, *194*, 5472.

Song, H., Liu, B., Huai, W., Yu, Z., Wang, W., Zhao, J., et al. (2016). The E3 ubiquitin ligase TRIM31 attenuates NLRP3 inflammasome activation by promoting proteasomal degradation of NLRP3. *Nature Communications*, *7*, 13727.

Song, N., Liu, Z. S., Xue, W., Bai, Z. F., Wang, Q. Y., Dai, J., et al. (2017). NLRP3 phosphorylation is an essential priming event for inflammasome activation. *Molecular Cell*, *68*, 185.

Spalinger, M. R., Kasper, S., Gottier, C., Lang, S., Atrott, K., Vavricka, S. R., et al. (2016). NLRP3 tyrosine phosphorylation is controlled by protein tyrosine phosphatase PTPN22. *The Journal of Clinical Investigation*, *126*, 1783.

Spalinger, M. R., Lang, S., Gottier, C., Dai, X., Rawlings, D. J., Chan, A. C., et al. (2017). PTPN22 regulates NLRP3-mediated IL1B secretion in an autophagy-dependent manner. *Autophagy*, *13*, 1590.

Stienstra, R., Joosten, L. A., Koenen, T., van Tits, B., van Diepen, J. A., van den Berg, S. A., et al. (2010). The inflammasome-mediated caspase-1 activation controls adipocyte differentiation and insulin sensitivity. *Cell Metabolism*, *12*, 593.

Strowig, T., Henao-Mejia, J., Elinav, E., & Flavell, R. (2012). Inflammasomes in health and disease. *Nature*, *481*, 278.

Tanabe, Y., Suehara, Y., Kohsaka, S., Hayashi, T., Akaike, K., Mukaihara, K., et al. (2018). IRE1alpha-XBP1 inhibitors exerted anti-tumor activities in Ewing's sarcoma. *Oncotarget*, *9*, 14428.

Tang, T., Lang, X., Xu, C., Wang, X., Gong, T., Yang, Y., et al. (2017). CLICs-dependent chloride efflux is an essential and proximal upstream event for NLRP3 inflammasome activation. *Nature Communications*, *8*, 202.

Tapia-Abellan, A., Angosto-Bazarra, D., Martinez-Banaclocha, H., de Torre-Minguela, C., Ceron-Carrasco, J. P., Perez-Sanchez, H., et al. (2019). MCC950 closes the active conformation of NLRP3 to an inactive state. *Nature Chemical Biology*, *15*, 560.

Timmermans, K., van der Wal, S. E., Vaneker, M., van der Laak, J. A., Netea, M. G., Pickkers, P., et al. (2013). IL-1beta processing in mechanical ventilation-induced inflammation is dependent on neutrophil factors rather than caspase-1. *Intensive Care Medicine Experimental*, *1*, 27.

Torres, J., Mehandru, S., Colombel, J. F., & Peyrin-Biroulet, L. (2017). Crohn's disease. *Lancet*, *389*, 1741.

Triantafilou, K., Hughes, T. R., Triantafilou, M., & Morgan, B. P. (2013). The complement membrane attack complex triggers intracellular Ca2+ fluxes leading to NLRP3 inflammasome activation. *Journal of Cell Science*, *126*, 2903.

Ungaro, R., Mehandru, S., Allen, P. B., Peyrin-Biroulet, L., & Colombel, J. F. (2017). Ulcerative colitis. *Lancet*, *389*, 1756.

van de Veerdonk, F. L., Smeekens, S. P., Joosten, L. A., Kullberg, B. J., Dinarello, C. A., van der Meer, J. W., et al. (2010). Reactive oxygen species-independent activation of the IL-1beta inflammasome in cells from patients with chronic granulomatous disease. *Proceedings of the National Academy of Sciences of the United States of America*, *107*, 3030.

van der Heijden, T., Kritikou, E., Venema, W., van Duijn, J., van Santbrink, P. J., Slutter, B., et al. (2017). NLRP3 inflammasome inhibition by MCC950 reduces atherosclerotic lesion development in apolipoprotein E-deficient mice-brief report. *Arteriosclerosis, Thrombosis, and Vascular Biology*, *37*, 1457.

Vandanmagsar, B., Youm, Y. H., Ravussin, A., Galgani, J. E., Stadler, K., Mynatt, R. L., et al. (2011). The NLRP3 inflammasome instigates obesity-induced inflammation and insulin resistance. *Nature Medicine*, *17*, 179.

Voet, S., Srinivasan, S., Lamkanfi, M., & van Loo, G. (2019). Inflammasomes in neuroinflammatory and neurodegenerative diseases. *EMBO Molecular Medicine*, *11*, e10248.

Walle, L. V., Van Opdenbosch, N., Jacques, P., Fossoul, A., Verheugen, E., Vogel, P., et al. (2014). Negative regulation of the NLRP3 inflammasome by A20 protects against arthritis. *Nature*, *512*, 69.

Wang, Y., Han, Z., Fan, Y., Zhang, J., Chen, K., Gao, L., et al. (2017). MicroRNA-9 inhibits NLRP3 inflammasome activation in human atherosclerosis inflammation cell models through the JAK1/STAT signaling pathway. *Cellular Physiology and Biochemistry*, *41*, 1555.

Wang, X., Jiang, W., Yan, Y., Gong, T., Han, J., Tian, Z., et al. (2014). RNA viruses promote activation of the NLRP3 inflammasome through a RIP1-RIP3-DRP1 signaling pathway. *Nature Immunology*, *15*, 1126.

Wannamaker, W., Davies, R., Namchuk, M., Pollard, J., Ford, P., Ku, G., et al. (2007). (S)-1-((S)-2-{[1-(4-amino-3-chloro-phenyl)-methanoyl]-amino}-3,3-dimethyl-butanoyl)-pyrrolidine-2-carboxylic acid ((2R,3S)-2-ethoxy-5-oxo-tetrahydro-furan-3-yl)-amide (VX-765), an orally available selective interleukin (IL)-converting enzyme/caspase-1 inhibitor, exhibits potent anti-inflammatory activities by inhibiting the release of IL-1beta and IL-18. *The Journal of Pharmacology and Experimental Therapeutics*, *321*, 509.

Yan, Y., Jiang, W., Liu, L., Wang, X., Ding, C., Tian, Z., et al. (2015). Dopamine controls systemic inflammation through inhibition of NLRP3 inflammasome. *Cell*, *160*, 62.

Yan, Y., Jiang, W., Spinetti, T., Tardivel, A., Castillo, R., Bourquin, C., et al. (2013). Omega-3 fatty acids prevent inflammation and metabolic disorder through inhibition of NLRP3 inflammasome activation. *Immunity*, *38*, 1154.

Yang, X. M., Downey, J. M., Cohen, M. V., Housley, N. A., Alvarez, D. F., & Audia, J. P. (2017). The highly selective caspase-1 inhibitor VX-765 provides additive protection against myocardial infarction in rat hearts when combined with a platelet inhibitor. *Journal of Cardiovascular Pharmacology and Therapeutics*, *22*, 574.

Yang, D., He, Y., Munoz-Planillo, R., Liu, Q., & Nunez, G. (2015). Caspase-11 requires the pannexin-1 channel and the purinergic P2X7 pore to mediate pyroptosis and endotoxic shock. *Immunity*, *43*, 923.

Yang, C. S., Kim, J. J., Kim, T. S., Lee, P. Y., Kim, S. Y., Lee, H. M., et al. (2015). Small heterodimer partner interacts with NLRP3 and negatively regulates activation of the NLRP3 inflammasome. *Nature Communications*, *6*, 6115.

Yao, X., Zhang, C., Xing, Y., Xue, G., Zhang, Q., Pan, F., et al. (2017). Remodelling of the gut microbiota by hyperactive NLRP3 induces regulatory T cells to maintain homeostasis. *Nature Communications*, *8*, 1896.

Youm, Y. H., Nguyen, K. Y., Grant, R. W., Goldberg, E. L., Bodogai, M., Kim, D., et al. (2015). The ketone metabolite beta-hydroxybutyrate blocks NLRP3 inflammasome-mediated inflammatory disease. *Nature Medicine*, *21*, 263.

Yue, S., Zhu, J., Zhang, M., Li, C., Zhou, X., Zhou, M., et al. (2016). The myeloid heat shock transcription factor 1/beta-catenin axis regulates NLR family, pyrin domain-containing 3 inflammasome activation in mouse liver ischemia/reperfusion injury. *Hepatology*, *64*, 1683.

Zambon, A., & Cusi, K. (2007). The role of fenofibrate in clinical practice. *Diabetes & Vascular Disease Research*, *4*(Suppl. 3), S15.

Zanoni, I., Ostuni, R., Capuano, G., Collini, M., Caccia, M., Ronchi, A. E., et al. (2009). CD14 regulates the dendritic cell life cycle after LPS exposure through NFAT activation. *Nature*, *460*, 264.

Zhao, W. Y., Zhang, L., Sui, M. X., Zhu, Y. H., & Zeng, L. (2016). Protective effects of sirtuin 3 in a murine model of sepsis-induced acute kidney injury. *Scientific Reports*, *6*, 33201.

Zhong, Z., Liang, S., Sanchez-Lopez, E., He, F., Shalapour, S., Lin, X. J., et al. (2018). New mitochondrial DNA synthesis enables NLRP3 inflammasome activation. *Nature*, *560*, 198.

Zhong, Z., Sanchez-Lopez, E., & Karin, M. (2016). Autophagy, NLRP3 inflammasome and auto-inflammatory/immune diseases. *Clinical and Experimental Rheumatology*, *34*, 12.

Zhong, Z., Umemura, A., Sanchez-Lopez, E., Liang, S., Shalapour, S., Wong, J., et al. (2016). NF-kappaB restricts inflammasome activation via elimination of damaged mitochondria. *Cell*, *164*, 896.

Zhou, Y., Lu, M., Du, R. H., Qiao, C., Jiang, C. Y., Zhang, K. Z., et al. (2016). MicroRNA-7 targets Nod-like receptor protein 3 inflammasome to modulate neuroinflammation in the pathogenesis of Parkinson's disease. *Molecular Neurodegeneration*, *11*, 28.

Zhou, R., Tardivel, A., Thorens, B., Choi, I., & Tschopp, J. (2010). Thioredoxin-interacting protein links oxidative stress to inflammasome activation. *Nature Immunology*, *11*, 136.

Zhou, R., Yazdi, A. S., Menu, P., & Tschopp, J. (2011). A role for mitochondria in NLRP3 inflammasome activation. *Nature*, *469*, 221.

CHAPTER FOUR

Fine-tuning of antiviral innate immunity by ubiquitination

Yi Zheng, Chengjiang Gao*
State Key Laboratory of Microbial Technology, Key Laboratory of Infection and Immunity of Shandong Province & Department of Immunology, the School of Basic Medical Sciences, Shandong University, Jinan, Shandong, China
*Corresponding author: e-mail address: cgao@sdu.edu.cn

Contents

Abstract

The innate immune system represents the first defense line of the host following viral infection. The infection triggers the recognition of pathogen-associated molecular patterns (PAMPs) from the viruses by pattern recognition receptors (PRRs) of the host cell. The interaction between viral PAMPs and PRRs evokes a sophisticated signal transduction system and eventually promotes the expression of type I interferons (IFNs) and proinflammatory cytokines. Ubiquitination plays an indispensable role in fine-tuning almost every single step of this signaling cascade given on its versatile functions. Ubiquitin ligases and deubiquitinases (DUBs), which cooperatively and accurately regulate the dynamic and reversible ubiquitination process, are the master regulators of antiviral signaling. In this review, we concentrate on summarizing the ubiquitin ligases and DUBs that modulate the central signaling molecules in antiviral innate immunity. Especially, we emphasize the ones that were identified by the immunologists from China.

Advances in Immunology, Volume 145
ISSN 0065-2776
https://doi.org/10.1016/bs.ai.2019.11.004

1. The antiviral innate immune system

The very first step of innate immunity signaling is the sensing of PAMPs by the correspondent PRRs. The invading viruses possess different types of nucleic acids as the PAMPs, such as double-stranded RNA (dsRNA), positive or negative single-stranded RNA (ssRNA), and dsDNA (Akira, Uematsu, & Takeuchi, 2006). The viral PAMPs are mainly perceived by three types of PRRs, including Toll-like receptors (TLRs), RIG-I-like receptors (RLRs), and DNA sensors, such as cyclic GMP-AMP synthase (cGAS), IFI16, and recently identified hnRNPA2B1 (Wang, Wen, & Cao, 2019).

The recognition of the PAMPs by the PRRs elicits the signal transduction cascade. The PRRs are predominantly in the state of autorepression in the absence of the PAMPs. Binding of the viral nucleic acids trigger the conformational transition and subsequent activation of the PRRs, which leads to the interaction between PRRs and the adaptor proteins, such as Toll/interleukin-1 receptor domain-containing adaptor protein inducing interferon-beta (TRIF) (Yamamoto et al., 2003), myeloid differentiation factor-88 (MyD88) (Deguine & Barton, 2014), mitochondrial antiviral signaling protein (MAVS) (Seth, Sun, Ea, & Chen, 2005), and stimulator of interferon genes protein (STING) (Ishikawa & Barber, 2008). The activation of the adaptor proteins further results in the ensuing complex formation and activation of the kinases including inhibitor of nuclear factor kappa-B [IκB] kinase (IKK) family and TANK-binding kinase-1 (TBK1). IKK family and TBK1 are responsible for activating the transcription factors nuclear factor kappa-light-chain-enhancer of activated B cells (NF-κB) and interferon-regulatory factor 3 (IRF3), respectively (Fitzgerald et al., 2003; Woronicz, Gao, Cao, Rothe, & Goeddel, 1997). IKKβ within IKK family directly phosphorylates IκBα, promoting its phosphorylation, ubiquitination, and proteasomal degradation. Degradation of IκBα unleashes the sequestered NF-κB, which translocates from cytoplasm to the nucleus and then engages in stimulating the production of proinflammatory cytokines (Hayden & Ghosh, 2008). TBK1 collaborates with IKKε to phosphorylate IRF3, resulting in its dimerization and translocation to the nucleus. The translocated IRF3 induces the expression of the genes encoding type I IFNs and IFN regulatory factors in the nucleus (Sato et al., 2000).

2. Ubiquitination and its crosstalk with innate immunity

The conjugation of ubiquitin, an 8.5 kDa protein comprising of 76 amino acids, to a substrate protein is called ubiquitination. This ubiquitous post-translational modification (PTM) is completed through a cascade of three distinct classes of enzymes. Ubiquitin molecules are first activated by ubiquitin-activating enzymes (E1s), then conjugated by ubiquitin-conjugating enzymes (E2s), and are finally ligated to the substrate by ubiquitin ligases (E3s) (Pickart & Eddins, 2004).

Given on limited numbers of E1 and E2 enzymes, the specific recognition of substrate is largely dependent on the E3 ubiquitin ligase. E3s are categorized into three types according to their domain structure and the catalytic mechanisms: HECT (homologous to E6-associated protein C-terminus), RING (Really Interesting New Gene), and RBR (RING-IBR [in-between-RINGs]-RING) (Zheng & Shabek, 2017). Structurally, HECT type E3s have a unique and conserved C-terminal HECT domain, while the RING E3s are characterized by their RING or U-box fold catalytic domain. RBR E3s are defined by tripartite domain arrangement, including two predicted RING fingers (RING1 and RING2) and a central IBR zinc-binding domain (Zheng & Shabek, 2017). Besides the structural difference, the three types of E3 also distinguish each other from the mechanism of how they transfer the ubiquitin from E2 conjugating enzyme to substrate. RING-type E3 ligases adopt their RING finger domain to interact with E2 and mediate the direct transfer of the ubiquitin from E2 to the target protein, while an E3-ubiquitin thioester intermediate was observed in HECT-type E3 ligases (Zheng & Shabek, 2017). HECT type E3 ligase utilizes HECT domain and N-terminal domain to interact with E2 and substrate, respectively (Sluimer & Distel, 2018). The ubiquitin is transferred to an active cysteine residue in the HECT domain before conjugating to the substrate. For RBR type, it possesses the hybrid mechanistic feature of the RING and HECT types (Walden & Rittinger, 2018). The E2 conjugating enzyme binds with the RING1 domain of RBR E3, and the ubiquitin molecule conjugation must transit from the E2 to an active cysteine residue located within the RING2 domain. Within the three families, RING E3 comprises the largest number, with over 600 predicted members in the human genome (Zheng & Shabek, 2017). Compared to the large number of RING type E3 ligases, numbers of HECT and RBR types

E3s are relatively limited, with less than 20 were reported, respectively (Sluimer & Distel, 2018; Walden & Rittinger, 2018).

The release of conjugated ubiquitin from the substrate is catalyzed by DUBs. There are approximately 100 DUBs in human (Mevissen & Komander, 2017). To date, seven structurally distinct DUB families have been delineated, including six families of cysteine proteases: the ubiquitin-specific proteases (USPs), the ovarian tumor proteases (OTU), the ubiquitin C-terminal hydrolases (UCHs), the Josephin family, the motif interacting with ubiquitin (MIU)-containing novel DUB family [MINDYs], Zinc finger with UFM1-specific peptidase domain protein (ZUFSP), and a family of Zn-dependent JAB1/MPN/MOV34 metalloprotease DUBs (JAMMs, also known as MPN+). DUBs modulate ubiquitin modification in two distinct manners. One is directed toward the substrates through the protein-protein interaction, while the other shows the selectivity for the ubiquitin linkage architecture. Within the seven families, USPs is the largest family, comprising 54 members in the human genome.

Ubiquitination mainly occurs at lysine residues of the substrate proteins, which can be attached with a single ubiquitin moiety (monoubiquitination) or ubiquitin chains (polyubiquitination) (Malynn & Ma, 2010). Ubiquitin itself contains eight amino groups for another ubiquitin molecule to conjugate with: the ε-amino groups of seven lysine residues (K6, 11, 27, 29, 33, 48, and 63) and the α-amino group of the N-terminal methionine residue. Polyubiquitin chains with a single type of linkage are referred to homotypic, in which the K48- and K63-based chains are the best characterized. K48-based ubiquitin chains label the substrate for proteasome-dependent degradation, while K63-linked polyubiquitination of the substrate performs various non-degradative roles (Malynn & Ma, 2010). Recently, there are emerging studies investigating the functions of atypical polyubiquitin chains. For example, a recent study utilizing a phage-display-derived K6-specific affimer approach observed that K6 affimers mark damaged mitochondria upon activation of E3 ligase Parkin (Michel, Swatek, Hospenthal, & Komander, 2017), suggesting that K6-linked ubiquitination is closely related with the mitophagy. Besides, the ubiquitin chains with atypical linkage are tightly associated with the regulation of innate immunity. For example, M1-linked chains, which are catalyzed by an RBR type E3 ligase linear ubiquitin chain assembly complex (LUBAC), are essential for the activation of NF-κB and regulation of IFN production (Ikeda et al., 2011; Kirisako et al., 2006).

Besides these homotypic chains, heterotypic chains containing mixed lysine linkages also participate in a series of physiological processes through proteolytic degradation and non-proteolytic functions. For example, Ube2C and Ube2S cooperate and conjugate K11/K48-branched ubiquitin chains in APC/C for its proteasomal dependent degradation, while IL-1 stimulation of the cell triggers the formation of K63/M1-linked conjugates. These heterotypic chains add up the functional diversity and complexity of ubiquitination (Yau & Rape, 2016).

As shown in Fig. 1, ubiquitination of the receptor protein, adaptor protein, kinase, and effector protein are essential for potently activating the production of the type I IFN and proinflammatory cytokines to combat the pathogens (Zheng & Gao, 2019). Upon the infection of the RNA viruses, the K63-linked polyubiquitination of RIG-I is indispensable for its oligomerization and activation (Gack et al., 2007). At the meanwhile, some of the signaling molecules need to be upregulated to mount a robust antiviral response. For example, USP27x stabilizes cGAS dependent on its deubiquitinase activity during the viral infection (Guo et al., 2019). After eliminating the invading pathogens, the host cells need to shut off the signaling transduction to prevent the aberrant autoimmunity. In this case, ubiquitination can facilitate the degradation or deactivation of signaling molecules to dampen the immune response. For example, RNF125 upregulates the K48-linkage of RIG-I, and USP21 downregulates K63-linked polyubiquitination of RIG-I (Arimoto et al., 2007; Fan et al., 2014). Both E3 ubiquitin ligases and DUBs play indispensable roles in reaching the balance between eradicating pathogens and preventing risky collateral damage, as shown in Figs. 1 and 2.

3. Ubiquitination regulation of the innate immune system

3.1 TLR signaling

All TLRs belong to the type I transmembrane domain proteins comprising of tripartite sequences: an N-terminal leucine-rich repeat-containing ectodomain essential for sensing of the PAMPs, a single transmembrane spanning region, and a cytoplasmic C-terminal globular Toll/interleukin-1 (IL-1) receptor (TIR) domain responsible for binding with the adaptor proteins to transduce the downstream signaling (Lester & Li, 2014). Within all TLRs, TLR3/7/8/9 belongs to the intracellular TLRs and are responsible for detecting the viral nucleic acids in the

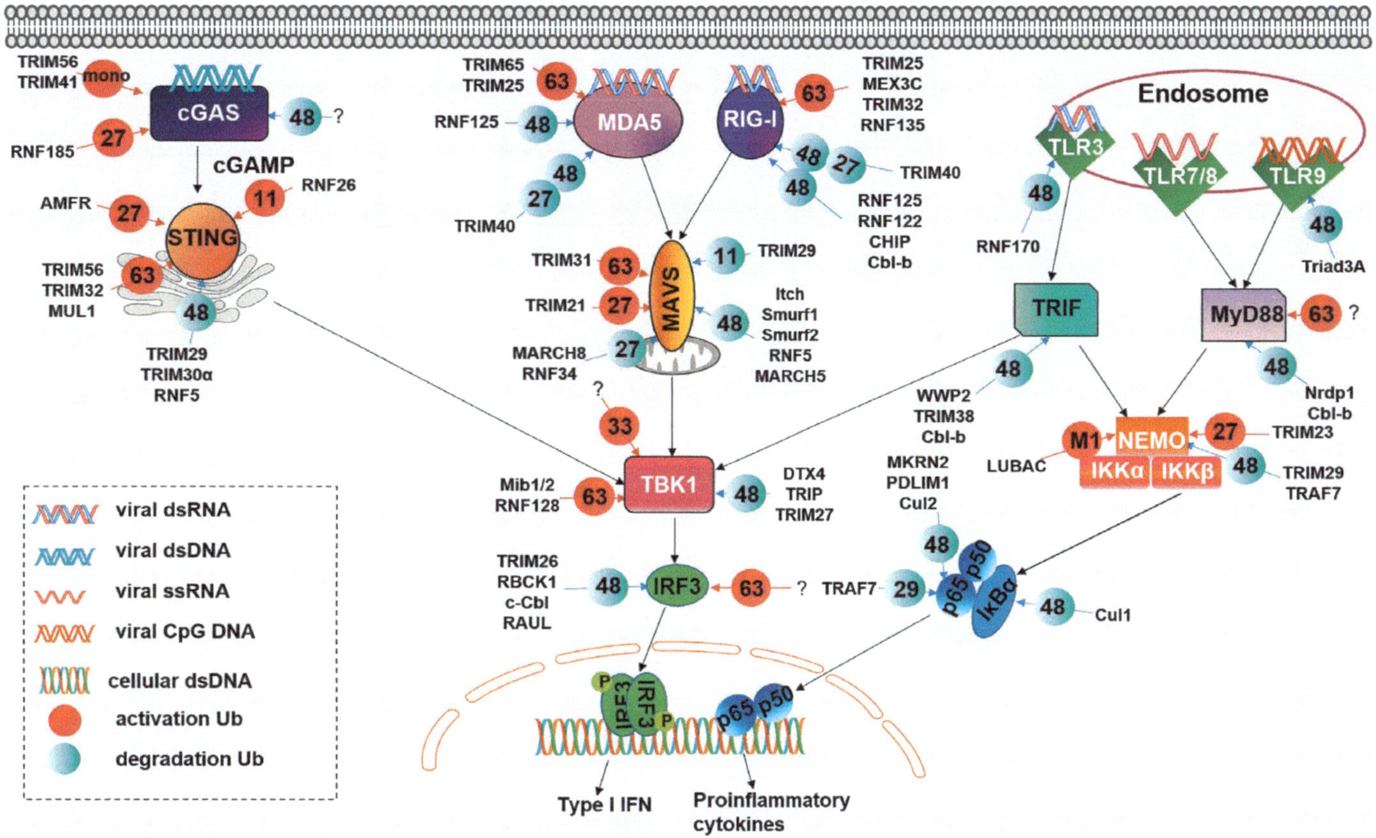

Fig. 1 Illustration of the E3 ubiquitin ligases which regulate the antiviral innate immunity signaling. The diagram depicts the components of type I interferon pathway and proinflammatory pathway during viral infection. And the E3 ubiquitin ligases responsible for the activation or degradation of the PRRs, adaptor proteins, kinases, and effector proteins are also listed besides them.

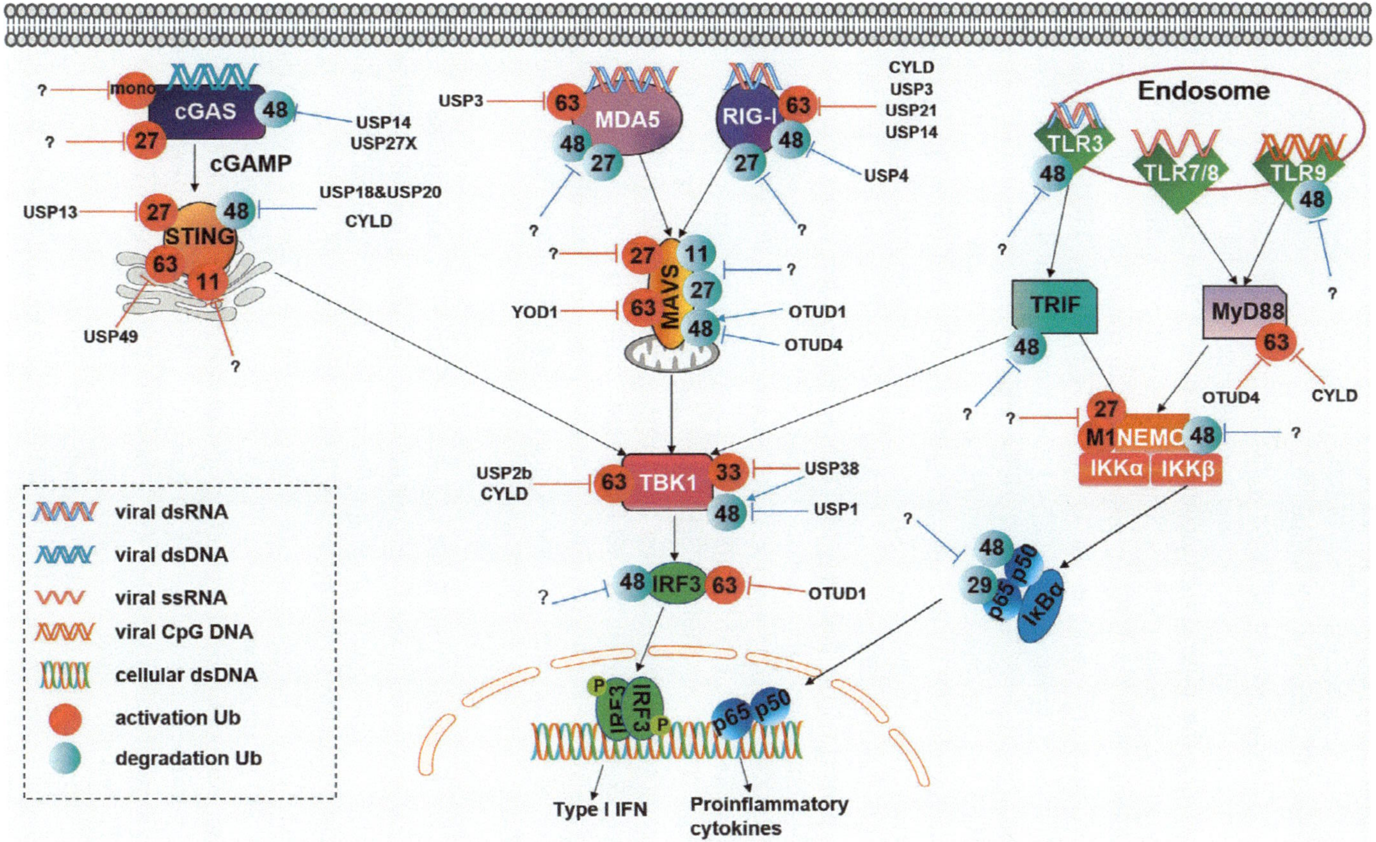

Fig. 2 Illustration of the DUBs which regulate the antiviral innate immunity signaling. And the DUBs accountable for modulating the activation or degradation of the PRRs, adaptor proteins, kinases, and effector proteins are also listed besides them.

endosomal compartment. TLR3 and TLR7/8 recognize dsRNA and ssRNA, respectively. For TLR9, it engages unmethylated CpG DNA species (Xagorari & Chlichlia, 2008).

The engagement of TLRs with the viral PAMPs triggers the interaction between the TIR domain and two adaptor proteins, TRIF and MyD88, relaying the distinct intracellular signaling. TLR3 interacts with TRIF to stimulate both the type I interferon and pro-inflammatory response, whereas TLR7/8/9 binds with MyD88 to trigger the production of pro-inflammatory cytokines. In TLR3-TRIF pathway, TRIF associates with Tumor Necrosis Factor (TNF) receptor-associated factor 3 (TRAF3) for activation of TBK1 and IKKε and subsequent phosphorylation of IRF3 to drive the expression of type I IFN (Lester & Li, 2014). In the meanwhile, TRIF also interacts with TRAF6 and Receptor-interacting serine/threonine-protein kinase 1 (RIP1), leading to the activation of TGF-β-activated kinase 1 (TAK1) and IKK complex. In MyD88-dependent TLR pathway, MyD88 recruits another subset of downstream molecules including kinases interleukin-1 receptor-associated kinase 4 (IRAK4), IRAK1, and TRAF6 for activation of TAK1 and IKK complex (Xagorari & Chlichlia, 2008). The activation of classical IKK complex from TRIF or MyD88 dependent pathway phosphorylates IκBα and promotes its ubiquitination and proteasomal degradation. Subsequently, the sequestration of NF-κB is released, causing it to translocate from the cytoplasm to the nucleus and eventually triggering the subsequent expression of pro-inflammatory cytokines such as TNF, interleukin 6 (IL-6), and IL-12.

3.1.1 E3 ligases and DUBs regulating TLRs, TRIF, and MyD88

TLR receptors have been identified to be the target of Triad3A and RNF170 for ubiquitination and degradation. Triad3A (RNF216) enhances the degradation of TLR4 and TLR9 but does not affect the protein level of TLR2 (Chuang & Ulevitch, 2004). Different from Triad3A, RNF170 specifically marks TLR3 for ubiquitination dependent degradation, supported by the observation that mRNA levels of IFN-β and IL-6 in peritoneal macrophages from Rnf170$^{-/-}$ mice were enhanced compared to those in cells from Rnf170$^{+/+}$ mice stimulated with poly(I:C) rather than LPS or CpG (Song et al., 2019).

The stability of TRIF is under the modulation of a couple of E3 ubiquitin ligases, including WWP2, TRIM38, and Cbl-b. WWP2 was identified as the E3 ubiquitin ligase for TRIF through a mass spectrometry study (Yang et al., 2013). Treatment with poly(I:C) enhanced the interaction between WWP2 and TRIF, resulting in K48-linked polyubiquitination and degradation of TRIF. Furthermore, the production of both IFN-β and pro-inflammatory cytokines were increased in *Wwp2*$^{-/-}$ bone marrow-derived macrophages (BMDMs) following the stimulation of poly(I:C). *In vivo* study observed that the concentration of IFN-β and pro-inflammatory cytokines in the serum from *Wwp2*$^{-/-}$ mice were significantly elevated responding to poly(I:C), causing an earlier inflammatory death. TRIM38 acts as another E3 ubiquitin ligase for TRIF (Xue et al., 2012). Treatment of HeLa cells with poly(I:C) induced the expression of TRIM38, causing the delivery of the K48-linked polymeric chains on TRIF and its proteasomal-dependent degradation. The interaction between Cbl-b and TRIF is mediated by the integrin CD11b and dependent on the phosphorylation of TRIF and MyD88 (Han et al., 2010). Besides TRIF, Cbl-b also promotes the ubiquitination and degradation of MyD88 (Han et al., 2010). Nrdp1 acts as another E3 ligase for K48-linked polyubiquitination and degradation of MyD88. Intriguingly, Ndrp1 also facilitates the K63-linked polyubiquitination of TBK1 and promotes the type I interferon response. This observation suggests that Ndrp1 plays a dual role in TLR induced immune response, inhibiting the pro-inflammatory response while enhancing the type I interferon response. Of note, E3 ligase Pellino in Drosophila also enhances the ubiquitination and induces a faster turnover of MyD88, functioning as a negative regulator in Toll-mediated innate immunity (Ji et al., 2014). Contrary to the abundant numbers of E3 ligases for TRIF and MyD88 have been identified, the DUBs responsible for cleaving the K48-linked chains from TRIF and MyD88 have not been reported yet.

The K63-linked polyubiquitination of MyD88 was enhanced following *nontypeable Haemophilus influenzae* infection, which is cleaved by the deubiquitinase CYLD (Lee, Miyata, Lim, & Li, 2016). K63-linked ubiquitination at K231 of MyD88 was required for the efficient production of proinflammatory cytokines upon bacterial infection. However, whether the same modification of MyD88 exists during viral infection and what is the E3 ubiquitin ligase for MyD88 need to be further investigated. Another study suggested that OTUD4 negatively regulates the activation of MyD88 dependent on its phosphorylation and UBD domain (Zhao et al., 2018). Mechanistically, phosphorylation-activated OTUD4 cleaves the K63-linked polyubiquitin chains from MyD88 and dampen the activation of downstream signaling dependent on MyD88.

3.2 RLRs-MAVS signaling

RLRs, a family of DExD/H-box RNA helicases, is involved in the sensing of viral RNA species. RLRs includes three members, retinoic acid-inducible gene-I (RIG-I), melanoma differentiation-associated protein 5 (MDA5), and LGP2 (laboratory of genetics and physiology 2). RIG-I and MDA5, the two well-characterized RLR members, harbor two tandem N-terminal caspase activation and recruitment domains (CARDs), a central helicase domain, and a C-terminal domain (CTD) (Schlee, 2013). CARD domain is essential for transducing downstream signaling. Since LGP2 lacks the CARD domain, it was previously suggested to be a negative regulator in the physiological condition (Yoneyama et al., 2005). But a recent study suggested that LGP2 may play a positive role in regulating MDA5-RNA interaction (Bruns, Leser, Lamb, & Horvath, 2014). Helicase domain and CTD recognize and bind with RNA. RIG-I and MDA5 are responsible for detecting distinct RNA species. RIG-I directly interacts with 5′ triphosphorylated ssRNA, 5′ triphosphorylated short dsRNA, whereas MDA5 is accountable for the recognition of long dsRNA (Kato et al., 2006). The *in vivo* functional studies have suggested that RIG-I is indispensable for sensing of paramyxoviruses, influenza virus, and Japanese encephalitis virus, whereas MDA5 is critical for picornavirus detection (Kato et al., 2006).

Two CARDs of RIG-I are disguised by the intramolecular interaction with the helicase domain in the absence of ligand RNA, showing the auto-inhibited state (Jiang et al., 2011; Kowalinski et al., 2011). Upon binding with viral RNA, tandem CARDs of RIG-I are unmasked and further oligomerized for activation. Unlike RIG-I, two CARDs of MDA5 were not sequestered in the absence of ligand RNA. Instead, MDA5 utilizes long dsRNA as a signaling platform to synergistically assemble into the core filament, which in turn promotes stochastic oligomerization of the tandem CARDs (Wu, Peisley, et al., 2013). The activated CARD domain of RIG-I or MDA5 interacts with the CARD domain of the MAVS (also known as Cardif, IPS-1 or VISA) on the mitochondria outer membrane (Kawai et al., 2005; Meylan et al., 2005; Seth et al., 2005; Xu et al., 2005), and this CARD-CARD interaction results in the conformational transition of MAVS and subsequent formation of a prion-like structure, which robustly activate the downstream signaling (Hou et al., 2011). The MAVS polymers act as a scaffold and recruit the TRAF2, 3, 5, and 6 as well as NEMO to activate kinases TBK1 and IKKε (Fang et al., 2017; Liu et al., 2013). The activated TBK1/IKKε phosphorylate and activate IRF3 to trigger transcriptional activation of type I IFN.

3.2.1 E3 ligases and DUBs regulating the activation of RLRs

In the past, a series of studies have particularly emphasized the importance of K63-linked polyubiquitination in activating RIG-I. TRIM25 is the first identified enzyme to facilitate the conjugation of K63-linked polyubiquitin chains at K172, which is located on the second CARD domain of RIG-I (Gack et al., 2007). Besides TRIM25, E3 ubiquitin ligases TRIM4 and MEX3C also catalyze the K63 linkage ubiquitination at the CARD domain of RIG-I (Kuniyoshi et al., 2014; Yan, Li, Mao, Hu, & Shu, 2014). Recent studies suggested that TRIM25, TRIM4, and MEX3C can cooperate to ubiquitinate multiple lysine residues in the CARD domain of RIG-I to potently activate the downstream signaling (Sun et al., 2016; Xian et al., 2017). Distinguishing from the above E3s, RNF135 (Riplet) promotes the K63-linked polyubiquitination at various lysine residues in the CTD domain of RIG-I (Oshiumi et al., 2010). RNF135 deficiency in multiple cell types, including MEFs, macrophages, and cDCs, showed a significantly decreased amount of IFN-β following viral infection of either influenza A virus or VSV. Furthermore, *Rnf135*$^{-/-}$ mice were less resistant to VSV infection compared with WT mice (Oshiumi et al., 2010). Notably, the ubiquitination in the CTD domain of RIG-I probably warrants for the ubiquitination of CARD domain, demonstrated by the phenomenon that knockout of RNF135 alone abrogated the polyubiquitination of endogenous RIG-I (Okamoto, Kouwaki, Fukushima, & Oshiumi, 2017; Oshiumi et al., 2010). A recent study indicated that RNF135 not only relies on its catalytic domain to play a ubiquitination-dependent role but also cross-bridges RIG-I filaments on dsRNAs, induces aggregate-like RIG-I assemblies and plays a ubiquitination-independent function (Cadena et al., 2019). This suggests the RNF135 plays a central role in modulating the activation of RIG-I mediated signaling pathway.

Given the structural similarity between MDA5 and RIG-I, K63-linked polyubiquitination of the CARD domain is supposed to be a prerequisite for the activation of MDA5. A previous study suggested that TRIM25 was not involved in catalyzing the K63-linked polyubiquitination of MDA5 (Gack et al., 2007), which is disputed by a recent study from Dr. Shu Hongbing group. Dr. Shu group indicated that a newly identified RNA *co*-sensor ZCCHC3 recruits TRIM25 to facilitate the K63-linked polyubiquitination of CARD domain in both RIG-I and MDA5, supported by the observation that both *Trim25*$^{-/-}$ and *Zcchc3*$^{-/-}$ cells displayed less K63-linked polyubiquitination of MDA5 (Lian et al., 2018). Another TRIM family member TRIM65 interacts with the helicase domain of MDA5 and facilitate

K63-linked polyubiquitination at K743 of helicase domain, which is essential for the aggregation and subsequent activation of MDA5 (Lang et al., 2017). Besides, deficiency of TRIM65 in both BMDMs and MEFs produced much less IFN-α/β following EMCV infection compared with the WT counterparts (Lang et al., 2017). A previous structural study indicated that the filament assembly of MDA5 along the dsRNA axis is essential for its dsRNA recognition since monomeric MDA5 binds to dsRNA with a poor affinity (del Toro Duany, Wu, & Hur, 2015). K743 is located on the surface of MDA5 monomer (Wu, Peisley, et al., 2013), and ubiquitination of this site is likely required for the formation and stability of MDA5 filament.

A couple of DUBs including USP21, USP3, and USP14 have been indicated to reverse this process given the importance of K63-linked polyubiquitination in the regulation of RIG-I and MDA5 activation. USP21 was identified to be a negative regulator through the IFN-β luciferase reporter assay (Fan et al., 2014). USP21 catalyzes the deubiquitination of RIG-I through interacting with it. Interestingly, this study found that USP21 can deubiquitinate the polyubiquitination of RIG-I mediated by both TRIM25 and RNF135, indicating USP21 presumably cleaves the K63-linked polyubiquitin chains from multiple lysine sites in either CARD or CTD domain. Furthermore, deficiency of USP21 in immune cells and mice were more resistant to the viral infection, confirming its negative regulation of the RIG-I activation (Fan et al., 2014). USP3, in another study, was identified to be another DUB for RIG-I (Cui et al., 2014). Knockdown of USP3 specifically enhanced K63-linked ubiquitination of RIG-I, upregulated the phosphorylation of IRF3 and augmented the production of type I interferon cytokines and antiviral immunity. Besides RIG-I, USP3 also facilitates the deubiquitination of MDA5 (Cui et al., 2014). USP14 interacts with RIG-I and catalyze the deubiquitination of RIG-I dependent on its USP domain (Li et al., 2019). Knockdown of USP14 or inhibition of USP14 enzymatic activity greatly enhanced the K63-linked polyubiquitination of RIG-I and the type I interferon response following infection of VSV, resulting in the limited spread of viral replication.

3.2.2 E3 ligases and DUBs modulating the activation of MAVS

MAVS, the downstream adaptor protein, is comprised of three functional domains: the N-terminal CARD domain, a middle proline-rich region, and a C-terminal transmembrane domain (TM) (Liu & Gao, 2018). The CARD domain mediates the interaction between MAVS and

RIG-I/MDA5, while the proline-rich domain of MAVS interacts with a plethora of protein involving in regulating the function of MAVS (Belgnaoui, Paz, & Hiscott, 2011). TM domain tethers MAVS on mitochondria or peroxisome, critical for MAVS-mediated IFN-β induction following viral infection (Dixit et al., 2010; Seth et al., 2005).

A previous study suggested that K63-linked ubiquitination of MAVS promoted the recruitment of IKKε to activate IRF3 and expression of IFN stimulated genes (ISGs) (Paz et al., 2009). However, the specific E3 ubiquitin ligase responsible for this modification was not investigated in this study. Recently, our lab identified TRIM31 as a *bona fide* E3 ubiquitin ligase for MAVS combining both *in vitro* and *in vivo* study (Liu et al., 2017). *In vitro* ubiquitination assay demonstrated that TRIM31 facilitates the conjugation of K63-linked not K48-linked ubiquitin chains on MAVS, which occurs at K10, K311, and K461 of MAVS. Furthermore, deficiency of TRIM31 or mutation of MAVS ubiquitination sites abrogated the prion-like aggregation of the MAVS, a prerequisite for robust activation of downstream signaling upon RNA virus infection. Consistently, $Trim31^{-/-}$ peritoneal macrophages secreted much fewer IFN-β following SeV or VSV infection instead of HSV infection, suggesting its specific regulation of RLR-mediated signaling. More importantly, *in vivo* study demonstrated that $Trim31^{-/-}$ mice were more susceptible to infection of RNA virus than were WT mice, confirming the positive role of TRIM31 in antiviral response (Liu et al., 2017). In addition to TRIM31, another TRIM family member TRIM21 facilitates the conjugation of K27-linked polymeric chains at K325 of MAVS (Xue et al., 2018). Subsequently, the K27-linked polyubiquitination of MAVS promotes the interaction between TBK1 and MAVS, consistent with the observation that TBK1 interacts with K27-linked instead of K63-linked di-ubiquitin chains *in vitro* (Wang, Liu, et al., 2014). Currently, YOD1 is the only identified DUB responsible for downregulating the K63-linked polyubiquitination of MAVS (Liu et al., 2019). Following viral infection, YOD1 is enriched in the mitochondria to interact with MAVS and removed the K63-linked polyubiquitin chains from MAVS, therefore abrogating the formation of prion-like aggregates of MAVS and attenuating the activation of IRF3 and the production of IFN-β. Intriguingly, both YOD1 and TRIM31 interact with the proline-rich domain of MAVS, suggesting competition for the interaction with MAVS likely adds up another layer of regulation of MAVS activation. Of note, the DUB accountable for the cleavage of K27-linked activation ubiquitin chains from MAVS needs further investigation.

3.2.3 E3 ligases and DUBs responsible for the stability of RLRs and MAVS

There is a long list of E3 ubiquitin ligases regulating the degradation of RIG-I and MDA5, indicating their physiological importance in the innate immunity. Two E3 ligases RNF125 and TRIM40 were identified to promote the degradation of both RIG-I and MDA5. RNF125 is the first identified E3 ligase responsible for ubiquitination-dependent degradation of RIG-I and MDA5 (Arimoto et al., 2007). TRIM40 conjugates both K27- and K48-linked polymeric chains at the first CARD domain of both RIG-I and MDA5 to facilitate their degradation (Zhao et al., 2017). Congruently, significantly increased amount of IFN-β, TNFα, and IL-6 were secreted from *Trim40*$^{-/-}$ peritoneal macrophages compared with WT counterparts following SeV or VSV infection. Also, *Trim40*$^{-/-}$ mice were less susceptible to viral infection compared with their WT littermates. Of note, the TRIM40 expression level was markedly downregulated following RNA virus infection, indicating the host cell may modulate its level to support the immune response. Besides RNF125 and TRIM40, other RING-type E3 ligases, including RNF122, CHIP, and c-Cbl, only target RIG-I for K48-linked polyubiquitination and proteasome-dependent degradation (Chen et al., 2013; Wang et al., 2016; Zhou et al., 2018). Different from the abundant numbers of E3s, USP4 is the only identified DUB for upregulating the stability of RIG-I. USP4 interacts with RIG-I and cleaves K48-linked polyubiquitin chains from RIG-I, supported by the observation that the overexpression of USP4 significantly enhanced RIG-I protein level, while knockdown of USP4 had an opposite effect (Wang et al., 2013). Congruently, overexpression of USP4 significantly promoted RIG-I-triggered IFN-β signaling and, at the meanwhile, inhibited the VSV replication.

Akin to RIG-I, extensive studies have been performed on the discovery of E3 ubiquitin ligases responsible for the degradation of MAVS, including AIP4 (Itch), Smurf1, Smurf2, RNF5, and MARCH5 (Pan et al., 2014; Wang, Tong, & Ye, 2012; Yoo et al., 2015; You et al., 2009; Zhong et al., 2010). Theses E3 ligases facilitate the K48-linked polyubiquitination and downregulate the stability of MAVS dependent on the proteasome pathway. In addition to the above E3s, TRIM29 triggers the proteasome-dependent degradation of MAVS through K11-linked instead of K48-linked polyubiquitination (Xing, Zhang, Minze, Li, & Zhang, 2018). Rather than promoting the degradation of MAVS dependent on proteasome like above E3s, MARCH8 and RNF34 facilitate the ubiquitination of MAVS for autophagic-dependent degradation. The interaction between MARCH8 and MAVS is mediated through BST2, an interferon-inducible antiviral factor known for tethering the viral particles on the cellular membranes (Jin et al., 2017). Therefore, knockout of BST2 also enhanced the expression of IFN, impairing the replication of viruses. Different from MARCH8, RNF34 directly interact with MAVS and promotes the K27-/K29-linked ubiquitination of MAVS at Lys 297, 311, 348, and 362, which serves as a recognition signal for NDP52-dependent autophagic degradation (He et al., 2019). Different from the vast numbers of E3 downregulating the level of MAVS, there are only two DUBs, OTUD4 and OTUD1, regulating the protein level of MAVS in distinctive mechanisms. OTUD4 directly targets MAVS to upregulate its stability, whereas OTUD1 marks Smurf1 for deubiquitination to indirectly modulate the level of MAVS (Liuyu et al., 2019; Zhang, Liu, et al., 2018). OTUD4 interacts with MAVS to cleave K48-linked polyubiquitin chains, thereby maintaining MAVS stability and promoting innate antiviral signaling (Liuyu et al., 2019). Knockout or knockdown of OTUD4 impairs RNA virus-triggered expression and production of type I interferon and promotes VSV replication *in vitro* and *in vivo*. OTUD1 removes the K48-linked ubiquitin chains from Smurf1, enhancing its stability. Since Smurf1 is the E3 ligase for degradation of MAVS, deficiency of OTUD1 leads to the increased stability of MAVS (Zhang, Liu, et al., 2018). Therefore, OTUD1 is a negative regulator of type I interferon response. Interestingly, the viral infection triggers the upregulation of both OTUD4 and OTUD1, which is dependent on IRF3/7 or NF-κB, respectively. This suggests that the host cell modulate multiple factors to fine-tune the innate immune response.

3.3 cGAS-STING signaling

In the past years, various proteins such as AIM2, DAI, RNA polymerase III, IFI16, and DDX41 were reported to recognize microbial DNA and regarded as CDSs (Shu & Wang, 2014). However, the functional roles of these proteins in sensing of various DNA pathogens were limited to specific cell type or mouse models. Distinctive from the DNA sensors above, cGAS recognizes cytosolic microbial or endogenous aberrant DNA in a variety of cell types (Cai, Chiu, & Chen, 2014). In the absence of ligand DNA, cGAS exists in an auto-repressed state (Li et al., 2013). The direct presentation of ligand DNA to cGAS induces it to undergo a conformational rearrangement, induce its enzymatic activity, and the consequent production of cGAMP (Li et al., 2013). Notably, the direct interaction between DNA and cGAS also promotes liquid-liquid phase separation and the formation of liquid-like droplets, where cGAS is activated and cGAMP is produced (Du & Chen, 2018). The endogenous cGAMP acts as a second messenger and binds to the endoplasmic reticulum (ER)-membrane adaptor protein STING (Wu, Sun, et al., 2013). The cGAMP binding triggers STING to go through a conformational change and form oligomers through side-by-side packing of dimeric STING molecules (Shang et al., 2012). In the resting cells, STING is anchored in the ER through associating with the Ca^{2+} sensor stromal interaction molecule 1 (STIM1) (Srikanth et al., 2019). cGAMP-driven conformational change induces STING to translocate to the ER–Golgi intermediate compartment (ERGIC) and the Golgi apparatus, which is dependent on the cytoplasmic coat protein complex II (COPII) and ADP-ribosylation factor (ARF) GTPases (Dobbs et al., 2015; Gui et al., 2019). Following its trafficking to the Golgi, STING interacts with TBK1, which leads to the activation of TBK1. Activated TBK1 further phosphorylate the C-terminal tail region of STING, in which the negatively charged surface serves as a docking site for IRF3, which is then phosphorylated and activated by TBK1 (Liu et al., 2015). Activated IRF3 dimerizes and translocates into the nucleus to modulate the expression of IFN-β.

3.3.1 E3 ligases accountable for cGAS activation

K27-linked polyubiquitination and monoubiquitination are responsible for upregulating the function of cGAS. RNF185 facilitates the conjugation of K27-linked polyubiquitin chains at K173 and K384 of cGAS and potentiating its catalytic activity. Decreased ubiquitination of cGAS by either mutation of these two lysine residues or the RING domain of RNF185 affected the production of cGMAP (Wang et al., 2017). Different from RNF185, TRIM56 and TRIM41 induce the monoubiquitination of cGAS. TRIM56 facilitates monoubiquitination at K335 of CTD domain (Seo et al., 2018), while the lysine residue marked by TRIM41 has not been identified (Liu et al., 2018). K335 is located on the interaction interface during the formation of the cGAS dimer (Li et al., 2013). And this study found that deficiency of TRIM56 affect the dimerization of cGAS (Seo et al., 2018), suggesting the monoubiquitination of K335 is crucial for the stability of cGAS oligomerization. Furthermore, monoubiquitination of cGAS mediated by TRIM56 and TRIM41 upregulated the enzymatic activity of cGAS displayed by the enhanced production of cGAMP

(Liu et al., 2018; Seo et al., 2018). Although a couple of E3 ligases activate cGAS, the DUBs responsible for reversing this process have yet to be identified.

3.3.2 E3 ligases and DUBs regulating STING activation

STING, also known as TMEM173, MPYS, MITA, and ERIS, was identified by four independent groups, including Dr. Shu Hongbing and Dr. Jiang Zhengfan (Ishikawa, Ma, & Barber, 2009; Jin et al., 2008; Sun et al., 2009; Zhong et al., 2008). The structure of human STING includes the N-terminal 4 transmembrane regions (TMs) and a C-terminal domain (CTD). The CTD domain is further separated into the dimerization domain (DD) and the carboxy-terminal tail (CTT), within which a PLPLRT/SD motif binds to the dimer interface of TBK1 (Zhao et al., 2019).

Until now, four E3 ubiquitin ligases, including TRIM56, TRIM32, MUL1, and AMFR, are indicated to upregulate the function of STING. Three of them, TRIM56, TRIM32, and MUL1, promote the K63-linked chains conjugation of STING, while AMFR facilitates the K27-linked polyubiquitination. TRIM56 binds to the CTD domain of STING to promote the polyubiquitination at K150 of STING, inducing the dimerization of STING and its interaction with TBK1 (Tsuchida et al., 2010). TRIM32 interacts with the transmembrane domain of STING and facilitates the ubiquitination at K20, K150, K224, and K236 of STING (Zhang, Hu, Wang, & Shu, 2012). MUL1 is responsible for the K63-linked polyubiquitination at K224 of STING (Ni, Konno, & Barber, 2017). AMFR, an ER membrane-associated E3 ubiquitin ligase, is identified as an interacting partner with STING following HSV-1 infection through a proteomic study (Wang, Liu, et al., 2014). AMFR, identified by Dr. Wang Chen group, catalyzes the formation of K27-linked polyubiquitin chain at K137, 150, 224, and 236 of STING, which serves as a scaffold to recruit TBK1 through interaction between K27 polyubiquitin chains and ULD domain of TBK1. Of note, the interaction between AMFR and STING was enhanced by another protein Insig1. Consequently, the deficiency of either AMFR or Insig1 in MEFs or BMDMs attenuated IRF3 activation as well as the subsequent production of IFN-β following HSV-1 infection (Wang, Liu, et al., 2014). Comparing these lysine residues that are modified by the E3s above, we observe that there is a certain extent of overlap between these E3s such as K150, K224, and K236, suggesting that robust STING activation presumably requires redundant and multiple layers of regulation.

There are two reported DUBs, USP13 and USP49, to counter the K27- and K63-linked polyubiquitination of STING, respectively. USP13 releases the K27-linked polyubiquitin chains from STING dependent on its enzymatic activity, resulting in the less recruitment of TBK1 following viral infection (Sun et al., 2017). Furthermore, knockdown or knockout of USP13 led to the enhanced activation of IRF3, higher expression of IFN-β following HSV-1 infection, and impaired replication of HSV-1. Viral infection stimulates the interaction between USP49 and STING and potentiates the deubiquitination of STING modified by K63 polymeric chains, which subsequently inhibits the aggregation of STING and the recruitment of TBK1 (Ye et al., 2019). Consequently, knockdown or knockout of USP49 resulted in significant higher HSV-1-induced production of IFNs, thereby limiting HSV-1 replication. Consistently, *Usp49*$^{-/-}$ mice were more resistant to lethal HSV-1 infection compared to *Usp49*$^{+/+}$ mice.

3.3.3 E3 ligases and DUBs responsible for the stability of cGAS and STING

According to our knowledge, a specific E3 ligase promoting the ubiquitination and subsequent degradation of cGAS is lacking until now. A study indicated that K48-linked ubiquitin chains at K414 of cGAS modulate its degradation through the autophagy-lysosome pathway (Chen et al., 2016). The interaction between cGAS modified by K48-linked polyubiquitin chains and the ubiquitin associated domain (UBA) of autophagy cargo protein p62 results in the transportation of ubiquitinated cGAS into the autophagosome for degradation. In this study, they also discovered that TRIM14 recruits USP14 to prevent the turnover of cGAS by removing the K48-linked ubiquitin chains and blocking the interaction between cGAS and p62 (Chen et al., 2016). Recently, USP27x was identified by our lab as another deubiquitinase to regulate the stability of cGAS (Guo et al., 2019). Different from USP14, USP27x directly interacts with cGAS to cleave the K48-linked polyubiquitin chains from it. Therefore, deficiency of USP27x in Raw264.7 cells resulted in increased ubiquitination and less stability of cGAS as well as subsequent impaired production of type I interferon.

A couple of E3 ubiquitin ligases, including RNF5, RNF26, TRIM29, and TRIM30α, are accountable for regulating the protein stability of STING. RNF5, identified by Dr. Shu Hongbing group, is the first reported E3 ligase for STING. RNF5 promotes the K48-linked polyubiquitination and proteasome degradation of STING (Zhong et al., 2009). RNF26 polyubiquitinates STING with K11-linked polymeric chains at K150, which prevents STING from K48-mediated degradation by RNF5 (Qin et al., 2014). Two research groups independently identified TRIM29 as an E3 ligase for STING. One group found that Epstein-Barr virus (EBV) hijacked TRIM29 to target STING for degradation in airway epithelial cells and myeloid dendritic cells, resulting in the less production of type I interferons for the persistent infection of EBV (Xing et al., 2017). Another group observed the similar phenomenon that deficiency of TRIM29 elevated the production of the type I interferon and proinflammatory cytokines upon viral infection, and *Trim29*$^{-/-}$ mice were less susceptible to lethal HSV-1 infection than WT counterparts (Li, Lin, et al., 2018). TRIM30α interacts with STING and leads to K48-linked ubiquitination at K275 of STING and its degradation. Furthermore, the production of type I IFN as well as IL-6 in *Trim30α*$^{-/-}$ BMDCs and peritoneal macrophages was elevated in responses to HSV-1 or transfected DNA compared with WT counterparts. Consistently, *Trim30α*$^{-/-}$ mice were less susceptible to HSV-1 infection than WT mice (Wang, Lian, et al., 2015), confirming its negative regulation of STING-mediated DNA virus-triggered signaling. Of note, a recent study indicated that the stability of STING is also under the regulation of p62-dependent autophagy (Prabakaran et al., 2018). They observed that the degradation of STING through autophagy pathway was accompanied by the enhanced polyubiquitination. However, the E3 ligase that links ubiquitinated STING to p62 for degradation was not investigated in this study.

A couple of deubiquitinases, such as USP20 and CYLD, are involved in reversing the turnover of STING during viral infection. USP20 cleaves the K48/K33-linked polyubiquitination of STING to enhance its stability following viral infection (Zhang et al., 2016). However, the interaction between USP20 and STING is not direct and mediated by another deubiquitinase USP18. Therefore, deficiency of either USP18 or USP20 affect the stability of STING and the subsequent production of type I IFN during viral infection. Notably, reconstitution of USP18 or its enzymatic mutant can identically enhance the stability of STING, confirming that USP18 recruits USP20 to release the ubiquitin from STING. In another study, CYLD was found to partially colocalizes with STING and bound specifically with K48-based polymeric chains on STING, resulting in selective cleavage of these chains from STING and ensuing enhanced protein level of STING (Zhang, Wei, et al., 2018). Consistently, deficiency of CYLD potentiated the degradation of STING, attenuating the induction of IRF3-responsive genes upon the viral infection. Additionally, CYLD knockout mice were less resistant to lethal HSV-1 than their WT littermates.

3.4 Downstream signaling molecules

The signaling molecules downstream of adaptor proteins, such as TRAF3 and 6, kinases TBK1 and IKK, transcriptional factors IRF3/p65, were shared between different antiviral pathways, even though distinctive receptors and adaptor proteins were utilized. The activation and turnover of these downstream signaling molecules are also under tight regulation of a series of E3 ubiquitin ligases and DUBs.

3.4.1 E3 ligases and DUBs for activation of downstream molecules

RNF166 and HECTD3 act as the E3 ligases catalyzing the K63-linked polyubiquitination of TRAF proteins under different stimuli. RNF166 specifically interacts with TRAF3 and TRAF6, which is enhanced following SeV infection. Furthermore, overexpression of RNF166 promoted the K63-linked polyubiquitination of both TRAF3 and TRAF6 and subsequent production of type I IFN during SeV infection, whereas knockdown of RNF166 had the opposite effect (Chen et al., 2015). HECTD3 promotes the conjugation of K63-linked polymeric chains at K138 of TRAF3 during bacterial infection, leading to the enhanced expression of the IFN-β (Li, Li, et al., 2018). Furthermore, *Hectd3*$^{-/-}$ BMDMs produced considerably less expression of IFN-β and ISGs compared with WT counterparts in response to poly(I:C), dsDNA, or the bacterial infection (Li, Li, et al., 2018). But the exact function of HECTD3 during viral infection still requires further examination. There are multiple DUBs, such as OTUB1, OTUB2, OTUD5, UCHL1, responsible for releasing the K63-linked polyubiquitin chains from TRAF3 and TRAF6 (Davis & Gack, 2015), suggesting the importance of tight regulation of activated TRAF3 and TRAF6.

Several E3 ubiquitin ligases, including Mib1, Mib2, and RNF128, promote the K63-linked polyubiquitination of TBK1 for its activation. These E3s regulate the activation of TBK1 under different stimuli. Mib1 and Mib2 modulate the ubiquitination of TBK1 following RNA virus infection (Li, Wang, Berman, Kong, & Dorf, 2011), whereas RNF128 is a general regulator of TBK1 against both DNA and RNA viral infection (Song et al., 2016). RNF128, identified by our lab, facilitates the conjugation of the K63-linked chains at K30 and K401 of TBK1 (Song et al., 2016). Decreased ubiquitination of TBK1, achieved by deletion of RNF128 or mutation of ubiquitination sites in TBK1, significantly impaired its phosphorylation and kinase activity upon viral infection. Furthermore, *Rnf128*$^{-/-}$ mice were more susceptible to viral infection than WT counterparts. Notably, viral infection significantly induced the protein level of RNF128, which indicates the host cells likely regulate its level to clear the viral infection. There are also a couple of DUBs related to the regulation of TBK1 activation. USP2b interacts with TBK1 and cleaves the K63-linked polyubiquitin chains from TBK1, resulting in the reduction of the kinase activity of TBK1 during viral infection (Zhang, Zhao, Zhang, Zhao, & Gao, 2014). Moreover, knockdown of USP2b in THP-1 cells enhances the expression of IFN-β following a broad spectrum of stimulation, including LPS, poly(I:C), and ISD. *In vivo* ubiquitination assay demonstrated that USP2b downregulated the ubiquitination level of TBK1 rather than RIG-I or MAVS, confirming the specific targeting of TBK1 by USP2b (Zhang et al., 2014). Of note, the interaction between USP2b and TBK1 is enhanced following the viral infection, suggesting this is likely negative feedback to avoid the excessive immune response. Distinct from the substrate specificity of USP2b, CYLD also targets RIG-I and IKKε for K63-linked deubiquitination in addition to TBK1, suggesting CYLD dampens the RLR-mediated type I interferon response through marking multiple substrates for deubiquitination (Friedman et al., 2008). In another independent study, OTUD1 was identified to cleave the K63-linked polyubiquitin chains from IRF3. Impaired K63-linked polyubiquitination of IRF3 by either deletion of OTUD1 or mutation of IRF3 ubiquitination sites affected the nuclear translocation of IRF3 and subsequentially its nuclear activity (Lu et al., 2018). However, the E3 ubiquitin ligase that is responsible for K63-linked ubiquitination of IRF3 was not examined in this study and requires further investigation.

E3 ligase TRIM23 regulates the activation of NEMO through atypical K27-linked polyubiquitination occurring at K105/309/325/326/344 (Arimoto et al., 2010). Moreover, knockdown of TRIM23 in MEFs affected the production of IFN-β with SeV infection and enhanced the production of viral particles following VSV infection (Arimoto et al., 2010). Besides K27-linked modification, a heterotrimeric RBR-family E3 ligase LUBAC complex, composed of HOIP, HOIL-1L, and Sharpin, catalyzes the linear ubiquitination of NEMO at K285 and K309 (Ikeda et al., 2011; Kirisako et al., 2006). The linear ubiquitination of NEMO plays a dual role in modulating the NF-κB pathway and type I IFN response. It plays a positive role in the regulation of NF-κB supported by the observation that mutations of K285 and K309 of NEMO abolished its activation in the NF-κB reporter assay (Tokunaga et al., 2009). However, the linear ubiquitination of NEMO exerts the negative effect on type I IFN response. Mechanistically, the linear ubiquitinated NEMO competes with MAVS to interact with TRAF3 and therefore affects the downstream signaling (Belgnaoui et al., 2012).

3.4.2 E3 ligases and DUBs responsible for the stability of downstream molecules

The protein level of TRAF3 and TRAF6 are regulated by the E3 ligases Triad3A and TRIM38 (Nakhaei et al., 2009; Zhao, Wang, Zhang, Yuan, & Gao, 2012). Triad3A promotes K48-linked polyubiquitination of TRAF3, leading to its proteasomal degradation (Nakhaei et al., 2009). Intriguingly, Triad3A was found to be induced in the late time point of infection by RNA viruses (Nakhaei et al., 2009), suggesting this is likely negative feedback to avoid the excessive immune response. TRIM38 facilitates the conjugation of the K48-linked polyubiquitin chains on TRAF6 (Zhao et al., 2012). Consistently, knockdown of TRIM38 in primary macrophages elevated the protein level of TRAF6 and the production of pro-inflammatory cytokines upon stimulation of TLR agonists. OTUD7B and USP25 have been indicated as the DUBs to maintain the protein levels of TRAF3 responding to the noncanonical NF-κB inducers or viral infections, respectively. The deficiency of OTUD7B led to a markedly enhanced degradation of TRAF3 in response to the noncanonical NF-κB inducers rather than the type I interferon pathway (Hu et al., 2013). The viral infection triggers the expression of USP25, which cleaves the K48-linked polyubiquitin chains from TRAF3 and TRAF6. Furthermore, deletion of USP25 resulted in enhanced ubiquitination and turnover of TRAF3 and TRAF6. Consistently, USP25 deficient mice were less resistant to H5N1 or HSV-1 infection compared with the wild-type mice (Lin et al., 2015).

A couple of E3 ubiquitin ligases, such as TRIP, DTX4, and TRIM27, are responsible for modulating the turnover of TBK1. TRIP, identified by our group, directly interacts with TBK1 and promotes K48-linked polyubiquitination as well as the subsequent degradation of TBK1 (Zhang, Wang, et al., 2012). DTX4, identified by Dr. Cui Jun group, conjugates the K48-linked polyubiquitin chains at K670 of TBK1 and promotes its proteasomal-dependent degradation (Cui et al., 2012). In this process, NLRP4 is indispensable for the interaction between DTX4 and TBK1, which is enhanced following the virus infection. Congruently, knockdown of either NLRP4 or DTX4 in THP-1 cells enhanced the stability of TBK1, inducing the expression of IFN-β and restricting viral infection (Cui et al., 2012). Akin to DTX4, the interaction between TRIM27 and TBK1 is mediated by a subset of proteins, including Siglec1, DAP12, and SHP2. TRIM27 facilitates the K48-linked polyubiquitination of TBK1, which occurs at K251 and K372 of TBK1 (Zheng et al., 2015). Until now, USP1 and USP38 are the two identified DUBs to regulate the stability of TBK1. USP1 forms a complex with UAF1 and promotes the removal of the K48-linked polyubiquitin chains from TBK1, resulting in the elevated stability of TBK1 in the physiological conditions (Yu et al., 2017). Consistently, knockdown of either USP1 or UAF1 significantly impairs the expression of IFN-β, causing the enhanced replication of viral infection. Besides, the same study found that a specific inhibitor of USP1/UAF1 ML323 promoted viral replication through *in vitro* and *in vivo* study, further confirming the positive regulation of TBK1 by USP1/UAF1 complex (Yu et al., 2017). Contrary to USP1, USP38 enhances the turnover of TBK1 (Lin et al., 2016). Mechanistically, USP38 facilitates the removal of K33-linked chains from TBK1, which protects TBK1 from degradation. The deubiquitination of TBK1 by USP38 leads to the NLRP4 and DTX4 mediated K48-linked polyubiquitination and degradation of TBK1. Consistent with this, depletion of USP38 enhanced the expression of IFN-β and subsequently restricted viral replication. Moreover, overexpression of USP38 resulted in the downregulation of TBK1 rather than IRF3 and IKK complex, suggesting targeting of TBK1 by USP38 is specific (Lin et al., 2016).

The E3 ligases TRIM29 and TRAF7 promote the turnover of NEMO through proteasome- and lysosome-dependent pathway, respectively. TRIM29 facilitates the K48-linked polyubiquitination at K183 of NEMO, inducing its proteasomal-dependent degradation (Xing et al., 2016). Distinct from TRIM29, TRAF7 conjugates K29-linked polyubiquitin in NEMO and triggers its lysosome-dependent degradation of NEMO (Zotti et al., 2011). Therefore, both TRIM29 and TRAF7 play a negative role in enhancing the proinflammatory response.

Various E3 ligases, including RBCK1, c-Cbl, TRIM26, and RAUL, are responsible for polyubiquitination and degradation of IRF3. RBCK1 and c-Cbl interact with IRF3 and promotes its ubiquitination and degradation (Zhang et al., 2008; Zhao et al., 2016). Different from RBCK1 and c-Cbl, TRIM26, identified by our group, specifically targets the nuclear IRF3 for K48-linked polyubiquitination and degradation

(Wang, Zhao, Zhao, Zhang, & Gao, 2015). Congruently, TRIM26 attenuated the activation of the IFN-β promoter and the production of IFN-β downstream of TLR3/4, RLR, and DNA sensing pathways. More importantly, TRIM26 transgenic mice showed much less IRF3 activation and IFN-β production, with increased virus replication (Wang, Zhao, et al., 2015). Interestingly, KSHV hijacks E3 ligase RAUL for the degradation of IRF3, therefore counteracting the antiviral response for the viral persistence (Yu & Hayward, 2010). Of note, two studies proposed the contradictory roles of TRIM21 on IRF3. One study claimed that TRIM21 promoted the ubiquitination and degradation of IRF3 (Higgs et al., 2008), while the other one found TRIM21 enhanced the stability of IRF3 during viral infection (Zhong et al., 2009). Therefore, the exact role and regulatory mechanism of TRIM21 in antiviral immunity require further investigation since TRIM21 also targets MAVS for K27-linked polyubiquitination (Xue et al., 2018). p65 is also targeted for degradation by a series of E3 ubiquitin ligases. Two nuclear E3 ligases, PDLIM2 and MKRN2, cooperatively promote the polyubiquitination and proteasomal degradation of nuclear p65 (Shin et al., 2017). CUL2 and COMMD1 facilitate the degradation of p65 dependent on its phosphorylation by CK1γ1 (Wang, Hu, Tong, & Ye, 2014). Besides, TRAF7 enhances the K29-linked polyubiquitination of p65, resulting in its lysosomal degradation (Zotti et al., 2011).

4. Conclusions and perspectives

Substantial studies, especially from the immunologists in China, have emphasized the fundamental roles of ubiquitination in fine-tuning of the antiviral immune response. Both monoubiquitination and polyubiquitination are indispensable regulatory mechanisms for effective initiating and terminating the innate immunity. An interesting phenomenon is unlike the designated roles of the canonical K48- and K63-linked chains, the same type of atypical chain conjugating to different lysine residues of the same substrate exert quite distinctive functions, demonstrating their functional complexity and diversity. Therefore, delineating the corresponding E3s and DUBs of the atypical chains in the specific circumstance will provide new therapeutic targets for the treatment of infectious as well as autoimmune diseases besides adding new knowledge for the innate immunity and other physiological signaling pathways. Another interesting phenomenon is that various E3s and DUBs determine the activation and stability of key signaling molecules. How these E3s and DUBs cooperate in a dynamic, temporal, and spatial manner to tightly modulate the immune defense requires further investigation. Lastly, compared with the vast numbers of E3s accountable for the important signaling molecules, the numbers of corresponding DUBs are relatively limited. Therefore, delineating the corresponding DUBs modulating the signaling pathway warrants for detailed examination.

Acknowledgments

We apologize to colleagues whose work and publications could not be referenced owing to space constraints. This work was supported in part by grants from the Natural Science Foundation of China (81930039, 31730026, 81525012, 81471538) awarded to Dr. Gao Chengjiang, and the Fundamental Research Funds of Shandong University (21510078614099), the Fundamental Research Funds of Cheeloo College of Medicine (21510089393109), China Postdoctoral Science Foundation (2018M642662), and the Natural Science Foundation of China (81901604) awarded to Dr. Zheng Yi.

Conflicts of interest

None declared.

References

Akira, S., Uematsu, S., & Takeuchi, O. (2006). Pathogen recognition and innate immunity. *Cell*, *124*(4), 783–801. https://doi.org/10.1016/j.cell.2006.02.015.

Arimoto, K., Funami, K., Saeki, Y., Tanaka, K., Okawa, K., Takeuchi, O., et al. (2010). Polyubiquitin conjugation to NEMO by triparite motif protein 23 (TRIM23) is critical in antiviral defense. *Proceedings of the National Academy of Sciences of the United States of America*, *107*(36), 15856–15861. https://doi.org/10.1073/pnas.1004621107.

Arimoto, K., Takahashi, H., Hishiki, T., Konishi, H., Fujita, T., & Shimotohno, K. (2007). Negative regulation of the RIG-I signaling by the ubiquitin ligase RNF125. *Proceedings of the National Academy of Sciences of the United States of America*, *104*(18), 7500–7505. https://doi.org/10.1073/pnas.0611551104.

Belgnaoui, S. M., Paz, S., & Hiscott, J. (2011). Orchestrating the interferon antiviral response through the mitochondrial antiviral signaling (MAVS) adapter. *Current Opinion in Immunology*, *23*(5), 564–572. https://doi.org/10.1016/j.coi.2011.08.001.

Belgnaoui, S. M., Paz, S., Samuel, S., Goulet, M. L., Sun, Q., Kikkert, M., et al. (2012). Linear ubiquitination of NEMO negatively regulates the interferon antiviral response through disruption of the MAVS-TRAF3 complex. *Cell Host & Microbe*, *12*(2), 211–222. https://doi.org/10.1016/j.chom.2012.06.009.

Bruns, A. M., Leser, G. P., Lamb, R. A., & Horvath, C. M. (2014). The innate immune sensor LGP2 activates antiviral signaling by regulating MDA5-RNA interaction and filament assembly. *Molecular Cell*, *55*(5), 771–781. https://doi.org/10.1016/j.molcel.2014.07.003.

Cadena, C., Ahmad, S., Xavier, A., Willemsen, J., Park, S., Park, J. W., et al. (2019). Ubiquitin-dependent and -independent roles of E3 ligase RIPLET in innate Immunity. *Cell*, *177*(5), 1187–1200, e1116. https://doi.org/10.1016/j.cell.2019.03.017.

Cai, X., Chiu, Y. H., & Chen, Z. J. (2014). The cGAS-cGAMP-STING pathway of cytosolic DNA sensing and signaling. *Molecular Cell, 54*(2), 289–296. https://doi.org/10.1016/j.molcel.2014.03.040.

Chen, W. L., Han, C. F., Xie, B., Hu, X., Yu, Q., Shi, L. Y., et al. (2013). Induction of siglec-G by RNA viruses inhibits the innate immune response by promoting RIG-I degradation. *Cell, 152*(3), 467–478. https://doi.org/10.1016/j.cell.2013.01.011.

Chen, M., Meng, Q., Qin, Y., Liang, P., Tan, P., He, L., et al. (2016). TRIM14 Inhibits cGAS degradation mediated by selective autophagy receptor p62 to promote innate immune responses. *Molecular Cell, 64*(1), 105–119. https://doi.org/10.1016/j.molcel.2016.08.025.

Chen, H. W., Yang, Y. K., Xu, H., Yang, W. W., Zhai, Z. H., & Chen, D. Y. (2015). Ring finger protein 166 potentiates RNA virus-induced interferon-beta production via enhancing the ubiquitination of TRAF3 and TRAF6. *Scientific Reports, 5*. 14770. https://doi.org/10.1038/srep14770.

Chuang, T. H., & Ulevitch, R. J. (2004). Triad3A, an E3 ubiquitin-protein ligase regulating toll-like receptors. *Nature Immunology, 5*(5), 495–502. https://doi.org/10.1038/ni1066.

Cui, J., Li, Y., Zhu, L., Liu, D., Songyang, Z., Wang, H. Y., et al. (2012). NLRP4 negatively regulates type I interferon signaling by targeting the kinase TBK1 for degradation via the ubiquitin ligase DTX4. *Nature Immunology, 13*(4), 387–395. https://doi.org/10.1038/ni.2239.

Cui, J., Song, Y., Li, Y., Zhu, Q., Tan, P., Qin, Y., et al. (2014). USP3 inhibits type I interferon signaling by deubiquitinating RIG-I-like receptors. *Cell Research, 24*(4), 400–416. https://doi.org/10.1038/cr.2013.170.

Davis, M. E., & Gack, M. U. (2015). Ubiquitination in the antiviral immune response. *Virology, 479–480*, 52–65. https://doi.org/10.1016/j.virol.2015.02.033.

Deguine, J., & Barton, G. M. (2014). MyD88: A central player in innate immune signaling. *F1000Prime Reports, 6*, 97. https://doi.org/10.12703/P6-97.

del Toro Duany, Y., Wu, B., & Hur, S. (2015). MDA5-filament, dynamics and disease. *Current Opinion in Virology, 12*, 20–25. https://doi.org/10.1016/j.coviro.2015.01.011.

Dixit, E., Boulant, S., Zhang, Y., Lee, A. S., Odendall, C., Shum, B., et al. (2010). Peroxisomes are signaling platforms for antiviral innate immunity. *Cell, 141*(4), 668–681. https://doi.org/10.1016/j.cell.2010.04.018.

Dobbs, N., Burnaevskiy, N., Chen, D., Gonugunta, V. K., Alto, N. M., & Yan, N. (2015). STING activation by translocation from the ER is associated with infection and autoinflammatory disease. *Cell Host & Microbe, 18*(2), 157–168. https://doi.org/10.1016/j.chom.2015.07.001.

Du, M., & Chen, Z. J. (2018). DNA-induced liquid phase condensation of cGAS activates innate immune signaling. *Science, 361*(6403), 704–709. https://doi.org/10.1126/science.aat1022.

Fan, Y., Mao, R., Yu, Y., Liu, S., Shi, Z., Cheng, J., et al. (2014). USP21 negatively regulates antiviral response by acting as a RIG-I deubiquitinase. *The Journal of Experimental Medicine, 211*(2), 313–328. https://doi.org/10.1084/jem.20122844.

Fang, R., Jiang, Q., Zhou, X., Wang, C., Guan, Y., Tao, J., et al. (2017). MAVS activates TBK1 and IKKepsilon through TRAFs in NEMO dependent and independent manner. *PLoS Pathogens, 13*(11), e1006720. https://doi.org/10.1371/journal.ppat.1006720.

Fitzgerald, K. A., McWhirter, S. M., Faia, K. L., Rowe, D. C., Latz, E., Golenbock, D. T., et al. (2003). IKKepsilon and TBK1 are essential components of the IRF3 signaling pathway. *Nature Immunology, 4*(5), 491–496. https://doi.org/10.1038/ni921.

Friedman, C. S., O'Donnell, M. A., Legarda-Addison, D., Ng, A., Cardenas, W. B., Yount, J. S., et al. (2008). The tumour suppressor CYLD is a negative regulator of RIG-I-mediated antiviral response. *EMBO Reports, 9*(9), 930–936. https://doi.org/10.1038/embor.2008.136.

Gack, M. U., Shin, Y. C., Joo, C. H., Urano, T., Liang, C., Sun, L., et al. (2007). TRIM25 RING-finger E3 ubiquitin ligase is essential for RIG-I-mediated antiviral activity. *Nature*, *446*(7138), 916–920. https://doi.org/10.1038/nature05732.

Gui, X., Yang, H., Li, T., Tan, X., Shi, P., Li, M., et al. (2019). Autophagy induction via STING trafficking is a primordial function of the cGAS pathway. *Nature*, *567*(7747), 262–266. https://doi.org/10.1038/s41586-019-1006-9.

Guo, Y., Jiang, F., Kong, L., Li, B., Yang, Y., Zhang, L., et al. (2019). Cutting edge: USP27X deubiquitinates and stabilizes the DNA sensor cGAS to regulate cytosolic DNA-mediated signaling. *Journal of Immunology*, *203*(8), 2049–2054. https://doi.org/10.4049/jimmunol.1900514.

Han, C., Jin, J., Xu, S., Liu, H., Li, N., & Cao, X. (2010). Integrin CD11b negatively regulates TLR-triggered inflammatory responses by activating Syk and promoting degradation of MyD88 and TRIF via Cbl-b. *Nature Immunology*, *11*(8), 734–742. https://doi.org/10.1038/ni.1908.

Hayden, M. S., & Ghosh, S. (2008). Shared principles in NF-kappaB signaling. *Cell*, *132*(3), 344–362. https://doi.org/10.1016/j.cell.2008.01.020.

He, X., Zhu, Y., Zhang, Y., Geng, Y., Gong, J., Geng, J., et al. (2019). RNF34 functions in immunity and selective mitophagy by targeting MAVS for autophagic degradation. *The EMBO Journal*, *38*(14), e100978. https://doi.org/10.15252/embj.2018100978.

Higgs, R., Ni Gabhann, J., Ben Larbi, N., Breen, E. P., Fitzgerald, K. A., & Jefferies, C. A. (2008). The E3 ubiquitin ligase Ro52 negatively regulates IFN-beta production post-pathogen recognition by polyubiquitin-mediated degradation of IRF3. *Journal of Immunology*, *181*(3), 1780–1786.

Hou, F., Sun, L., Zheng, H., Skaug, B., Jiang, Q. X., & Chen, Z. J. (2011). MAVS forms functional prion-like aggregates to activate and propagate antiviral innate immune response. *Cell*, *146*(3), 448–461. https://doi.org/10.1016/j.cell.2011.06.041.

Hu, H., Brittain, G. C., Chang, J. H., Puebla-Osorio, N., Jin, J., Zal, A., et al. (2013). OTUD7B controls non-canonical NF-kappaB activation through deubiquitination of TRAF3. *Nature*, *494*(7437), 371–374. https://doi.org/10.1038/nature11831.

Ikeda, F., Deribe, Y. L., Skanland, S. S., Stieglitz, B., Grabbe, C., Franz-Wachtel, M., et al. (2011). SHARPIN forms a linear ubiquitin ligase complex regulating NF-kappaB activity and apoptosis. *Nature*, *471*(7340), 637–641. https://doi.org/10.1038/nature09814.

Ishikawa, H., & Barber, G. N. (2008). STING is an endoplasmic reticulum adaptor that facilitates innate immune signalling. *Nature*, *455*(7213), 674–678. https://doi.org/10.1038/nature07317.

Ishikawa, H., Ma, Z., & Barber, G. N. (2009). STING regulates intracellular DNA-mediated, type I interferon-dependent innate immunity. *Nature*, *461*(7265), 788–792. https://doi.org/10.1038/nature08476.

Ji, S., Sun, M., Zheng, X., Li, L., Sun, L., Chen, D., et al. (2014). Cell-surface localization of pellino antagonizes toll-mediated innate immune signalling by controlling MyD88 turnover in Drosophila. *Nature Communications*, *5*, 3458. https://doi.org/10.1038/ncomms4458.

Jiang, F., Ramanathan, A., Miller, M. T., Tang, G. Q., Gale, M., Jr., Patel, S. S., et al. (2011). Structural basis of RNA recognition and activation by innate immune receptor RIG-I. *Nature*, *479*(7373), 423–427. https://doi.org/10.1038/nature10537.

Jin, S., Tian, S., Luo, M., Xie, W., Liu, T., Duan, T., et al. (2017). Tetherin suppresses type I interferon signaling by targeting MAVS for NDP52-mediated selective autophagic degradation in human cells. *Molecular Cell*, *68*(2), 308–322, e304. https://doi.org/10.1016/j.molcel.2017.09.005.

Jin, L., Waterman, P. M., Jonscher, K. R., Short, C. M., Reisdorph, N. A., & Cambier, J. C. (2008). MPYS, a novel membrane tetraspanner, is associated with major histocompatibility complex class II and mediates transduction of apoptotic signals. *Molecular and Cellular Biology, 28*(16), 5014–5026. https://doi.org/10.1128/MCB.00640-08.

Kato, H., Takeuchi, O., Sato, S., Yoneyama, M., Yamamoto, M., Matsui, K., et al. (2006). Differential roles of MDA5 and RIG-I helicases in the recognition of RNA viruses. *Nature, 441*(7089), 101–105. https://doi.org/10.1038/nature04734.

Kawai, T., Takahashi, K., Sato, S., Coban, C., Kumar, H., Kato, H., et al. (2005). IPS-1, an adaptor triggering RIG-I- and Mda5-mediated type I interferon induction. *Nature Immunology, 6*(10), 981–988. https://doi.org/10.1038/ni1243.

Kirisako, T., Kamei, K., Murata, S., Kato, M., Fukumoto, H., Kanie, M., et al. (2006). A ubiquitin ligase complex assembles linear polyubiquitin chains. *The EMBO Journal, 25*(20), 4877–4887. https://doi.org/10.1038/sj.emboj.7601360.

Kowalinski, E., Lunardi, T., McCarthy, A. A., Louber, J., Brunel, J., Grigorov, B., et al. (2011). Structural basis for the activation of innate immune pattern-recognition receptor RIG-I by viral RNA. *Cell, 147*(2), 423–435. https://doi.org/10.1016/j.cell.2011.09.039.

Kuniyoshi, K., Takeuchi, O., Pandey, S., Satoh, T., Iwasaki, H., Akira, S., et al. (2014). Pivotal role of RNA-binding E3 ubiquitin ligase MEX3C in RIG-I-mediated antiviral innate immunity. *Proceedings of the National Academy of Sciences of the United States of America, 111*(15), 5646–5651. https://doi.org/10.1073/pnas.1401674111.

Lang, X., Tang, T., Jin, T., Ding, C., Zhou, R., & Jiang, W. (2017). TRIM65-catalized ubiquitination is essential for MDA5-mediated antiviral innate immunity. *The Journal of Experimental Medicine, 214*(2), 459–473. https://doi.org/10.1084/jem.20160592.

Lee, B. C., Miyata, M., Lim, J. H., & Li, J. D. (2016). Deubiquitinase CYLD acts as a negative regulator for bacterium NTHi-induced inflammation by suppressing K63-linked ubiquitination of MyD88. *Proceedings of the National Academy of Sciences of the United States of America, 113*(2), E165–E171. https://doi.org/10.1073/pnas.1518615113.

Lester, S. N., & Li, K. (2014). Toll-like receptors in antiviral innate immunity. *Journal of Molecular Biology, 426*(6), 1246–1264. https://doi.org/10.1016/j.jmb.2013.11.024.

Li, F., Li, Y., Liang, H., Xu, T., Kong, Y., Huang, M., et al. (2018). HECTD3 mediates TRAF3 polyubiquitination and type I interferon induction during bacterial infection. *The Journal of Clinical Investigation, 128*(9), 4148–4162. https://doi.org/10.1172/JCI120406.

Li, Q., Lin, L., Tong, Y., Liu, Y., Mou, J., Wang, X., et al. (2018). TRIM29 negatively controls antiviral immune response through targeting STING for degradation. *Cell Discovery, 4*, 13. https://doi.org/10.1038/s41421-018-0010-9.

Li, X., Shu, C., Yi, G., Chaton, C. T., Shelton, C. L., Diao, J., et al. (2013). Cyclic GMP-AMP synthase is activated by double-stranded DNA-induced oligomerization. *Immunity, 39*(6), 1019–1031. https://doi.org/10.1016/j.immuni.2013.10.019.

Li, S., Wang, L., Berman, M., Kong, Y. Y., & Dorf, M. E. (2011). Mapping a dynamic innate immunity protein interaction network regulating type I interferon production. *Immunity, 35*(3), 426–440. https://doi.org/10.1016/j.immuni.2011.06.014.

Li, H., Zhao, Z., Ling, J., Pan, L., Zhao, X., Zhu, H., et al. (2019). USP14 promotes K63-linked RIG-I deubiquitination and suppresses antiviral immune responses. *European Journal of Immunology, 49*(1), 42–53. https://doi.org/10.1002/eji.201847603.

Lian, H., Zang, R., Wei, J., Ye, W., Hu, M. M., Chen, Y. D., et al. (2018). The zinc-finger protein ZCCHC3 binds RNA and facilitates viral RNA sensing and activation of the RIG-I-like receptors. *Immunity, 49*(3), 438–448, e435. https://doi.org/10.1016/j.immuni.2018.08.014.

Lin, D., Zhang, M., Zhang, M. X., Ren, Y., Jin, J., Zhao, Q., et al. (2015). Induction of USP25 by viral infection promotes innate antiviral responses by mediating the stabilization of TRAF3 and TRAF6. *Proceedings of the National Academy of Sciences of the United States of America*, *112*(36), 11324–11329. https://doi.org/10.1073/pnas.1509968112.

Lin, M., Zhao, Z., Yang, Z., Meng, Q., Tan, P., Xie, W., et al. (2016). USP38 inhibits type I interferon signaling by editing TBK1 ubiquitination through NLRP4 signalosome. *Molecular Cell*, *64*(2), 267–281. https://doi.org/10.1016/j.molcel.2016.08.029.

Liu, S., Cai, X., Wu, J., Cong, Q., Chen, X., Li, T., et al. (2015). Phosphorylation of innate immune adaptor proteins MAVS, STING, and TRIF induces IRF3 activation. *Science*, *347*(6227), aaa2630. https://doi.org/10.1126/science.aaa2630.

Liu, S., Chen, J., Cai, X., Wu, J., Chen, X., Wu, Y. T., et al. (2013). MAVS recruits multiple ubiquitin E3 ligases to activate antiviral signaling cascades. *eLife2*, e00785. https://doi.org/10.7554/eLife.00785.

Liu, B., & Gao, C. (2018). Regulation of MAVS activation through post-translational modifications. *Current Opinion in Immunology*, *50*, 75–81. https://doi.org/10.1016/j.coi.2017.12.002.

Liu, C., Huang, S., Wang, X., Wen, M., Zheng, J., Wang, W., et al. (2019). The otubain YOD1 suppresses aggregation and activation of the signaling adaptor MAVS through Lys63-linked deubiquitination. *Journal of Immunology*, *202*(10), 2957–2970. https://doi.org/10.4049/jimmunol.1800656.

Liu, Z. S., Zhang, Z. Y., Cai, H., Zhao, M., Mao, J., Dai, J., et al. (2018). RINCK-mediated monoubiquitination of cGAS promotes antiviral innate immune responses. *Cell & Bioscience*, *8*, 35, https://doi.org/10.1186/s13578-018-0233-3.

Liu, B., Zhang, M., Chu, H., Zhang, H., Wu, H., Song, G., et al. (2017). The ubiquitin E3 ligase TRIM31 promotes aggregation and activation of the signaling adaptor MAVS through Lys63-linked polyubiquitination. *Nature Immunology*, *18*(2), 214–224. https://doi.org/10.1038/ni.3641.

Liuyu, T., Yu, K., Ye, L., Zhang, Z., Zhang, M., Ren, Y., et al. (2019). Induction of OTUD4 by viral infection promotes antiviral responses through deubiquitinating and stabilizing MAVS. *Cell Research*, *29*(1), 67–79. https://doi.org/10.1038/s41422-018-0107-6.

Lu, D., Song, J., Sun, Y., Qi, F., Liu, L., Jin, Y., et al. (2018). Mutations of deubiquitinase OTUD1 are associated with autoimmune disorders. *Journal of Autoimmunity*, *94*, 156–165. https://doi.org/10.1016/j.jaut.2018.07.019.

Malynn, B. A., & Ma, A. (2010). Ubiquitin makes its mark on immune regulation. *Immunity*, *33*(6), 843–852. https://doi.org/10.1016/j.immuni.2010.12.007.

Mevissen, T. E. T., & Komander, D. (2017). Mechanisms of deubiquitinase specificity and regulation. *Annual Review of Biochemistry*, *86*, 159–192. https://doi.org/10.1146/annurev-biochem-061516-044916.

Meylan, E., Curran, J., Hofmann, K., Moradpour, D., Binder, M., Bartenschlager, R., et al. (2005). Cardif is an adaptor protein in the RIG-I antiviral pathway and is targeted by hepatitis C virus. *Nature*, *437*(7062), 1167–1172. https://doi.org/10.1038/nature04193.

Michel, M. A., Swatek, K. N., Hospenthal, M. K., & Komander, D. (2017). Ubiquitin linkage-specific affimers reveal insights into K6-linked ubiquitin signaling. *Molecular Cell*, *68*(1), 233–246, e235. https://doi.org/10.1016/j.molcel.2017.08.020.

Nakhaei, P., Mesplede, T., Solis, M., Sun, Q., Zhao, T., Yang, L., et al. (2009). The E3 ubiquitin ligase Triad3A negatively regulates the RIG-I/MAVS signaling pathway by targeting TRAF3 for degradation. *PLoS Pathogens*, *5*(11), e1000650. https://doi.org/10.1371/journal.ppat.1000650.

Ni, G., Konno, H., & Barber, G. N. (2017). Ubiquitination of STING at lysine 224 controls IRF3 activation. *Science Immunology*, *2*(11), eaah7119. https://doi.org/10.1126/sciimmunol.aah7119.

Okamoto, M., Kouwaki, T., Fukushima, Y., & Oshiumi, H. (2017). Regulation of RIG-I activation by K63-linked polyubiquitination. *Frontiers in Immunology*, *8*, 1942. https://doi.org/10.3389/fimmu.2017.01942.

Oshiumi, H., Miyashita, M., Inoue, N., Okabe, M., Matsumoto, M., & Seya, T. (2010). The ubiquitin ligase Riplet is essential for RIG-I-dependent innate immune responses to RNA virus infection. *Cell Host & Microbe*, *8*(6), 496–509. https://doi.org/10.1016/j.chom.2010.11.008.

Pan, Y., Li, R., Meng, J. L., Mao, H. T., Zhang, Y., & Zhang, J. (2014). Smurf2 negatively modulates RIG-I-dependent antiviral response by targeting VISA/MAVS for ubiquitination and degradation. *Journal of Immunology*, *192*(10), 4758–4764. https://doi.org/10.4049/jimmunol.1302632.

Paz, S., Vilasco, M., Arguello, M., Sun, Q., Lacoste, J., Nguyen, T. L., et al. (2009). Ubiquitin-regulated recruitment of IkappaB kinase epsilon to the MAVS interferon signaling adapter. *Molecular and Cellular Biology*, *29*(12), 3401–3412. https://doi.org/10.1128/MCB.00880-08.

Pickart, C. M., & Eddins, M. J. (2004). Ubiquitin: Structures, functions, mechanisms. *Biochimica et Biophysica Acta*, *1695*(1–3), 55–72. https://doi.org/10.1016/j.bbamcr.2004.09.019.

Prabakaran, T., Bodda, C., Krapp, C., Zhang, B. C., Christensen, M. H., Sun, C., et al. (2018). Attenuation of cGAS-STING signaling is mediated by a p62/SQSTM1-dependent autophagy pathway activated by TBK1. *The EMBO Journal*, *37*(8), e97858. https://doi.org/10.15252/embj.201797858.

Qin, Y., Zhou, M. T., Hu, M. M., Hu, Y. H., Zhang, J., Guo, L., et al. (2014). RNF26 temporally regulates virus-triggered type I interferon induction by two distinct mechanisms. *PLoS Pathogens*, *10*(9), e1004358. https://doi.org/10.1371/journal.ppat.1004358.

Sato, M., Suemori, H., Hata, N., Asagiri, M., Ogasawara, K., Nakao, K., et al. (2000). Distinct and essential roles of transcription factors IRF-3 and IRF-7 in response to viruses for IFN-alpha/beta gene induction. *Immunity*, *13*(4), 539–548.

Schlee, M. (2013). Master sensors of pathogenic RNA—RIG-I like receptors. *Immunobiology*, *218*(11), 1322–1335. https://doi.org/10.1016/j.imbio.2013.06.007.

Seo, G. J., Kim, C., Shin, W. J., Sklan, E. H., Eoh, H., & Jung, J. U. (2018). TRIM56-mediated monoubiquitination of cGAS for cytosolic DNA sensing. *Nature Communications*, *9*(1). 613https://doi.org/10.1038/s41467-018-02936-3.

Seth, R. B., Sun, L., Ea, C. K., & Chen, Z. J. (2005). Identification and characterization of MAVS, a mitochondrial antiviral signaling protein that activates NF-kappaB and IRF 3. *Cell*, *122*(5), 669–682. https://doi.org/10.1016/j.cell.2005.08.012.

Shang, G., Zhu, D., Li, N., Zhang, J., Zhu, C., Lu, D., et al. (2012). Crystal structures of STING protein reveal basis for recognition of cyclic di-GMP. *Nature Structural & Molecular Biology*, *19*(7), 725–727. https://doi.org/10.1038/nsmb.2332.

Shin, C., Ito, Y., Ichikawa, S., Tokunaga, M., Sakata-Sogawa, K., & Tanaka, T. (2017). MKRN2 is a novel ubiquitin E3 ligase for the p65 subunit of NF-kappaB and negatively regulates inflammatory responses. *Scientific Reports*, 7, 46097. https://doi.org/10.1038/srep46097.

Shu, H. B., & Wang, Y. Y. (2014). Adding to the STING. *Immunity*, *41*(6), 871–873. https://doi.org/10.1016/j.immuni.2014.12.002.

Sluimer, J., & Distel, B. (2018). Regulating the human HECT E3 ligases. *Cellular and Molecular Life Sciences*, *75*(17), 3121–3141. https://doi.org/10.1007/s00018-018-2848-2.

Song, G., Liu, B., Li, Z., Wu, H., Wang, P., Zhao, K., et al. (2016). E3 ubiquitin ligase RNF128 promotes innate antiviral immunity through K63-linked ubiquitination of TBK1. *Nature Immunology*, *17*(12), 1342–1351. https://doi.org/10.1038/ni.3588.

Song, X., Liu, S., Wang, W., Ma, Z., Cao, X., & Jiang, M. (2019). E3 ubiquitin ligase RNF170 inhibits innate immune responses by targeting and degrading TLR3 in murine cells. *Cellular & Molecular Immunology*. https://doi.org/10.1038/s41423-019-0236-y.

Srikanth, S., Woo, J. S., Wu, B., El-Sherbiny, Y. M., Leung, J., Chupradit, K., et al. (2019). The Ca(2+) sensor STIM1 regulates the type I interferon response by retaining the signaling adaptor STING at the endoplasmic reticulum. *Nature Immunology*, *20*(2), 152–162. https://doi.org/10.1038/s41590-018-0287-8.

Sun, W., Li, Y., Chen, L., Chen, H., You, F., Zhou, X., et al. (2009). ERIS, an endoplasmic reticulum IFN stimulator, activates innate immune signaling through dimerization. *Proceedings of the National Academy of Sciences of the United States of America*, *106*(21), 8653–8658. https://doi.org/10.1073/pnas.0900850106.

Sun, X., Xian, H., Tian, S., Sun, T., Qin, Y., Zhang, S., et al. (2016). A hierarchical mechanism of RIG-I ubiquitination provides sensitivity, robustness and synergy in antiviral immune responses. *Scientific Reports*, *6*, 29263. https://doi.org/10.1038/srep29263.

Sun, H., Zhang, Q., Jing, Y. Y., Zhang, M., Wang, H. Y., Cai, Z., et al. (2017). USP13 negatively regulates antiviral responses by deubiquitinating STING. *Nature Communications*, *8*, 15534. https://doi.org/10.1038/ncomms15534.

Tokunaga, F., Sakata, S., Saeki, Y., Satomi, Y., Kirisako, T., Kamei, K., et al. (2009). Involvement of linear polyubiquitylation of NEMO in NF-kappaB activation. *Nature Cell Biology*, *11*(2), 123–132. https://doi.org/10.1038/ncb1821.

Tsuchida, T., Zou, J., Saitoh, T., Kumar, H., Abe, T., Matsuura, Y., et al. (2010). The ubiquitin ligase TRIM56 regulates innate immune responses to intracellular double-stranded DNA. *Immunity*, *33*(5), 765–776. https://doi.org/10.1016/j.immuni.2010.10.013.

Walden, H., & Rittinger, K. (2018). RBR ligase-mediated ubiquitin transfer: A tale with many twists and turns. *Nature Structural & Molecular Biology*, *25*(6), 440–445. https://doi.org/10.1038/s41594-018-0063-3.

Wang, Y., Hu, L., Tong, X., & Ye, X. (2014). Casein kinase 1gamma1 inhibits the RIG-I/TLR signaling pathway through phosphorylating p65 and promoting its degradation. *Journal of Immunology*, *192*(4), 1855–1861. https://doi.org/10.4049/jimmunol.1302552.

Wang, Q., Huang, L., Hong, Z., Lv, Z., Mao, Z., Tang, Y., et al. (2017). The E3 ubiquitin ligase RNF185 facilitates the cGAS-mediated innate immune response. *PLoS Pathogens*, *13*(3), e1006264. https://doi.org/10.1371/journal.ppat.1006264.

Wang, W., Jiang, M., Liu, S., Zhang, S., Liu, W., Ma, Y., et al. (2016). RNF122 suppresses antiviral type I interferon production by targeting RIG-I CARDs to mediate RIG-I degradation. *Proceedings of the National Academy of Sciences of the United States of America*, *113*(34), 9581–9586. https://doi.org/10.1073/pnas.1604277113.

Wang, Y., Lian, Q., Yang, B., Yan, S., Zhou, H., He, L., et al. (2015). TRIM30alpha is a negative-feedback regulator of the intracellular DNA and DNA virus-triggered response by targeting STING. *PLoS Pathogens*, *11*(6), e1005012. https://doi.org/10.1371/journal.ppat.1005012.

Wang, Q., Liu, X., Cui, Y., Tang, Y., Chen, W., Li, S., et al. (2014). The E3 ubiquitin ligase AMFR and INSIG1 bridge the activation of TBK1 kinase by modifying the adaptor STING. *Immunity*, *41*(6), 919–933. https://doi.org/10.1016/j.immuni.2014.11.011.

Wang, Y., Tong, X., & Ye, X. (2012). Ndfip1 negatively regulates RIG-I-dependent immune signaling by enhancing E3 ligase Smurf1-mediated MAVS degradation. *Journal of Immunology*, *189*(11), 5304–5313. https://doi.org/10.4049/jimmunol.1201445.

Wang, L., Wen, M., & Cao, X. (2019). Nuclear hnRNPA2B1 initiates and amplifies the innate immune response to DNA viruses. *Science*, *365*(6454), eaav0758. https://doi.org/10.1126/science.aav0758.

Wang, L., Zhao, W., Zhang, M., Wang, P., Zhao, K., Zhao, X., et al. (2013). USP4 positively regulates RIG-I-mediated antiviral response through deubiquitination and stabilization of RIG-I. *Journal of Virology*, *87*(8), 4507–4515. https://doi.org/10.1128/JVI.00031-13.

Wang, P., Zhao, W., Zhao, K., Zhang, L., & Gao, C. (2015). TRIM26 negatively regulates interferon-beta production and antiviral response through polyubiquitination and degradation of nuclear IRF3. *PLoS Pathogens*, *11*(3), e1004726. https://doi.org/10.1371/journal.ppat.1004726.

Woronicz, J. D., Gao, X., Cao, Z., Rothe, M., & Goeddel, D. V. (1997). IkappaB kinase-beta: NF-kappaB activation and complex formation with IkappaB kinase-alpha and NIK. *Science*, *278*(5339), 866–869. https://doi.org/10.1126/science.278.5339.866.

Wu, B., Peisley, A., Richards, C., Yao, H., Zeng, X., Lin, C., et al. (2013). Structural basis for dsRNA recognition, filament formation, and antiviral signal activation by MDA5. *Cell*, *152*(1–2), 276–289. https://doi.org/10.1016/j.cell.2012.11.048.

Wu, J., Sun, L., Chen, X., Du, F., Shi, H., Chen, C., et al. (2013). Cyclic GMP-AMP is an endogenous second messenger in innate immune signaling by cytosolic DNA. *Science*, *339*(6121), 826–830. https://doi.org/10.1126/science.1229963.

Xagorari, A., & Chlichlia, K. (2008). Toll-like receptors and viruses: Induction of innate antiviral immune responses. *Open Microbiol Journal*, *2*, 49–59. https://doi.org/10.2174/1874285800802010049.

Xian, H., Xie, W., Yang, S., Liu, Q., Xia, X., Jin, S., et al. (2017). Stratified ubiquitination of RIG-I creates robust immune response and induces selective gene expression. *Science Advances*, *3*(9), e1701764. https://doi.org/10.1126/sciadv.1701764.

Xing, J., Weng, L., Yuan, B., Wang, Z., Jia, L., Jin, R., et al. (2016). Identification of a role for TRIM29 in the control of innate immunity in the respiratory tract. *Nature Immunology*, *17*(12), 1373–1380. https://doi.org/10.1038/ni.3580.

Xing, J., Zhang, A., Minze, L. J., Li, X. C., & Zhang, Z. (2018). TRIM29 negatively regulates the type I IFN production in response to RNA virus. *Journal of Immunology*, *201*(1), 183–192. https://doi.org/10.4049/jimmunol.1701569.

Xing, J., Zhang, A., Zhang, H., Wang, J., Li, X. C., Zeng, M. S., et al. (2017). TRIM29 promotes DNA virus infections by inhibiting innate immune response. *Nature Communications*, *8*(1), 945. https://doi.org/10.1038/s41467-017-00101-w.

Xu, L. G., Wang, Y. Y., Han, K. J., Li, L. Y., Zhai, Z., & Shu, H. B. (2005). VISA is an adapter protein required for virus-triggered IFN-beta signaling. *Molecular Cell*, *19*(6), 727–740. https://doi.org/10.1016/j.molcel.2005.08.014.

Xue, B., Li, H., Guo, M., Wang, J., Xu, Y., Zou, X., et al. (2018). TRIM21 promotes innate immune response to RNA viral infection through Lys27-linked polyubiquitination of MAVS. *Journal of Virology*, *92*(14), e00321-18. https://doi.org/10.1128/JVI.00321-18.

Xue, Q., Zhou, Z., Lei, X., Liu, X., He, B., Wang, J., et al. (2012). TRIM38 negatively regulates TLR3-mediated IFN-beta signaling by targeting TRIF for degradation. *PLoS One*, *7*(10), e46825. https://doi.org/10.1371/journal.pone.0046825.

Yamamoto, M., Sato, S., Hemmi, H., Hoshino, K., Kaisho, T., Sanjo, H., et al. (2003). Role of adaptor TRIF in the MyD88-independent toll-like receptor signaling pathway. *Science*, *301*(5633), 640–643. https://doi.org/10.1126/science.1087262.

Yan, J., Li, Q., Mao, A. P., Hu, M. M., & Shu, H. B. (2014). TRIM4 modulates type I interferon induction and cellular antiviral response by targeting RIG-I for K63-linked ubiquitination. *Journal of Molecular Cell Biology*, *6*(2), 154–163. https://doi.org/10.1093/jmcb/mju005.

Yang, Y., Liao, B., Wang, S., Yan, B., Jin, Y., Shu, H. B., et al. (2013). E3 ligase WWP2 negatively regulates TLR3-mediated innate immune response by targeting TRIF for ubiquitination and degradation. *Proceedings of the National Academy of Sciences of the United States of America, 110*(13), 5115–5120. https://doi.org/10.1073/pnas.1220271110.

Yau, R., & Rape, M. (2016). The increasing complexity of the ubiquitin code. *Nature Cell Biology, 18*(6), 579–586. https://doi.org/10.1038/ncb3358.

Ye, L., Zhang, Q., Liuyu, T., Xu, Z., Zhang, M. X., Luo, M. H., et al. (2019). USP49 negatively regulates cellular antiviral responses via deconjugating K63-linked ubiquitination of MITA. *PLoS Pathogens, 15*(4), e1007680. https://doi.org/10.1371/journal.ppat.1007680.

Yoneyama, M., Kikuchi, M., Matsumoto, K., Imaizumi, T., Miyagishi, M., Taira, K., et al. (2005). Shared and unique functions of the DExD/H-box helicases RIG-I, MDA5, and LGP2 in antiviral innate immunity. *Journal of Immunology, 175*(5), 2851–2858.

Yoo, Y. S., Park, Y. Y., Kim, J. H., Cho, H., Kim, S. H., Lee, H. S., et al. (2015). The mitochondrial ubiquitin ligase MARCH5 resolves MAVS aggregates during antiviral signalling. *Nature Communications, 6*, 7910. https://doi.org/10.1038/ncomms8910.

You, F., Sun, H., Zhou, X., Sun, W., Liang, S., Zhai, Z., et al. (2009). PCBP2 mediates degradation of the adaptor MAVS via the HECT ubiquitin ligase AIP4. *Nature Immunology, 10*(12), 1300–1308. https://doi.org/10.1038/ni.1815.

Yu, Y., & Hayward, G. S. (2010). The ubiquitin E3 ligase RAUL negatively regulates type i interferon through ubiquitination of the transcription factors IRF7 and IRF3. *Immunity, 33*(6), 863–877. https://doi.org/10.1016/j.immuni.2010.11.027.

Yu, Z., Song, H., Jia, M., Zhang, J., Wang, W., Li, Q., et al. (2017). USP1-UAF1 deubiquitinase complex stabilizes TBK1 and enhances antiviral responses. *The Journal of Experimental Medicine, 214*(12), 3553–3563. https://doi.org/10.1084/jem.20170180.

Zhang, J., Hu, M. M., Wang, Y. Y., & Shu, H. B. (2012). TRIM32 protein modulates type I interferon induction and cellular antiviral response by targeting MITA/STING protein for K63-linked ubiquitination. *The Journal of Biological Chemistry, 287*(34), 28646–28655. https://doi.org/10.1074/jbc.M112.362608.

Zhang, L., Liu, J., Qian, L., Feng, Q., Wang, X., Yuan, Y., et al. (2018). Induction of OTUD1 by RNA viruses potently inhibits innate immune responses by promoting degradation of the MAVS/TRAF3/TRAF6 signalosome. *PLoS Pathogens, 14*(5), e1007067. https://doi.org/10.1371/journal.ppat.1007067.

Zhang, M., Tian, Y., Wang, R. P., Gao, D., Zhang, Y., Diao, F. C., et al. (2008). Negative feedback regulation of cellular antiviral signaling by RBCK1-mediated degradation of IRF3. *Cell Research, 18*(11), 1096–1104. https://doi.org/10.1038/cr.2008.277.

Zhang, M., Wang, L., Zhao, X., Zhao, K., Meng, H., Zhao, W., et al. (2012). TRAF-interacting protein (TRIP) negatively regulates IFN-beta production and antiviral response by promoting proteasomal degradation of TANK-binding kinase 1. *The Journal of Experimental Medicine, 209*(10), 1703–1711. https://doi.org/10.1084/jem.20120024.

Zhang, L., Wei, N., Cui, Y., Hong, Z., Liu, X., Wang, Q., et al. (2018). The deubiquitinase CYLD is a specific checkpoint of the STING antiviral signaling pathway. *PLoS Pathogens, 14*(11), e1007435. https://doi.org/10.1371/journal.ppat.1007435.

Zhang, M., Zhang, M. X., Zhang, Q., Zhu, G. F., Yuan, L., Zhang, D. E., et al. (2016). USP18 recruits USP20 to promote innate antiviral response through deubiquitinating STING/MITA. *Cell Research, 26*(12), 1302–1319. https://doi.org/10.1038/cr.2016.125.

Zhang, L., Zhao, X., Zhang, M., Zhao, W., & Gao, C. (2014). Ubiquitin-specific protease 2b negatively regulates IFN-beta production and antiviral activity by targeting TANK-binding kinase 1. *Journal of Immunology, 193*(5), 2230–2237. https://doi.org/10.4049/jimmunol.1302634.

Zhao, B., Du, F., Xu, P., Shu, C., Sankaran, B., Bell, S. L., et al. (2019). A conserved PLPLRT/SD motif of STING mediates the recruitment and activation of TBK1. *Nature, 569*(7758), 718–722. https://doi.org/10.1038/s41586-019-1228-x.

Zhao, C., Jia, M., Song, H., Yu, Z., Wang, W., Li, Q., et al. (2017). The E3 ubiquitin ligase TRIM40 attenuates antiviral immune responses by targeting MDA5 and RIG-I. *Cell Reports, 21*(6), 1613–1623. https://doi.org/10.1016/j.celrep.2017.10.020.

Zhao, Y., Mudge, M. C., Soll, J. M., Rodrigues, R. B., Byrum, A. K., Schwarzkopf, E. A., et al. (2018). OTUD4 is a phospho-activated K63 deubiquitinase that regulates MyD88-dependent signaling. *Molecular Cell, 69*(3), 505–516, e505. https://doi.org/10.1016/j.molcel.2018.01.009.

Zhao, W., Wang, L., Zhang, M., Yuan, C., & Gao, C. (2012). E3 ubiquitin ligase tripartite motif 38 negatively regulates TLR-mediated immune responses by proteasomal degradation of TNF receptor-associated factor 6 in macrophages. *Journal of Immunology, 188*(6), 2567–2574. https://doi.org/10.4049/jimmunol.1103255.

Zhao, X., Zhu, H., Yu, J., Li, H., Ge, J., & Chen, W. (2016). c-Cbl-mediated ubiquitination of IRF3 negatively regulates IFN-beta production and cellular antiviral response. *Cellular Signalling, 28*(11), 1683–1693. https://doi.org/10.1016/j.cellsig.2016.08.002.

Zheng, Y., & Gao, C. (2019). E3 ubiquitin ligases, the powerful modulator of innate antiviral immunity. *Cellular Immunology, 340,* 103915. https://doi.org/10.1016/j.cellimm.2019.04.003.

Zheng, Q., Hou, J., Zhou, Y., Yang, Y., Xie, B., & Cao, X. (2015). Siglec1 suppresses antiviral innate immune response by inducing TBK1 degradation via the ubiquitin ligase TRIM27. *Cell Research, 25*(10), 1121–1136. https://doi.org/10.1038/cr.2015.108.

Zheng, N., & Shabek, N. (2017). Ubiquitin ligases: Structure, function, and regulation. *Annual Review of Biochemistry, 86*, 129–157. https://doi.org/10.1146/annurev-biochem-060815-014922.

Zhong, B., Yang, Y., Li, S., Wang, Y. Y., Li, Y., Diao, F., et al. (2008). The adaptor protein MITA links virus-sensing receptors to IRF3 transcription factor activation. *Immunity, 29*(4), 538–550. https://doi.org/10.1016/j.immuni.2008.09.003.

Zhong, B., Zhang, L., Lei, C., Li, Y., Mao, A. P., Yang, Y., et al. (2009). The ubiquitin ligase RNF5 regulates antiviral responses by mediating degradation of the adaptor protein MITA. *Immunity, 30*(3), 397–407. https://doi.org/10.1016/j.immuni.2009.01.008.

Zhong, B., Zhang, Y., Tan, B., Liu, T. T., Wang, Y. Y., & Shu, H. B. (2010). The E3 ubiquitin ligase RNF5 targets virus-induced signaling adaptor for ubiquitination and degradation. *Journal of Immunology, 184*(11), 6249–6255. https://doi.org/10.4049/jimmunol.0903748.

Zhou, P., Ding, X., Wan, X., Liu, L., Yuan, X., Zhang, W., et al. (2018). MLL5 suppresses antiviral innate immune response by facilitating STUB1-mediated RIG-I degradation. *Nature Communications, 9*(1), 1243. https://doi.org/10.1038/s41467-018-03563-8.

Zotti, T., Uva, A., Ferravante, A., Vessichelli, M., Scudiero, I., Ceccarelli, M., et al. (2011). TRAF7 protein promotes Lys-29-linked polyubiquitination of IkappaB kinase (IKKgamma)/NF-kappaB essential modulator (NEMO) and p65/RelA protein and represses NF-kappaB activation. *The Journal of Biological Chemistry, 286*(26), 22924–22933. https://doi.org/10.1074/jbc.M110.215426.

CHAPTER FIVE

Metabolic regulation of innate immunity

Shaonan Liang[a,b,†], Liangliang Ji[a,b,c,†], Lan Kang[a,b,d,†], Xiaoyu Hu[a,b,*]
[a]Institute for Immunology and School of Medicine, Tsinghua University, Beijing, China
[b]Beijing Key Laboratory for Immunological Research on Chronic Diseases, Tsinghua University, Beijing, China
[c]Tsinghua-Peking Center for Life Sciences, School of Life Sciences, Tsinghua University, Beijing, China
[d]Joint Graduate Program of Peking-Tsinghua-NIBS, School of Life Sciences, Tsinghua University, Beijing, China
*Corresponding author: e-mail address: xiaoyuhu@tsinghua.edu.cn

Contents

Abstract

Immune responses are often accompanied by radical changes of cellular metabolism of immune cells. On the other hand, an ever increasing number of metabolic pathways and products have been found to possess immune regulatory functions. The field of immunometabolism that investigates the interplay between metabolism and immunity has developed rapidly during the past decade. In this chapter, we attempt to summarize the recent progresses by scientists in China on metabolic regulation of innate immunity

† These authors contributed equally.

Advances in Immunology, Volume 145
ISSN 0065-2776
https://doi.org/10.1016/bs.ai.2019.11.005

from the following three perspectives: metabolic regulation of myeloid cell functions, metabolic adaptations of tissue resident myeloid cells, and metabolism and immunity at the mucosal surfaces.

Metabolism and immune defense are two essential processes ensuring survival of individual organisms and propagation of any given animal species. During the course of approximately 610 million years of evolution of the biological kingdom Animalia, for almost all species with few exceptions of a subpopulation of *Homo sapiens* and a limited number of domesticated livestock, animals spend significant amounts of time and energy on food gathering yet constantly face dreadful challenges of food shortage nutrient and deprivation. Meanwhile, the world that most animals reside in is not equivalent to specific pathogen free (SPF) facilities but filled with pathogens. One could postulate that animals that could better cope with microbes would gain evolutionary advantages over those that easily succumb to infectious threats under circumstances of nutrient fluctuations. Therefore, it is not surprising that after millions of years of natural selection, metabolism and immunity are intimately intertwined with the purpose of achieving maximal protection of host with minimal energy expenditure. In recent years, a subfield of immunology named "immunometabolism" with the goal of studying the interplay between metabolism and immunity has grown rapidly, which grasped attention from scientists all over the globe. Immunologists based in China have been similarly attracted to the immunometabolism arena and began to make important contributions toward uncovering the once-hidden connections between metabolic processes and immune responses. In this chapter, we attempt to review recent progresses on immunometabolic studies performed in China with a focus on several key cell types in innate immunity and host defense including macrophages, dendritic cells, and intestinal epithelium. Due to the space constraint and inevitably limited scope of knowledge by the authors, we apologize in advance if we have omitted any studies in this field that should be otherwise mentioned here.

1. Metabolic regulation of myeloid cell functions

The function of myeloid cells is regulated by a plethora of molecular mechanisms, among which metabolites or metabolic pathways are playing critical roles. A number of studies have supported that metabolic modules

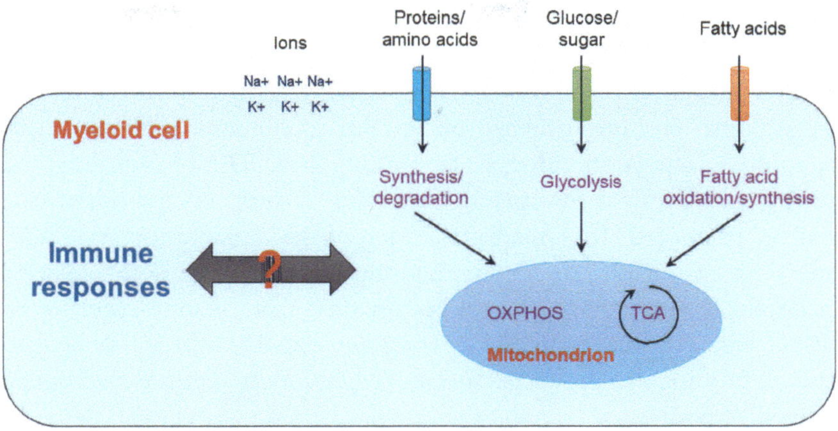

Fig. 1 Interactions between immune responses and metabolic pathways in myeloid cells. Amino acids, glucose and fatty acids within myeloid cells go through various metabolic pathways. Many of those pathways converge at the TCA cycle and fulfill the process of oxidative phosphorylation (OXPHOS) in mitochondrion. Ion influx and efflux form the membrane potential. A number of studies have identified the connections between immune responses and metabolic pathways in myeloid cells. Nevertheless, there remain plentiful open questions to be addressed in this field.

including amino acids, glucose, fatty acids, TCA cycle, ions and so on, play critical roles in regulating the immune responses of myeloid cells (Fig. 1). During the past two decades, Chinese scientists have made significant contributions to uncovering the functions and mechanisms of the interaction between metabolism and innate immunity.

1.1 Amino acid metabolism

Proteins in organisms are composed of 20 amino acids, of which metabolism is vital to maintain the physiological function of most biological processes including immune responses. In addition to protein synthesis, metabolic fates of some amino acids are reported to play important roles in regulating immune functions of myeloid cells. One example is that the iNOS- or arginase 1-mediated L-arginine metabolism is activated during IFN-γ/LPS- or IL-4-mediated macrophage polarization, respectively, and thus drive macrophages to bactericidal or wound repairing state (Bronte & Zanovello, 2005). Another example is that IDO-mediated tryptophan metabolism in myeloid cells suppresses T cell activation and therefore facilitates tumor growth (Munn & Mellor, 2016). There are still plentiful unrevealed amino acid pathways that may exert critical functions during myeloid cell immune responses.

In 2019, Xiaoyu Hu's group (Institute for Immunology at Tsinghua University) added new dimension to the L-arginine metabolism pathways in macrophages (Ji et al., 2019). They found that the third metabolic fate of L-arginine, creatine pathway, on one hand, inhibited IFN-γ-mediated macrophage activation through suppressing JAK-STAT1 signaling, and thereby compromised the bactericidal ability of host; on the other hand, creatine promoted IL-4-mediated macrophage polarization via ATP-dependent chromatin remodeling, and thus enhanced the host's ability of eosinophil recruitment. Their studies revealed that creatine regulates the iNOS- and arginase 1-mediated L-arginine metabolism in a feedback manner, forming a sophisticated metabolic network to regulate macrophage immune responses.

At the same year, Di Wang's group (Zhejiang University) collaborating with Yingliang Wu's group (Wuhan University) reported that serine and glucose metabolism in macrophages is synergistically integrated into the methionine metabolic cycle via de novo ATP synthesis and fuels the production of S-adenosylmethionine (SAM) during LPS stimulation (Yu et al., 2019). Mechanistically, SAM generation maintains a high ratio of SAM: S-adenosylhomocysteine and then promotes histone H3 lysine 36 trimethylation for IL-1β production. They clarified the importance of serine and methionine metabolism in pro-inflammatory macrophage activation, and identified a synergistic manner of amino acid and glucose metabolism in orchestrating SAM availability that is closely connected to the epigenetic state and inflammation.

Exemplified by the above studies, Chinese immunologists have contributed new knowledge toward better understanding of amino acid metabolism including L-arginine, serine and methionine pathways in regulating macrophage immune responses.

1.2 Hypoxia and glucose metabolism

Glucose metabolic pathways provide major energy sources for a number of cellular processes. Many immune cells including myeloid lineage cells require glucose metabolism to support their physiological activities. It has been well established that glycolysis is necessary for both pro- and anti-inflammatory activation in macrophages (Stienstra, Netea-Maier, Riksen, Joosten, & Netea, 2017). In addition, the hypoxia microenvironment will increase the cellular glycolysis by up-regulating a number of glycolytic genes. The expression of glucose transporter 1 (GLUT1) is highly induced by inflammatory stimuli including toll-like receptor (TLR) ligand LPS, which leads to the induction of cellular glycolysis despite the fact that the cells are placed in normal oxygen microenvironment, a process analogous to cancer Warburg effect. The increased glycolysis will stabilize the protein expression of HIF-1α and then promote the production of many inflammatory factors such as IL-1β, iNOS and IL-12 (O'Neill & Pearce, 2016). In addition, expression levels of some glycolytic enzymes including pyruvate dehydrogenase kinase 1 (PDK1), pyruvate kinase M2 (PKM2) and hexokinase II also contribute to the processes of macrophage activation (Van den Bossche, O'Neill, & Menon, 2017).

During the past 10 years, studies from China have made notable contributions to investigating the role of hypoxia in regulating myeloid cell function. Xun Qu's group (Shandong University) reported that hypoxia affected the biological activities of dendritic cells (DCs) by inducing their differentiation toward a Th2 polarizing phenotype, which displayed increased expression of IL-10 but decreased expression of TNF-α and IL-12p70 (Yang et al., 2009). The mechanistic studies revealed that hypoxia markedly altered cellular metabolism, led to the accumulation of extracellular adenosine and thereby triggered cellular responses via adenosine receptor A2b of which expression depended on HIF-1α (Yang et al., 2010). The downstream signaling of A2b significantly inhibited the expression of TNF-α and IL-12p70 through targeting cAMP in LPS-induced mature DCs. Qu's studies uncovered that unlike in macrophages, hypoxia in mDCs inhibited the expression of inflammatory factors and then promoted the type 2 immunity. However, Ruifu Yang's group (Beijing Institute of Microbiology and Epidemiology) reported that HIF-1α inhibition or deficiency in LPS-stimulated DCs would lead to decreased expression of IL-12p40 but increased levels of TGF-β (Liu et al., 2015). This observation is contrary to Qu's data that hypoxia inhibits the expression of IL-12p70 in DCs. Thus, the roles of hypoxia and HIF-1α in DCs should be further clarified and discussed.

In 2019, Xuetao Cao's group (Second Military Medical University) expanded the role of HIF-1α-dependent glycolysis in modulating DC migration and immune response (Liu, Zhang, et al., 2019). They reported that CCR7 stimulation would activate the HIF-1α transcription factor pathway and promote the glycolysis in DCs. A long non-coding RNA lnc-Dpf3 directly bound to HIF-1α and suppressed the expression of HIF-1α-dependent glycolytic gene *Ldha*, and thus inhibited DC glycolysis and migration. Cao's group also reported that HIF-1α-deficient DCs exhibited impaired migratory capacity in vitro and in vivo. In addition, they showed the evidence that inhibition of glycolysis in DCs impaired both the early and late stage of DC migration to draining lymph nodes in vivo. Thus, HIF-1α-dependent glycolysis is critical to CCR7-mediated DC migration and DC-based T cell immune responses.

Daolin Tang's group (The Third Affiliated Hospital of Guangzhou Medical University) explored the function of PKM2-dependent glycolysis in promoting the formation of NLRP3 inflammasome (Xie et al., 2016). They found that PKM2-mediated glycolysis promoted inflammasome activation by modulating EIF2AK2 phosphorylation in macrophages. Pharmacological and genetic inhibition of PKM2 or EIF2AK2 impaired the formation of NLRP3 and AIM2 inflammasomes, and consequently inhibited the production of IL-1β, IL-18 and HMGB1 by macrophages. In vivo data showed that conditional ablation of PKM2 in myeloid cells protected mice from septic death induced by NLRP3 and AIM2 inflammasome activation. Thus, they stressed the importance of PKM2-mediated glycolysis in regulating the macrophage inflammasome activation.

Overall, Chinese scientists have introduced new knowledge in the field regarding how hypoxia and glucose metabolism regulate the immune function of myeloid cells. They found various roles of hypoxia or HIF-1α in DCs, and renewed the role of glycolysis in promoting macrophage inflammasome activation. These findings re-emphasize the importance of hypoxia and glucose metabolism in the innate immune system.

1.3 Fatty acid and cholesterol metabolism

Fatty acids are another domain of crucial metabolites in maintaining host fitness and cellular activities. Fatty acid metabolism pathways can be categorized into fatty acid synthesis and fatty acid oxidation, which are highly activated in IFN-γ/LPS- and IL-4-induced macrophages, respectively. Fatty acid oxidation promotes the oxidative phosphorylation in mitochondrion and is necessary for IL-4-induced macrophage activation (Nomura et al., 2016). Short-chain fatty acid butyrate is reported to enhance bactericidal capacity of colonic macrophages (Schulthess et al., 2019). Cholesterol metabolism in macrophage is well-known for its function in atherosclerosis during which inflammatory macrophages display impaired ability of cholesterol transport and thus promote the formation of foam cells (Geeraerts, Bolli, Fendt, & Van Ginderachter, 2017).

In 2016, Di Wang's group found that bile acids suppressed NLRP3 inflammasome activation through the TGR5-cAMP-PKA axis (Guo et al., 2016). Bile acids are a diverse class of cholesterol-derived, amphipathic molecules that work as detergents to facilitate the digestion and absorption of dietary fatty acids. Bile acids could activate the cell membrane receptor TGR5, which transduce downstream signaling into cellular compartments. Di Wang's group identified that bile acid could activate the macrophage intracellular cAMP-PKA signaling and subsequently suppressed NLRP3 inflammasome activation and IL-1β release. This study provides an intriguing example about how cholesterol-related metabolites affect the function of myeloid cells.

In 2018, Yonghui Zhang's group (Tsinghua University) revealed that mevalonate pathway is a druggable target for vaccine adjuvants and cancer immunotherapies (Xia et al., 2018). The mevalonate pathway utilizes the HMG-CoA as raw materials and synthesizes mevalonic acids, which is a core metabolic pathway for multiple cellular processes including cholesterol biosynthesis and protein post-translational prenylation. Statins inhibit HMG-CoA reductase, an early stage enzyme in the mevalonate pathway. The downstream metabolite of the mevalonate pathway is geranylgeranyl diphosphate (GGPP). Zhang's group found that simvastatin prominently increased antigen presentation of bone marrow-derived DCs (BMDCs) to both $CD4^+$ and $CD8^+$ T cells, while GGPP abolished simvastatin's ability to enhance antigen presentation of BMDCs. These data indicated that the mevalonate pathway acts as an endogenous suppressor of antigen retention and presentation in BMDCs, and also an inhibitor of DC-based T cell activation.

There are still a large number of fatty acid- and cholesterol-related metabolites enriched in myeloid cells with unknown immune regulatory functions. Thus more work is needed to comprehensively understand the roles of these metabolites in the processes of innate immunity.

1.4 TCA cycle and its derivatives

Tricarboxylic acid (TCA) cycle, also named Krebs cycle, is a central hub of amino acid, glucose and fatty acid metabolism, and is crucial to mitochondrial and energy metabolism. Many metabolites involved in TCA cycle are found to be important to innate immune responses. Citrate promotes the production of an array of inflammatory factors including NO, ROS and PGE2 in macrophages. Accumulation of itaconate occurs in IFN-γ/LPS-activated macrophages and inhibits the expression of certain pro-inflammatory genes such as *Nos2*, *Il6* and *Il1b*. Succinate could stabilize the transcription factor HIF-1α and then promote the expression of IL-1β. Fumarate promotes while α-ketoglutarate (α-KG) attenuates inflammatory activation of macrophages. These findings indicate that metabolites in TCA cycle play essential yet distinct roles in regulating innate immunity (Williams & O'Neill, 2018). A number of Chinese research groups also uncovered important roles of certain TCA cycle-related metabolites in regulation of innate immune responses.

In 2019, Xuetao Cao's group reported that the first rate-limiting enzyme in the TCA cycle α-KG dehydrogenase (OGDH) increased the cellular abundance of itaconate that is required for viral replication in macrophages (Liu, You, et al., 2019). Their data showed that pharmacological inhibition of OGDH by succinyl phosphonate (SP) and CPI-613 dose-dependently inhibited viral replication in macrophages, while OGDH overexpression rescued this phenotype. Upon viral infection, one of most significantly down-regulated metabolites in OGDH-silenced macrophages is itaconate. In addition, treatment of macrophages with itaconate derivative dimethyl itaconate (DMI) also dose-dependently increased viral replication. Their work identified that TCA cycle-related metabolic pathway OGDH-itaconate axis promoted viral replication in an interferon-independent manner in macrophages.

In the same year, Chu Wang's group (Peking University) elucidated new functional insights for the anti-inflammatory metabolite itaconate in macrophages by developing an activity-based protein profiling technology (Qin et al., 2019). They used a specific thiol-reactive probe, 1-OH-Az, for quantitative chemoproteomic profiling of cysteine modifications by itaconate, and provided a global portrait of its proteome reactivity. By using 1-OH-Az, they systematically detected itaconate modified proteins in macrophages and found that itaconate modified and inhibited three key glycolytic enzymes including fructose-bisphosphate aldolase A (ALDOA), glyceraldehyde-3-phosphate dehydrogenase (GAPDH) and L-lactate dehydrogenase A (LDHA). Further analysis showed that itaconate modifications on cysteines of ALDOA and LDHA substantially inhibited their enzymatic activities and led to impaired overall glycolysis in macrophages. Their work implies that itaconate exerts anti-inflammatory function in macrophages through inhibition of glycolytic flux by modifying ALDOA and LDHA, which is independent of the previously reported KEAP1-NRF2 pathway.

Thus, the research from Chinese groups renewed the functions and mechanisms of TCA cycle, especially itaconate in myeloid cells. They employed new technologies to explore the underlying mechanisms regarding how metabolites affect the immune function of myeloid cells. In the foreseeable future, development and application of new cutting-edge technologies would be expected to aid in solving more scientific mysteries in the immunometabolism arena.

1.5 Ion metabolism

Ions are small chemical elements with pleiotropic properties. Ions play crucial roles in various cellular activities and functions such as maintenance of intracellular pH and membrane potential as well as functioning as enzyme co-factors. The function of ions in innate immunity had been inadequately explored until recently. In macrophages, intracellular potassium (K^+) efflux is a common trigger of NLRP3 inflammasome activation by bacterial toxins and particulate matter (Munoz-Planillo et al., 2013). Extracellular iron (Fe^{2+}) and heme induced macrophage necrosis through TLR4-dependent expression of TNF and TLR4-independent generation of ROS (Fortes et al., 2012). These are typical examples of how ions regulate the functions of myeloid cells while some Chinese scientists also made important contributions to this field.

Fudi Wang's group (Zhejiang University) reported that ferroportin (Fpn1)-mediated iron (Fe^{2+}) release inhibited the expression of TNF-α and IL-6 in LPS-induced macrophages (Zhang et al., 2011). Their data showed that depletion of Fpn1 in macrophages resulted in iron accumulation not only in macrophages, but also in spleen and liver. In addition, loss of Fpn1 led to increased expression of TNF-α and IL-6 in LPS-activated macrophage in vitro while reduction of intracellular iron levels inhibited the expression of those cytokines. Their studies demonstrated that Fpn1 played a critical role in macrophage iron release in vivo and in modulating innate immune responses. Thus, these findings from Wang's group implied the importance of intracellular iron in promoting macrophage inflammatory activation.

In 2018, Zhengfan Jiang's group (Peking University) discovered that manganese (Mn^{2+}) is critical for anti-viral responses in macrophages (Wang et al., 2018). They showed that upon virus infection, Mn^{2+} is released from organelles and accumulates in the cytosol, which primes the macrophages into an anti-viral state. In addition, Mn^{2+} markedly induced type I-IFN production and ISG expression in the absence of infection. Mechanistically, Mn^{2+} activated cGAS-STING pathway by increasing the sensitivity of cGAS to dsDNA and then promoting STING activation, which is independent of mtDNA release. In vivo data also showed that Mn^{2+} is required for the host defense against DNA virus. For the first time, Jiang's group uncovered the role of Mn^{2+} in innate immunity and clarified the importance of Mn^{2+} in cGAS-STING-mediated anti-viral responses in macrophages.

In recent years, despite of the efforts from Chinese research groups such as elucidation of the activities of Fe^{2+} and Mn^{2+} in the macrophage-mediated immune responses, there is still a long way to go in order to fully clarify the regulatory functions of ion molecules in the innate immune system.

1.6 Other metabolic factors and pathways

Plenty of other unclassified metabolic elements such as hormones and metabolic signals are also important to the function of myeloid cells. In 2019, Yufang Shi's group (Shanghai Institute of Nutrition and Health) in collaboration with Ying Wang (Shanghai Jiao Tong University) identified the role of insulin-like growth factor 2 (IGF-2) in macrophages (Du et al., 2019). They found that mesenchymal stem and/or stromal cells (MSCs)-produced IGF-2 exerted anti-inflammatory effects under low-oxygen condition. In vitro data showed that addition of IGF-2 in maturing but not matured macrophages significantly reduced the expression of IL-1β and increased the generation of PD-L1 upon LPS stimulation. Consistently, in vivo data demonstrated that IGF-2-preprogrammed macrophages promoted regulatory T cell differentiation and ameliorated EAE through PD-L1-dependent mechanisms. Metabolically, IGF-2 reprogrammed macrophages to commit to oxidative phosphorylation that determined an anti-inflammatory phenotype. In addition, metabolomics and epigenetics analyses revealed that IGF-2 markedly altered the cellular metabolism and histone modifications in macrophages.

Mechanistic target of rapamycin (mTOR) signaling pathway has been recognized as one of the most pivotal metabolic pathways in immune cells. In 2014, Yong Zhao's group (Institute of Zoology, Chinese Academy of Sciences) reported that tuberous sclerosis complex 1 (TSC1) acted as a critical regulator of macrophage polarization (Zhu et al., 2014). Molecular studies indicated that TSC1 inhibited inflammatory macrophage activation by suppressing the Ras GTPase-Raf1-MEK-ERK pathway in mTOR-independent manner, whereas TSC1 promoted anti-inflammatory macrophage polarization by mTOR-dependent pathways. In addition, in 2019, Hui Xiao's group (Institute Pasteur of Shanghai, Chinese Academy of Sciences) found that TSC1-mTOR pathway is important for homeostatic DC function through mechanisms involving metabolic-epigenetic coupling (Shi et al., 2019). The data from Xiao group demonstrated that TSC1-mTOR controlled the de novo fatty acid synthesis, diverted acetyl-CoA for histone acetylation, promoted the expression of MHC-1 on steady-state DCs, and thereby enhanced the responses of antigen-specific $CD8^+$ T cells. Thus, the work from these two groups provided mechanistic insights into the involvement of TSC1-mTOR pathway in regulation of myeloid cell function.

2. Metabolic adaptations of tissue resident myeloid cells

Innate immune cells are located in a variety of tissues within the body and contribute to maintenance of tissue homeostasis as well as host defense against infections and tumors. Macrophages and dendritic cells establish residence in various tissues and adapt to the environmental niche. There is accumulating evidence suggesting that metabolic fine-tuning is a prominent feature of niche adaptation (Caputa, Castoldi, & Pearce, 2019). Recently, an increased number of immunologists are considering metabolic processes in the functions of immune cells. The questions of how immune cells especially macrophages and DCs are able to metabolically adapt to distinct tissue niches will be the focus of this chapter. The multifaceted roles of cellular metabolism, including lipid metabolism and glucose metabolism, are tightly coupled to the functional requirements of macrophages within specific tissue niches.

2.1 Tissue-specific metabolic adaptations of macrophages and DCs

Alveolar macrophages (AMs) are positioned in the lumens of airway spaces in close contact with lung epithelium and are involved in cellular debris clearance and pathological situations such as pathogen invasion or tissue damages. The myeloid growth factors GM-CSF and TGF-β induce peroxisome proliferator-activated receptor gamma (PPARγ) expression in lung AMs to regulate their development and surfactant clearance function (Schneider et al., 2014; Yu et al., 2017). PPARγ controls the expression of genes encoding molecules that mediate aspects of lipid metabolism, including storage, lipolysis and cholesterol efflux to endow the AMs with the ability to degrade surfactant. It plays important roles not only in the generation of AMs by controlling differentiation of fetal lung monocyte precursors, but also in the lung allergic inflammation by licensing lung dendritic cell Th2 priming capacity. In addition, studies have shown that the lung environment controls AM responsiveness during type 2 inflammation via modulation of their metabolic activities and abilities to take up and metabolize glucose (Svedberg et al., 2019).

Yun-Cai Liu (Institute for Immunology at Tsinghua University) has a long-standing interest in the ubiquitin system in immune regulation and tolerance induction. Recently, his group has shed light on the VHL-HIF1α-glycolysis axis in controlling the function of AMs and the development of type 2 inflammation (Zhang et al., 2018). The transcription factor hypoxia inducible factor 1 (HIF-1) is understood to be the most important regulator of cellular response to hypoxia, which is essential for myeloid cell-mediated inflammation, antibacterial defense responses and anti-inflammatory repair/fibrotic responses. It is hydroxylated and then ubiquitinated by the E3 ligase von Hippel-Lindau protein (VHL) (Ohh et al., 2000). Liu group used mice with myeloid cell-restricted deletion of VHL and examined pulmonary type 2 and fibrotic response upon papain and bleomycin challenges. They found that VHL deficiency resulted in attenuated inflammatory and fibrotic responses via regulating glycolytic metabolism, mitochondrial respiration capacity and signature genes of AMs in a HIF1α-dependent manner. Moreover, they found that osteopontin, which was regulated by VHL in epigenetic modification-dependent manner, mediated the crosstalk between AMs and ILC2s for the type 2 inflammation and fibrosis. Interestingly, they identified the glycolytic metabolite 3-PG as a checkpoint regulator for osteopontin expression in AMs, which revealed new therapeutic targets for treating pulmonary allergy and fibrosis via metabolic manipulation.

2.2 Gut-resident myeloid cells adapt to the intestinal niche

Intestinal myeloid cells are located in a unique environment characterized by the exposure to not only tissue-intrinsic signals but also commensal microbiota. Several studies have shown that short chain fatty acids (SCFAs) butyrate, propionate and acetate, which are derived from anaerobic bacterial fermentation in the intestine, are key mediators of host-microbe cross talk, promoting intestinal epithelial barrier function and regulating the host mucosal immune system (Rooks & Garrett, 2016). Fiona Powrie's group identified that butyrate induced metabolic and transcriptional changes in intestinal macrophages via histone deacetylase 3 (HDAC3) inhibition, which enhanced their bactericidal function (Schulthess et al., 2019). Moreover, SCFA regulates the function of DCs, subsequently interacting with T cells to regulate immune responses. In addition, a vitamin A metabolite retinoic acid (RA) is instrumental in the initial phase of secondary lymphoid organ formation, and consequently is involved in orchestrating immune responses. Intestinal myeloid cells are the major source of RA and play important roles in the migratory and functional properties of T cells, B cells, and ILCs (Erkelens & Mebius, 2017).

Yan Shi (Institute for Immunology at Tsinghua University) revealed that retinaldehyde dehydrogenase (RALDH)$^+$ CD11b$^+$CD103$^+$ DCs from the gut lamina propria served to maintain the volume of secondary lymphoid organs (Zhang et al., 2016). They demonstrated that RALDH$^+$CD11b$^+$CD103$^+$DCs in the gut responded to commensal fungal colonization and migrated to the periphery. Subsequently, these DCs initiated peripheral lymph nodes development via imprinting peripheral lymphocytes for their homing to the gut in a RA-dependent manner. This work addressed the dependence of postnatal pLN development on gut microbiota and pointed out the exact subsets of cells responsible for pLN development and adult pLN maintenance. Furthermore, they observed the role of gut commensal fungi, *C. tropicalis* in neonatal LN development, although identification of the exact biochemical products that drive the migration of DCs awaits future investigation.

In addition to the role in the local gut environment, the metabolites could also contribute to the spatiotemporal regulation of innate immune interorgan communications that underpin systemic immunity. Lei Pan group (Chinese Academy of Sciences) unveiled how gut-fat body immunological communication (GFIC) relied on the intermediate activation of the polyol pathway in hemolymph and demonstrated that aldose reductase (AR) provided a critical metabolic checkpoint in the global inflammatory response in *Drosophila melanogaster* (Yang et al., 2019). Hyperactivation of immune deficiency (IMD) signaling in the gut was sufficient to trigger systemic IMD response in hemocytes and the fat body. Mechanistically, they found that sugar alcohols of the polyol pathway, an alternative pathway of glucose metabolism, served as alarmins to mediate this GFIC in a pathogen-independent way.

2.3 Myeloid cells adaption within adipose tissue

Adipose tissue (AT) is composed of multiple types of tissues, including white, brown and beige fat and homeostasis of white adipose tissue (WAT) requires an anti-inflammatory environment. Adipose tissue macrophages (ATMs), exhibiting an anti-inflammatory alternatively activated phenotype induced by IL-4 and IL-13, are critical in orchestrating metabolic homeostasis in WAT at steady state. However, during obesity characterized by chronic and low-level inflammation of AT, ATMs can switch into a pro-inflammatory phenotype and support to the development of type 1 inflammatory responses (McNelis & Olefsky, 2014). The endoplasmic reticulum (ER) is a critical organelle responsible for protein folding, maturation, quality control, and trafficking. Several studies have shown that obesity is associated with ER stress, which underlies the emergence of the stress and inflammatory responses in obesity (Ozcan et al., 2004).

Yong Liu (Chinese Academy of Sciences) uncovered a key role of the macrophage IRE1α pathway in mediating metabolic ER stress-induced obesity and metabolic syndrome through impairing brown adipose tissue (BAT) activity and WAT browning (Shan et al., 2017). They generated myeloid-specific IRE1α-knockout ($Ern1^{f/f}Lyz2$-Cre) mice and found that ablation of myeloid inositol-requiring enzyme 1α (IRE1α), the most conserved ER stress sensor, prevented diet-induced obesity and increased energy expenditure. To identify the role of IRE1α in macrophages, they analyzed ATMs and suggested that IRE1α pathway, which was activated by IL-4 in macrophages, suppressed M2 and enhanced M1 polarization in a negative feedback loop. They explained the correlation between metabolic ER stress and the obesity dependent on macrophage IRE1α pathway and proposed a new therapeutic target to treat obesity and metabolic disease.

2.4 Kupffer cells and non-alcoholic fatty liver disease

Non-alcoholic fatty liver disease (NAFLD) and alcoholic liver disease (ALD) are major causes of liver-related morbidity and mortality. Liver Kupffer cells, originated from yolk sac, are resident macrophages within the liver and the broad spectrum of their activation and polarization are suggested to contribute to the progression of NAFLD. In NAFLD, macrophages can be activated by various stimuli such as endotoxins, fatty acids, cholesterol and their metabolites, which are capable of direct pro-inflammatory macrophage activation (Kazankov et al., 2019).

Jing Hua (Shanghai Jiao Tong University) found that modulation of PPARγ activation had the potential to shift lipid-induced macrophage M1/M2 polarization through direct interaction with NF-κB pathway (Luo, Xu, Wang, Wu, & Hua, 2017). PPARγ, which is abundant in macrophages and induced by lipid, exerts important functions in macrophage M2-polarization. They used PPARγ agonists to shift macrophages toward an anti-inflammatory phenotype, identifying that PPARγ agonists could attenuate inflammation and downregulate the pro-inflammatory functions of macrophages, which suggested a new therapeutic approach for NAFLD.

2.5 Myeloid cells in tumor microenvironment

The homeostasis and evolution of the tumor microenvironment (TME) are governed by an intimate crosstalk among all cellular compartments. Tumor-associated macrophages (TAM) are one of the most abundant components of TME, and are involved in multiple processes leading to local growth and progression of the primary tumor and promotion of metastasis. Understanding how the TAM metabolism changes and how the altered metabolism regulates TAMs is of great interest and vital for developing effective therapies to treat cancer (Netea-Maier, Smit, & Netea, 2018). Recently, Chinese immunologists are making substantial efforts to investigate metabolic reprogramming of TAMs and their roles in modulating the functional phenotypes of these cells in the context of cancer development and progression.

2.5.1 Tumor cell metabolism shapes the development and function of TAMs

Several lines of evidence indicate that adjustments of the metabolic program regulate the differentiation, survival and function of TAMs. TME is typically hypoxic, as the uncontrolled cell proliferation prevails the blood supply, leading to the limited oxygen and nutrition. Tumor cells undergo metabolic adaptations, including a switch to aerobic glycolysis, termed the "Warburg effect," which leads to enhanced glycolysis and increased lactate production. To study the signals involved in the communication between lactate and macrophages, Qiang You (Nanjing Medical University) group identified that lactate could educate macrophage differentiation toward an alternatively activated (M2) phenotype to promote breast cancer proliferation, migration and angiogenesis (Mu et al., 2018). Mechanistically, they found that the activation of ERK1/2 and STAT3 signaling pathways was of importance in macrophage M2-polarization induced by lactate.

Their findings identified the lactate signaling cascade as a potential new therapeutic target for breast cancer treatment. In addition, another group, Xiang-Ping Yang (Huazhong University of Science and Technology) also studied how tumor-derived lactate primed TAMs into a pro-tumorigenic phenotype (Liu, Luo, et al., 2019). They demonstrated that lactate could downregulate the expression of macrophage-specific vacuolar ATPase (V-ATPases) subunit ATP6V0d2 via mTOR-dependent inhibition of the transcription factor regulator of lysosomal proteins, TFEB. To investigate the potential role of macrophage ATP6V0d2 in tumor growth and metastasis, they used $Atp6v0d2^{-/-}$ mice and found that KO mice were susceptible to tumor growth, which suggested that macrophage-expressed ATP6V0d2 inhibited tumor growth and suppressed tumor metastasis in vivo. Furthermore, they identified that $Atp6v0d2^{-/-}$ mice displayed enhanced pro-tumoral macrophage polarization and tumorigenesis with reduced lysosomal degradation of HIF-2α independently of oxygen level. In tumor samples from patients, the expression of ATP6V0d2 inversely correlated with HIF-2α expression in TAMs and postoperative survival of lung cancer patients, suggesting a critical role of the macrophage lactate/ATP6V0d2/HIF-2α axis in maintaining tumor growth in human patients. Rufu Chen group (Sun Yat-sen University) also found VCAM-1-induced lactate production from pancreatic cancer cells facilitated the M2-like polarization of macrophages in a dose-dependent manner (Ye et al., 2018). In addition to the alteration of functional phenotypes in TAM driven by metabolism, the mechanisms mobilizing TAMs into the chronically hypoxic compartments in tumor was studied by Xun Qu group (Shandong University). They found that the expression of 5-lipoxygenase (5-LOX) in ovarian cancer cells strongly correlated with the density of TAMs in hypoxic areas of human ovarian tumor tissues (Wen et al., 2015). Increased 5-LOX metabolites promoted migration and invasion of macrophages mediated by the upregulation of matrix metalloproteinase (MMP)-7 expression. To investigate the high-throughput and large-scale information of the differentiation mechanisms and intrinsic signals of TAMs regulated by the tumor microenvironment, Li Tang group (Beijing Institute of Radiation Medicine) constructed an in vitro TAM cell model, TES-TAMs, which was from tumor-extract-stimulated bone-marrow-derived macrophages (Liu et al., 2017). By using relatively comprehensive proteomics analysis, they found that the signal pathways in up-regulated expressed proteins of TAMs were enriched in glycolysis and inositol phosphate metabolism, which demonstrated their important roles in TAM differentiation.

2.5.2 TAM metabolism affects tumor progression and metastasis

The impact of TAMs on the metabolic profile of the TME also has a major influence on tumor progression and metastasis. Tumors contain distinct subpopulations of TAMs in different tumor regions which display distinct metabolic profiles. The classically activated macrophages exhibit highly glycolytic metabolism and reactive oxygen species (ROS) generation, while alternative activated macrophages are associated with increased oxidative phosphorylation (OXPHOS) and decreased lactate release. Recent literature suggests that TAMs have activated aerobic glycolysis, which also contributes to their functional reprogramming. In addition to glucose metabolism, TAMs undergo lipid metabolism including enhanced fatty acid biosynthesis, uptake and storage. Chinese immunologists have identified the lipid reprogramming metabolic pathways in TAMs and their roles in the development of tumor cells.

The group of Houjie Liang (The Third Military Medical University) demonstrated that AB-hydrolase containing 5 (ABHD5), a lipolytic co-activator, was expressed in TAMs and potentiated the growth of tumor cells through suppressing spermidine synthase (SRM)-dependent spermidine production in colorectal cancer (CRC) (Miao et al., 2016). They used CD11b promoter-driven myeloid-cell-specific ABHD5 transgenic and SRM transgenic mouse models to provide genetic evidence for validation of the ABHD5/SRM axis in vivo. In addition, they identified that ABHD5 suppressed ROS-dependent C/EBPε expression, which could activate transcription of the *srm* gene in macrophages in vitro. Their findings not only provided the first evidence that ABDH5 expression was increased in TAMs, but also revealed a novel mechanism linking a lipolytic factor to polyamine metabolism in TAMs and the growth of CRC, and shed light on therapeutic strategies to treat this malignancy.

Three years after the above discussed publication, the group of the first author, Hongming Miao (The Third Military Medical University), went on to demonstrate that ABHD5 expression was heterogeneous in TAMs and that ABHD5^{low} macrophages potentially facilitated tumor cell migration and cancer metastasis (Shang et al., 2019). They identified that macrophage ABHD5 inhibited cancer metastasis via suppression of NF-κB-dependent metalloproteinase (MMPs). For future investigation, it would be important to decipher the ontogeny of TAM subpopulation with distinct expression of ABHD5 to manage the cancer metastasis. In addition to identifying the role of ABHD5 in tumor progression and metastasis, the same group also studied lipid accumulation and its functional implications in TAMs

(Xiang et al., 2018). They implicated monoacylglycerol lipase (MGLL) as a regulator of lipid accumulation. MGLL deficiency promoted CB2 cannabinoid receptor/TLR4-dependent alternative activation of TAMs, subsequently suppressed the function of tumor-associated $CD8^+$ T cells and promoted tumor progression both in inoculated and genetic cancer models. Moreover, they verified that the expression of macrophage MGLL was decreased in cancer tissues and positively correlated with the survival of cancer patients. In summary, their studies implied that in response to microenvironmental cues, TAMs could alter their lipid metabolic profiles, which may augment their tumoricidal and inflammatory capacity.

Another group, Pingping Shen (Nanjing University) focused on how distinct metabolic pathways in TAMs were integrated into a coherent program that directed their gene expression (Niu et al., 2017). They found that caspase-1 inactivated medium-chain acyl-CoA dehydrogenase (MCAD) by cleaving PPARγ at Asp64. This truncated PPARγ translocated to mitochondria and bound with MCAD to attenuate its activity, inhibit fatty acid oxidation and lead to lipid accumulation, which promoted TAM differentiation. Furthermore, administration of caspase-1 inhibitors or infusion of macrophages overexpressing MCAD suppressed tumor growth in mouse models, supporting potential clinical applications for targeting the caspase-1/PPARγ/MCAD pathway in TAM differentiation and tumor progression. In addition to PPARs, liver X receptors (LXRs) are also receptors activated by lipids. Duyun Ye group (Huazhong University of Science and Technology) demonstrated the involvement of formyl peptide receptor-2 (FPR2, also termed lipoxin-A_4 receptor ALX) in tumorigenesis (Li et al., 2011). They observed that FPR2 activation by structurally distinct agonists regulated polarization of macrophages and tumor microenvironment, identifying FPR2 as an appreciable pleiotropic regulator role in tumor immunoediting. 20-Hydroxyeicosatetraenoic acid (20-HETE), a novel lipid mediator and 20-HETE-producing enzymes of cytochrome P450 (CYP) 4A families contribute to tumor growth and angiogenesis. Jing Yang group (Wuhan University) studied the correlations between CYP4A expression in TAMs and clinical outcome of patients with invasive breast carcinoma or melanoma (Chen et al., 2017). They identified that CYP4A in TAMs initiated pre-metastatic niche formation and promoted metastasis in breast cancer and melanoma through cytokines such as TGF-β, SDF-1 and VEGF. Mechanistically, CYP4A/20-HETE induced polarization of macrophages via STAT3 signaling. Their findings suggested that CYP4A may serve as a potential target for prevention and treatment of metastasis.

Several studies also report on implications of amino acids metabolism for functional reprogramming of the TAMs. Limin Zheng group (Sun Yat-sen University) focused on the regulatory mechanisms of indoleamine-2,3-dioxygenase (IDO), a rate-limiting enzyme for tryptophan catabolism, in TAMs (Zhao et al., 2012). They found that IDO selectively expressed at high levels in macrophages in situ in several types of human solid tumors induced by IFN-γ producing $CD69^+$ T cells. Upon encountering autologous T cells, TAMs produced IL-12 to activate T cells, which in turn led to IDO expression and promoted tumor progression.

In summary, current evidence in the literature has clearly demonstrated that metabolism plays a powerful role in defining the functions of myeloid cells. Different tissues provide signals which influence the nature of metabolic reprogramming and thereby adjust the function of resident myeloid cells. Undoubtedly, understanding how myeloid cells metabolically adapt to distinct tissues may allow new tissue-specific therapeutics to control immune responses and restore homeostasis.

3. Mucosal immunity and metabolism

Surface tissues of the body such as skin and gastrointestinal tract directly interface with the external environment, and are periodically exposed to pathogens including bacteria, fungi, viruses and parasites. In addition, these tissues also continuously encounter indigenous communities of commensal microorganisms. Thus, surface tissues are faced with the enormous challenges of maintaining homeostasis with the complex commensal species while constraining pathogen invasion. To cope with these microbial threats, epithelium acts as the first layer of physical barrier segregating microbiota from intestinal tissues. In addition, mucus and a diverse arsenal of antimicrobial proteins (AMPs), produced by epithelial cells, cover epithelial surfaces and limit the activities of microorganisms, thereby preventing microorganisms from disseminating into systemic infections (Gallo & Hooper, 2012; Perez-Lopez, Behnsen, Nuccio, & Raffatellu, 2016). The epithelial cells, mucus layer and immune cells residing in the gut constitute the intestinal mucosal barrier that is important for providing the defense against infections and maintaining intestinal homeostasis.

In addition to their barrier functions, the intestinal epithelial cells (IECs) are also essential for sensing nutritional fluctuations and regulating host metabolism. Metabolic programs and immune defense are evolutionarily integrated to ensure proper immune responses under various stress conditions, yet how these systems are coordinated at the intestinal surface is still not fully understood. Such integration also attracts Chinese immunologists' attention and they have undertaken studies to shed new light on the interactions between epithelial defense and metabolism in recent years.

AMPs are natural antibiotics and play an essential role in protecting host against infections through directly killing or inhibiting activities of microorganisms. Given the critical role of AMPs in host defense, the expression, secretion and maturation of AMPs are tightly controlled by multiple regulatory mechanisms. For example, the production of some AMPs such as Reg3 family is dependent on microbiota through IL-22-STAT3 signaling and the Toll-like receptor (TLR)-MyD88 axis (Mukherjee & Hooper, 2015), while whether AMP function is regulated by metabolism-related signals remains obscure. During the course of investigating intestinal mucosal immunity in response to nutrient fluctuations, Xiaoyu Hu's group found that many AMPs are significantly decreased such as Reg3 family and Saa1 during nutrient deprivation, while the anti-microbial peptide α-defensin is functionally sustained. Sustained α-defensin is due to the regulation of sustained defensin-processing enzyme matrix MMP7 by microbiota- and host-derived factors, which protects host against enteric pathogens during nutrient fluctuations. Furthermore, the expression of MMP7 is maintained by de-repression of the transcription activator Atoh1 upon attenuation of the transcriptional repressor Hes1 that is translationally regulated via mTOR signaling in IECs. The mTOR-Hes1-MMP7-α-defensin axis constitutes a regulatory loop that couples host nutrient status to epithelial antimicrobial immunity, which plays a vital role in maintaining proper mucosal immune functions under various nutritional conditions (Liang et al., 2019).

Not only can AMPs be regulated by metabolic programs but also are involved in modulation of host metabolism. Previous studies have shown that intestinal commensal microbes play an important role in regulating host metabolism by communicating with distant extra-intestinal organs while the mechanisms of the long-range crosstalk are not well understood (Schroeder & Backhed, 2016). It has been found that acetate, a bacterial metabolite, stimulates the vagus nerve to promote insulin secretion from pancreatic beta cells and to maintain glucose homeostasis (Perry et al., 2016), yet whether beta cells can directly sense microbial signaling molecules remains undefined. Zhihua Liu's group (Institute of Biophysics, Chinese Academy of Sciences) has found that the signals from commensal bacteria can be sensed directly in islet beta cells and modulate insulin distribution. Intestinal lysozyme from Paneth cells is required for releasing Nod1 ligands from commensal bacteria. Nod1 expressed in islet beta cells senses the intestine-derived Nod1 ligands and translocates to insulin granules. Activated Nod1 signaling recruits downstream Rip2 and Rab1a to drive insulin intracellular trafficking and promote insulin secretion. Furthermore, defects in the intestine-islet axis impair glucose tolerance via compromising glucose-stimulated insulin secretion (GSIS), which uncovers a physiological role of crosstalk between intestine and islets in promoting glucose homeostasis (Zhang et al., 2019).

The work from several Chinese groups also significantly contributed to our understanding of regulatory networks governing the expression of AMPs at tissue surface. IL-17A and IL-17F belong to the IL-17 family, which also includes IL-17B, IL-17C, IL-17D and IL-17E. IL-17A (also called IL17) and IL-17F are well-characterized cytokines contributing to the pathogenesis of a variety of autoimmune diseases and host defenses against extracellular pathogens (Gaffen, 2009). Furthermore, IL-17A or IL-17F acts with IL-22 to synergistically or additively induce AMPs in keratinocytes (Liang et al., 2006). Tuft cells-derived IL-17E (IL-25) initiates mucosal type 2 responses and promotes differentiation of tuft and goblet cells following infection with helminthes (Gerbe et al., 2016; Howitt et al., 2016; Jakob von Moltke, Ji, Liang, & Locksley, 2016). However, the roles of other members of the IL17 family in mucosal immunity are relatively poorly understood. Youcun Qian's group (Institute of Health Sciences, Chinese Academy of Sciences) has conducted a series of studies delineating the functions of IL-17 family cytokines in intestinal mucosal immunity and autoimmune inflammation. Qian's group has identified that IL-17C induces production of AMPs (S100A8/9, Lcn2 and Reg3β/γ) and inflammatory molecules through activating downstream IL-17RE-IL-17RA heterodimeric complex, which is important for host defense against bacterial infection. The orphan receptor IL-17RE is a functional receptor for IL-17C and is specifically required for IL-17C-mediated induction of genes. Because of the loss of IL-17C-mediated functions, IL-17RE deficient mice showed much lower expression of genes encoding antibacterial molecules, greater bacterial burdens, enhanced colon pathology and eventually mortality after *C. rodentium* infection. IL-17C, induced substantially in colonic epithelial cells (CECs) after challenge with *C. rodentium,* acts in concert with IL-22 to synergistically induce antibacterial peptides and plays an essential role in host mucosal immunity to intestinal pathogens (Song et al., 2011). In the following studies, Qian's group found that IL-17C is also involved in microbiota-mediated regulation of tumorigenesis. A dysregulated microbiota drives the upregulation of IL-17C specifically in IECs through

Toll-like receptor (TLR)-MyD88 dependent signaling during intestinal tumorigenesis. IL-17C in turn promotes intestinal tumor development by protecting IECs from apoptosis, which demonstrated that the microbiota can mediate cancer pathogenesis through the regulation of IL-17C (Song et al., 2014).

In addition to being induced by IL17C-IL17RE axis in CECs, the expression of AMPs can also be directly triggered by the damage of epidermal structures through releasing STA-2 from *C. elegans* hemidesmosomes (CeHDs) (Zhang, Li, et al., 2015). Previous studies showed that epidermis actively responds to wounding and infection via eliciting epidermal innate defense and inflammation. For example, upon sterile mechanical wounding of the skin, human and *Caenorhabditis elegans* can trigger an innate immune response, which results in elevated production of AMPs by epidermal cells (Pujol et al., 2008; Sorensen et al., 2006). However, the links between architectural damage and epidermal innate immune defense are not fully understood. The *C. elegans* epidermis provides an excellent model for understanding innate defense of the epithelial tissue, in which G protein signaling, p38-MAPK signaling, and STA-2 are all required for induction of the AMPs after mechanical wounding (Dierking et al., 2011; Ziegler et al., 2009). However, what are the signals produced by epidermal physical injury and how they can be recognized by innate immune system are still unclear. Huimin Zhang's group (Soochow University) utilized *C. elegans* epidermis as the model system and found that CeHDs are involved in the damage-induced innate immune response. The apical CeHD receptor MUP-4 tethers STA-2 protein and localizes it to CeHD attachment structures at the apical membrane under normal conditions. When the epidermis is structurally disturbed by internal or external insults, the apical CeHDs are disintegrated and lose the restriction upon STA-2 function and eventually activate the production of AMPs. The association between hemidesmosomes and STA-2 enables the epidermis to sense the stable adhesion structures and to quickly respond to extensive physical damage, efficiently triggering innate defense machinery (Zhang, Li, et al., 2015).

Paneth cells, located at the base of small intestinal crypts, play a critical role in maintaining the function of epithelial barrier by synthesizing and secreting substantial quantities of AMPs including α-defensin, Reg3 family, lysozyme and others. Dysfunction of Paneth cells contributes to the pathogenesis of inflammatory bowel disease (IBD) (Clevers & Bevins, 2013). Within Paneth cells, the AMPs are sorted after synthesis into specialized secretary granules called dense core vesicles (DCVs) while the mechanisms by which cargos are selectively sorted and transported into DCVs in mammalian cells are not fully understood. Zhihua Liu's group discovered that the symbiotic bacteria direct the DCV cargo-sorting process of lysozyme, which results in lysozyme secretion in Paneth cells rather than degradation. Nod2 is responsible for sensing commensal microbiota and recruits LRRK2 that participates in cargo-sorting by recruiting Rab2a onto the DCV surface. Rab2a, as a binding partner of LRRK2, is required for lysozyme sorting in Paneth cells. Furthermore, LRRK2 deficiency causes a specific deprivation of lysozyme in Paneth cells and lrrk2$^{-/-}$ mice are more susceptible to intestinal *Listeria monocytogenes* infection, which indicates that the lysozyme sorting directed by commensal bacteria through NOD2-LRRK2-Rab2a axis is important in controlling intestinal infection (Zhang, Pan, et al., 2015).

The innate host defense helps maintain intestinal homeostasis and fight against enteropathogens by forming a chemical barrier that segregates the bacteria from host epithelium to limit tissue inflammation and microbial translocation (Peterson & Artis, 2014). However, the host defense factors can also become important contributors to pathogenesis when exploited by pathogens. Epithelial adhesion is a crucial early event for intestinal colonization and invasion in the pathogenesis of many enteropathogens. Most enterobacteria use fimbriae, an adhesive filamentous organelle, while how *Shigella*, lacking of such adhesion machinery, invades the epithelium and elicits inflammation with low infectious inoculum is unclear. Wuyuan Lu (Xi'an Jiaotong University) discovered that *Shigella* targets human enteric α-defensin 5 (HD5), an abundant host protective AMP produced by Paneth cells, to augment its colonization and infectivity through interactions with multiple bacterial membrane proteins (Xu et al., 2018). The study uncovers an unusual mechanism that microbial pathogen subverts innate host defense through exploiting host components to colonize and destroy the intestinal epithelium. Similarly, MMP-10, previously known as an MMP that protects against pathogens, has a pro-colonization and pro-inflammatory role in *Helicobacter pylori* (*H. pylori*) infection (Lv et al., 2019). MMP-10 produced by gastric epithelial cells in response to infection protects against pathogens and also can contribute to pathology in infectious diseases (Kassim et al., 2007). However, the regulation, function, and clinical relevance of MMP-10 during *H. pylori* infection are unknown. Yuan Zhuang's group (The Third Military Medical University) found that MMP-10 is induced in gastric epithelial cells by *H. pylori* and interleukin-22 (IL-22) via the extracellular signal-regulated kinase (ERK) pathway. Increased MMP-10 promotes CD8^{+} T migration and accumulation via

CXCL16, and inhibits the expression of Reg3a, epithelial cadherin (E-cadherin) and zonula occludens-1 (ZO-1) that impairs host defense and promotes *H. pylori* colonization. Moreover, MMP-10$^{-/-}$, IL-22$^{-/-}$, and MMP-10$^{-/-}$ IL-22$^{-/-}$ mice showed effectively reduced gastric inflammation during *H. pylori* infection when compared to that in WT mice, which identified a previously unrecognized role for MMP-10 on the nature of infection (Lv et al., 2019).

In summary, it is getting clearer that the interactions between mucosal immunity and metabolism play an essential role in mucosal homeostasis and metabolic adaptions under various stress conditions while the mechanisms need to be further unraveled.

4. Concluding remarks

Despite of the tremendous progresses in the field of immunometabolism thanking to the efforts of scientists including those based in China, there remain critical unanswered questions and daunting challenges. For example, what are the metabolic profiles of innate immune cells in vivo within tissue microenvironments? How do innate immune cells from the same origins metabolically adapt to various tissue niches? Do metabolic features of the innate immune cells alter during the developmental and aging processes? What are the contributions of metabolites from commensal microbes residing in organs including but not limited to intestines? Are the observations obtained with animal models applicable to humans and if so, how do we utilize this knowledge to treat patients with metabolism and immune-related disorders? The future may appear capricious and unpredictable yet one predictable fact is that scientists in China will continue to make contributions to enrich our understanding of metabolic regulation of innate immune responses.

References

Bronte, V., & Zanovello, P. (2005). Regulation of immune responses by L-arginine metabolism. *Nature Reviews. Immunology*, *5*, 641–654.

Caputa, G., Castoldi, A., & Pearce, E. J. (2019). Metabolic adaptations of tissue-resident immune cells. *Nature Immunology*, *20*, 793–801.

Chen, X. W., Yu, T. J., Zhang, J., Li, Y., Chen, H. L., Yang, G. F., et al. (2017). CYP4A in tumor-associated macrophages promotes pre-metastatic niche formation and metastasis. *Oncogene*, *36*, 5045–5057.

Clevers, H. C., & Bevins, C. L. (2013). Paneth cells: Maestros of the small intestinal crypts. *Annual Review of Physiology*, *75*, 289–311.

Dierking, K., Polanowska, J., Omi, S., Engelmann, I., Gut, M., Lembo, F., et al. (2011). Unusual regulation of a STAT protein by an SLC6 family transporter in *C. elegans* epidermal innate immunity. *Cell Host & Microbe*, *9*, 425–435.

Du, L., Lin, L., Li, Q., Liu, K., Huang, Y., Wang, X., et al. (2019). IGF-2 preprograms maturing macrophages to acquire oxidative phosphorylation-dependent anti-inflammatory properties. *Cell Metabolism*, *29*, 1363–1375.e1368.

Erkelens, M. N., & Mebius, R. E. (2017). Retinoic acid and immune homeostasis: A balancing act. *Trends in Immunology*, *38*, 168–180.

Fortes, G. B., Alves, L. S., de Oliveira, R., Dutra, F. F., Rodrigues, D., Fernandez, P. L., et al. (2012). Heme induces programmed necrosis on macrophages through autocrine TNF and ROS production. *Blood*, *119*, 2368–2375.

Gaffen, S. L. (2009). Structure and signalling in the IL-17 receptor family. *Nature Reviews. Immunology*, *9*, 556–567.

Gallo, R. L., & Hooper, L. V. (2012). Epithelial antimicrobial defence of the skin and intestine. *Nature Reviews. Immunology*, *12*, 503–516.

Geeraerts, X., Bolli, E., Fendt, S. M., & Van Ginderachter, J. A. (2017). Macrophage metabolism as therapeutic target for cancer, atherosclerosis, and obesity. *Frontiers in Immunology*, *8*, 289.

Gerbe, F., Sidot, E., Smyth, D. J., Ohmoto, M., Matsumoto, I., Dardalhon, V., et al. (2016). Intestinal epithelial tuft cells initiate type 2 mucosal immunity to helminth parasites. *Nature*, *529*, 226–230.

Guo, C., Xie, S., Chi, Z., Zhang, J., Liu, Y., Zhang, L., et al. (2016). Bile acids control inflammation and metabolic disorder through inhibition of NLRP3 inflammasome. *Immunity*, *45*, 944.

Howitt, M. R., Lavoie, S., Michaud, M., Blum, A. M., Tran, S. V., Weinstock, J. V., et al. (2016). Tuft cells, taste-chemosensory cells orchestrate parasite type 2 immunity in the gut. *Science*, *351*, 1329–1333.

Jakob von Moltke, J., Ji, M., Liang, H. E., & Locksley, R. M. (2016). Tuft-cell-derived IL-25 regulates an intestinal ILC2-epithelial response circuit. *Nature*, *529*, 221–225.

Ji, L., Zhao, X., Zhang, B., Kang, L., Song, W., Zhao, B., et al. (2019). Slc6a8-mediated creatine uptake and accumulation reprogram macrophage polarization via regulating cytokine responses. *Immunity*, *51*, 272–284.e277.

Kassim, S. Y., Gharib, S. A., Mecham, B. H., Birkland, T. P., Parks, W. C., & McGuire, J. K. (2007). Individual matrix metalloproteinases control distinct transcriptional responses in airway epithelial cells infected with Pseudomonas aeruginosa. *Infection and Immunity*, *75*, 5640–5650.

Kazankov, K., Jorgensen, S. M. D., Thomsen, K. L., Moller, H. J., Vilstrup, H., George, J., et al. (2019). The role of macrophages in nonalcoholic fatty liver disease and nonalcoholic steatohepatitis. *Nature Reviews. Gastroenterology & Hepatology*, *16*, 145–159.

Li, Y., Cai, L., Wang, H., Wu, P., Gu, W., Chen, Y., et al. (2011). Pleiotropic regulation of macrophage polarization and tumorigenesis by formyl peptide receptor-2. *Oncogene*, *30*, 3887–3899.

Liang, S., Guo, X. K., Ou, J., Huang, R., Xue, Q., Zhang, B., et al. (2019). Nutrient sensing by the intestinal epithelium orchestrates mucosal antimicrobial defense via translational control of Hes1. *Cell Host & Microbe*, *25*, 706–718.e707.

Liang, S. C., Tan, X. Y., Luxenberg, D. P., Karim, R., Dunussi-Joannopoulos, K., Collins, M., et al. (2006). Interleukin (IL)-22 and IL-17 are coexpressed by Th17 cells and cooperatively enhance expression of antimicrobial peptides. *The Journal of Experimental Medicine*, *203*, 2271–2279.

Liu, G., Bi, Y., Xue, L., Zhang, Y., Yang, H., Chen, X., et al. (2015). Dendritic cell SIRT1-HIF1α axis programs the differentiation of CD4+ T cells through IL-12 and TGF-β1. *Proceedings of the National Academy of Sciences of the United States of America*, *112*, E957–E965.

Liu, D., Chang, C., Lu, N., Wang, X., Lu, Q., Ren, X., et al. (2017). Comprehensive proteomics analysis reveals metabolic reprogramming of tumor-associated macrophages stimulated by the tumor microenvironment. *Journal of Proteome Research*, *16*, 288–297.

Liu, N., Luo, J., Kuang, D., Xu, S., Duan, Y., Xia, Y., et al. (2019). Lactate inhibits ATP6V0d2 expression in tumor-associated macrophages to promote HIF-2α-mediated tumor progression. *The Journal of Clinical Investigation*, *129*, 631–646.

Liu, Y., You, Y., Lu, Z., Yang, J., Li, P., Liu, L., et al. (2019). N (6)-methyladenosine RNA modification-mediated cellular metabolism rewiring inhibits viral replication. *Science*, *365*, 1171–1176.

Liu, J., Zhang, X., Chen, K., Cheng, Y., Liu, S., Xia, M., et al. (2019). CCR7 chemokine receptor-inducible lnc-Dpf3 restrains dendritic cell migration by inhibiting HIF-1α-mediated glycolysis. *Immunity*, *50*, 600–615.e615.

Luo, W., Xu, Q., Wang, Q., Wu, H., & Hua, J. (2017). Effect of modulation of PPAR-gamma activity on Kupffer cells M1/M2 polarization in the development of non-alcoholic fatty liver disease. *Scientific Reports*, *7*, 44612.

Lv, Y. P., Cheng, P., Zhang, J. Y., Mao, F. Y., Teng, Y. S., Liu, Y. G., et al. (2019). Helicobacter pylori-induced matrix metallopeptidase-10 promotes gastric bacterial colonization and gastritis. *Science Advances*, *5*, eaau6547.

McNelis, J. C., & Olefsky, J. M. (2014). Macrophages, immunity, and metabolic disease. *Immunity*, *41*, 36–48.

Miao, H., Ou, J., Peng, Y., Zhang, X., Chen, Y., Hao, L., et al. (2016). Macrophage ABHD5 promotes colorectal cancer growth by suppressing spermidine production by SRM. *Nature Communications*, *7*, 11716.

Mu, X., Shi, W., Xu, Y., Xu, C., Zhao, T., Geng, B., et al. (2018). Tumor-derived lactate induces M2 macrophage polarization via the activation of the ERK/STAT3 signaling pathway in breast cancer. *Cell Cycle*, *17*, 428–438.

Mukherjee, S., & Hooper, L. V. (2015). Antimicrobial defense of the intestine. *Immunity*, *42*, 28–39.

Munn, D. H., & Mellor, A. L. (2016). IDO in the tumor microenvironment: Inflammation, counter-regulation, and tolerance. *Trends in Immunology*, *37*, 193–207.

Munoz-Planillo, R., Kuffa, P., Martinez-Colon, G., Smith, B. L., Rajendiran, T. M., & Nunez, G. (2013). K(+) efflux is the common trigger of NLRP3 inflammasome activation by bacterial toxins and particulate matter. *Immunity*, *38*, 1142–1153.

Netea-Maier, R. T., Smit, J. W. A., & Netea, M. G. (2018). Metabolic changes in tumor cells and tumor-associated macrophages: A mutual relationship. *Cancer Letters*, *413*, 102–109.

Niu, Z., Shi, Q., Zhang, W., Shu, Y., Yang, N., Chen, B., et al. (2017). Caspase-1 cleaves PPARγ for potentiating the pro-tumor action of TAMs. *Nature Communications*, *8*, 766.

Nomura, M., Liu, J., Rovira, I. I., Gonzalez-Hurtado, E., Lee, J., Wolfgang, M. J., et al. (2016). Fatty acid oxidation in macrophage polarization. *Nature Immunology*, *17*, 216–217.

Ohh, M., Park, C. W., Ivan, M., Hoffman, M. A., Kim, T. Y., Huang, L. E., et al. (2000). Ubiquitination of hypoxia-inducible factor requires direct binding to the beta-domain of the von Hippel-Lindau protein. *Nature Cell Biology*, *2*, 423–427.

O'Neill, L. A., & Pearce, E. J. (2016). Immunometabolism governs dendritic cell and macrophage function. *Journal of Experimental Medicine*, *213*, 15–23.

Ozcan, U., Cao, Q., Yilmaz, E., Lee, A. H., Iwakoshi, N. N., Ozdelen, E., et al. (2004). Endoplasmic reticulum stress links obesity, insulin action, and type 2 diabetes. *Science*, *306*, 457–461.

Perez-Lopez, A., Behnsen, J., Nuccio, S. P., & Raffatellu, M. (2016). Mucosal immunity to pathogenic intestinal bacteria. *Nature Reviews. Immunology*, *16*, 135–148.

Perry, R. J., Peng, L., Barry, N. A., Cline, G. W., Zhang, D., Cardone, R. L., et al. (2016). Acetate mediates a microbiome-brain-beta-cell axis to promote metabolic syndrome. *Nature, 534*, 213–217.

Peterson, L. W., & Artis, D. (2014). Intestinal epithelial cells: Regulators of barrier function and immune homeostasis. *Nature Reviews. Immunology, 14*, 141–153.

Pujol, N., Cypowyj, S., Ziegler, K., Millet, A., Astrain, A., Goncharov, A., et al. (2008). Distinct innate immune responses to infection and wounding in the *C. elegans* epidermis. *Current Biology, 18*, 481–489.

Qin, W., Qin, K., Zhang, Y., Jia, W., Chen, Y., Cheng, B., et al. (2019). S-glycosylation-based cysteine profiling reveals regulation of glycolysis by itaconate. *Nature Chemical Biology, 15*, 983–991.

Rooks, M. G., & Garrett, W. S. (2016). Gut microbiota, metabolites and host immunity. *Nature Reviews. Immunology, 16*, 341–352.

Schneider, C., Nobs, S. P., Kurrer, M., Rehrauer, H., Thiele, C., & Kopf, M. (2014). Induction of the nuclear receptor PPAR-gamma by the cytokine GM-CSF is critical for the differentiation of fetal monocytes into alveolar macrophages. *Nature Immunology, 15*, 1026–1037.

Schroeder, B. O., & Backhed, F. (2016). Signals from the gut microbiota to distant organs in physiology and disease. *Nature Medicine, 22*, 1079–1089.

Schulthess, J., Pandey, S., Capitani, M., Rue-Albrecht, K. C., Arnold, I., Franchini, F., et al. (2019). The short chain fatty acid butyrate imprints an antimicrobial program in macrophages. *Immunity, 50*, 432–445.e437.

Shan, B., Wang, X., Wu, Y., Xu, C., Xia, Z., Dai, J., et al. (2017). The metabolic ER stress sensor IRE1α suppresses alternative activation of macrophages and impairs energy expenditure in obesity. *Nature Immunology, 18*, 519–529.

Shang, S., Ji, X., Zhang, L., Chen, J., Li, C., Shi, R., et al. (2019). Macrophage ABHD5 suppresses NF-κB-dependent matrix metalloproteinase expression and cancer metastasis. *Cancer Research, 79*, 5513–5526.

Shi, L., Chen, X., Zang, A., Li, T., Hu, Y., Ma, S., et al. (2019). TSC1/mTOR-controlled metabolic-epigenetic cross talk underpins DC control of CD8+ T-cell homeostasis. *PLoS Biology, 17*, e3000420.

Song, X., Gao, H., Lin, Y., Yao, Y., Zhu, S., Wang, J., et al. (2014). Alterations in the microbiota drive interleukin-17C production from intestinal epithelial cells to promote tumorigenesis. *Immunity, 40*, 140–152.

Song, X., Zhu, S., Shi, P., Liu, Y., Shi, Y., Levin, S. D., et al. (2011). IL-17RE is the functional receptor for IL-17C and mediates mucosal immunity to infection with intestinal pathogens. *Nature Immunology, 12*, 1151–1158.

Sorensen, O. E., Thapa, D. R., Roupe, K. M., Valore, E. V., Sjobring, U., Roberts, A. A., et al. (2006). Injury-induced innate immune response in human skin mediated by trans-activation of the epidermal growth factor receptor. *The Journal of Clinical Investigation, 116*, 1878–1885.

Stienstra, R., Netea-Maier, R. T., Riksen, N. P., Joosten, L. A. B., & Netea, M. G. (2017). Specific and complex reprogramming of cellular metabolism in myeloid cells during innate immune responses. *Cell Metabolism, 26*, 142–156.

Svedberg, F. R., Brown, S. L., Krauss, M. Z., Campbell, L., Sharpe, C., Clausen, M., et al. (2019). The lung environment controls alveolar macrophage metabolism and responsiveness in type 2 inflammation. *Nature Immunology, 20*, 571–580.

Van den Bossche, J., O'Neill, L. A., & Menon, D. (2017). Macrophage immunometabolism: Where are we (going)? *Trends in Immunology, 38*, 395–406.

Wang, C., Guan, Y., Lv, M., Zhang, R., Guo, Z., Wei, X., et al. (2018). Manganese increases the sensitivity of the cGAS-STING pathway for double-stranded DNA and is required for the host defense against DNA viruses. *Immunity, 48*, 675–687.e677.

Wen, Z., Liu, H., Li, M., Li, B., Gao, W., Shao, Q., et al. (2015). Increased metabolites of 5-lipoxygenase from hypoxic ovarian cancer cells promote tumor-associated macrophage infiltration. *Oncogene*, *34*, 1241–1252.

Williams, N. C., & O'Neill, L. A. J. (2018). A Role for the Krebs cycle intermediate citrate in metabolic reprogramming in innate immunity and inflammation. *Frontiers in Immunology*, *9*, 141.

Xia, Y., Xie, Y., Yu, Z., Xiao, H., Jiang, G., Zhou, X., et al. (2018). The mevalonate pathway is a druggable target for vaccine adjuvant discovery. *Cell*, *175*, 1059–1073.e1021.

Xiang, W., Shi, R., Kang, X., Zhang, X., Chen, P., Zhang, L., et al. (2018). Monoacylglycerol lipase regulates cannabinoid receptor 2-dependent macrophage activation and cancer progression. *Nature Communications*, *9*, 2574.

Xie, M., Yu, Y., Kang, R., Zhu, S., Yang, L., Zeng, L., et al. (2016). PKM2-dependent glycolysis promotes NLRP3 and AIM2 inflammasome activation. *Nature Communications*, *7*, 13280.

Xu, D., Liao, C., Zhang, B., Tolbert, W. D., He, W., Dai, Z., et al. (2018). Human enteric alpha-defensin 5 promotes Shigella infection by enhancing bacterial adhesion and invasion. *Immunity*, *48*, 1233–1244.e1236.

Yang, M., Ma, C., Liu, S., Shao, Q., Gao, W., Song, B., et al. (2010). HIF-dependent induction of adenosine receptor A2b skews human dendritic cells to a Th2-stimulating phenotype under hypoxia. *Immunology and Cell Biology*, *88*, 165–171.

Yang, M., Ma, C., Liu, S., Sun, J., Shao, Q., Gao, W., et al. (2009). Hypoxia skews dendritic cells to a T helper type 2-stimulating phenotype and promotes tumour cell migration by dendritic cell-derived osteopontin. *Immunology*, *128*, e237–e249.

Yang, S., Zhao, Y., Yu, J., Fan, Z., Gong, S. T., Tang, H., et al. (2019). Sugar alcohols of polyol pathway serve as alarmins to mediate local-systemic innate immune communication in drosophila. *Cell Host & Microbe*, *26*, 240–251.e248.

Ye, H., Zhou, Q., Zheng, S., Li, G., Lin, Q., Wei, L., et al. (2018). Tumor-associated macrophages promote progression and the Warburg effect via CCL18/NF-kB/VCAM-1 pathway in pancreatic ductal adenocarcinoma. *Cell Death & Disease*, *9*, 453.

Yu, X., Buttgereit, A., Lelios, I., Utz, S. G., Cansever, D., Becher, B., et al. (2017). The cytokine TGF-beta promotes the development and homeostasis of alveolar macrophages. *Immunity*, *47*, 903–912.e904.

Yu, W., Wang, Z., Zhang, K., Chi, Z., Xu, T., Jiang, D., et al. (2019). One-carbon metabolism supports S-adenosylmethionine and histone methylation to drive inflammatory macrophages. *Molecular Cell*, *75*, 1147–1160.e1145.

Zhang, W., Li, Q., Li, D., Li, J., Aki, D., & Liu, Y. C. (2018). The E3 ligase VHL controls alveolar macrophage function via metabolic-epigenetic regulation. *The Journal of Experimental Medicine*, *215*, 3180–3193.

Zhang, Y., Li, W., Li, L., Li, Y., Fu, R., Zhu, Y., et al. (2015). Structural damage in the *C. elegans* epidermis causes release of STA-2 and induction of an innate immune response. *Immunity*, *42*, 309–320.

Zhang, Z., Li, J., Zheng, W., Zhao, G., Zhang, H., Wang, X., et al. (2016). Peripheral lymphoid volume expansion and maintenance are controlled by gut microbiota via $RALDH^+$ dendritic cells. *Immunity*, *44*, 330–342.

Zhang, Q., Pan, Y., Yan, R., Zeng, B., Wang, H., Zhang, X., et al. (2015). Commensal bacteria direct selective cargo sorting to promote symbiosis. *Nature Immunology*, *16*, 918–926.

Zhang, Q., Pan, Y., Zeng, B., Zheng, X., Wang, H., Shen, X., et al. (2019). Intestinal lysozyme liberates Nod1 ligands from microbes to direct insulin trafficking in pancreatic beta cells. *Cell Research*, *29*, 516–532.

Zhang, Z., Zhang, F., An, P., Guo, X., Shen, Y., Tao, Y., et al. (2011). Ferroportin1 deficiency in mouse macrophages impairs iron homeostasis and inflammatory responses. *Blood*, *118*, 1912–1922.

Zhao, Q., Kuang, D. M., Wu, Y., Xiao, X., Li, X. F., Li, T. J., et al. (2012). Activated CD69+ T cells foster immune privilege by regulating IDO expression in tumor-associated macrophages. *Journal of Immunology*, *188*, 1117–1124.

Zhu, L., Yang, T., Li, L., Sun, L., Hou, Y., Hu, X., et al. (2014). TSC1 controls macrophage polarization to prevent inflammatory disease. *Nature Communications*, *5*, 4696.

Ziegler, K., Kurz, C. L., Cypowyj, S., Couillault, C., Pophillat, M., Pujol, N., et al. (2009). Antifungal innate immunity in *C. elegans*: PKCdelta links G protein signaling and a conserved p38 MAPK cascade. *Cell Host & Microbe*, *5*, 341–352.

CHAPTER SIX

Regulation of MHC class I-independent NK cell education by SLAM family receptors

Shasha Chen*, Dan Li, Yuande Wang, Qiaozhen Li, Zhongjun Dong*
School of Medicine and Institute for Immunology, Beijing Key Lab for Immunological Research on Chronic Diseases, Tsinghua University, Beijing, China
*Corresponding authors: e-mail address: css0206@mail.tsinghua.edu.cn; dongzj@mail.tsinghua.edu.cn

Contents

Abstract

Seven members of signaling lymphocytic activation molecule (SLAM) family receptors (SFRs) are ubiquitously expressed on hematopoietic cells and they play critical roles in immune cell differentiation and activation. The engagement of these receptors transmits intracellular signaling mainly by recruiting SLAM-associated protein (SAP) and its related adaptors, EWS-FLI1-activated transcript-2 (EAT-2) and EAT-2-related transducer (ERT). The critical roles of SFRs and SAP-family adaptors are highlighted by the discovery that SAP is mutated in human X-linked lymphoproliferative (XLP1) disease in which the contact between T and B cells in germinal center and cytotoxic lymphocytes (NK cells and CD8$^+$ T cells) function are severely compromised. These immune defects are closely associated with the defective antibody production and the high incidence of lymphoma in the patients with XLP1. In addition to these well-known functions,

Advances in Immunology, Volume 145
ISSN 0065-2776
https://doi.org/10.1016/bs.ai.2019.11.006

SLAM-SAP family is involved in NK cell education, a process describing NK cell functional competence. In this chapter, we will mainly discuss these unappreciated roles of SAP-dependent and SAP-independent SFR signaling in regulating MHC-I-independent NK cell education.

Human X-linked lymphoproliferative (XLP) is a severe primary immunodeficiency, which is generally characterized by a fatal response to infection with the Epstein-Barr virus (EBV). This disease can be divided into two kinds, XLP1 and XLP2. XLP1 is caused by the genetic mutation in *SH2D1A,* while XLP2 is caused by the deficiency of X-linked inhibitor of apoptosis protein (XIAP, encoded by *BIRC4*). There are three main clinical symptoms in XLP1 disease, that is, fulminant infectious mononucleosis, B-cell lymphomas (in 30% of XLP1 patients) and defective antibody production. The XLP1 disease-causing gene *SH2D1A* encodes signaling lymphocytic activation molecule (SLAM)-associated protein (SAP), an adaptor protein that is recruited to SFRs. Using mice lacking SAP or SFRs, a few recent studies have disclosed that the XLP1 symptoms are highly associated with the defective immune responses in natural killer (NK) cell cytotoxicity, $CD8^{+}$ T cell activation and humoral immunity. However, many other discoveries have also highlighted the important roles of SFRs and SAP in regulating the development and functional maturation of innate immune cells. Here we will mainly introduce the unappreciated roles of SLAM-SAP family molecules in NK cell education, a process designated as NK cell functional competence.

1. SLAM family receptors

1.1 SLAM family receptors are self-ligands

There are seven SFR members, that is, SLAMF1 (SLAM), SLAMF2 (CD48), SLAMF3 (Ly9), SLAMF4 (2B4), SLAMF5 (CD84), SLAMF6 (Ly108 in mouse; NKT-B-antigen (NTB-A) in human), and SLAMF7 (CD2-like receptor activating cytotoxic cells, CRACC). All the genes encoding SFRs are closely linked and positioned in chromosome 1. These receptors are widely but solely expressed on hematopoietic lineage cells. For examples, SLAM was ubiquitously expressed on T cells, B cells, NK cells, macrophages, dendritic cells (DCs), and platelets. Intriguingly, SLAM is frequently used as a marker of hematopoietic stem cells (HSCs) (Kiel et al., 2005; Oguro, Ding, & Morrison, 2013). Ly9 is also abundant in all lymphoid and myeloid cells.

In contrast, 2B4 distribution is mainly limited to NK cells and part of activated $CD8^+$ T cells (Angulo, Cuenca, Martinez-Vicente, & Engel, 2019; de la Fuente et al., 2001; Hagberg et al., 2013; Romero et al., 2004). The expression profile of other SFR members refer to Table 1 (Cannons, Tangye, & Schwartzberg, 2011; Romero, Sintes, & Engel, 2014).

SFRs are type I transmembrane glycoproteins. This family are also assigned to CD2 superfamily immunoglobulin that typically consist of an N-terminal Ig-like V-type (IgV) domain and a single C-terminal Ig-like C2-type (IgC) domain, with one exception that Ly9 possesses four Ig-like domains that bearing two tandem repeats of the IgV-IgC set (Angulo et al., 2019). IgV domain determines the specificity of SFR recognition. Interestingly, SFR members are self-ligands, that is, they recognize themselves (Table 1). For examples, Ly9 mutations at the amino acids glutamic acid 27 (E^{27}), E^{29} or arginine 89 (R^{89}) will disrupt the homophilic interaction, whereas the arginine44-to-alanine ($R^{44}A$) mutation plays a contrast role (Romero et al., 2005). The highly polymorphic ligand-binding domains of Ly9 suggests the variability of favored selection and functions (Limaye et al., 2008). By contrast, CRACC is a glycosylated self-ligand receptor (Ishibashi et al., 2018; Postelnek et al., 2016).

There is one exception that 2B4 binds to CD48, which is widely expressed on nearly all hematopoietic cells but not mouse neutrophils and a subpopulation of long-term HSC (LT-HSC) (McArdel, Terhorst, & Sharpe, 2016). CD48 is a glycosylphosphatidylinositol (GPI) linked protein and the soluble form has been detected in human serum, especially the patients with EBV infection, arthritis, leukemia or lymphoma (Cabrero, Freeman, Lane, & Reiser, 1993; Calpe et al., 2008; Smith, Biggs, Norris, Anderson-Stewart, & Ward, 1997). CD48 can bind to both 2B4 and CD2. However, by using nuclear magnetic resonance analyses, it has been shown that the FG-loop of 2B4 is dynamically disordered but might be stabilized by the binding of CD48 which is different from CD2 (Ames, Vyas, Lusin, & Mariuzza, 2005; Wang et al., 1999). The affinity of CD48 binding to 2B4 is higher than CD48 binding to CD2 both in mouse and human, whereas CD58, sharing homology with CD48, binding with higher affinity to CD2 comparing to CD48 (Arulanandam et al., 1993; Brown et al., 1998; Davis & van der Merwe, 1996; Dustin, Sanders, Shaw, & Springer, 1987; McArdel et al., 2016; Sandrin, Mouhtouris, Vaughan, Warren, & Parish, 1993; van der Merwe et al., 1994). After binding with 2B4 or CD2, CD48 itself appears to be no signal. Thus, whether CD48 is considered as a member of SFRs is largely debatable.

Table 1 SLAM family members and the downstream signal transduction pathways.

Members	Synonym	Ligand	ITSM	Tyrosine sites in ITSM	Expression	Effectors
SLAMF1	CD150 SLAM	SLAMF1	Human: 3 Mouse: 3	Human: Y^{281}, Y^{327} Mouse: Y^{281}, Y^{327}	HSC, T, B, NK, NKT, Macrophages, DC, platelets	SAP, EAT-2, SHIP-1, SHP-1, SHP-2, Fyn, Lck, Dok1, PKC-θ, Akt
SLAMF2	CD48	None	None	None	Widely expressed on hematopoietic cells (except of mouse neutrophils and subpopulation of LT-HSC)	LAT
SLAMF3	CD229 Ly9	SLAMF3	Human: 2 Mouse: 2	Human: Y^{603}, Y^{626} Mouse: Y^{587}, Y^{624}	Thymocytes, T, B, NK, macrophages, DC	SAP, EAT-2, Fyn, SHP-2, Lck, ERK, AP2, Grb2
SLAMF4	CD244 2B4	SLAMF2	Human: 4 Mouse: 4	Human: Y^{266}, Y^{292}, Y^{312}, Y^{337} Mouse: Y^{266}, Y^{325}, Y^{344}, Y^{369}	Activated $CD8^+$ T cells, NK, monocytes, basophils, eosinophils, DCs and mast cells in mouse but not human	SAP, EAT-2, Fyn, Lck, LAT, PI3K, Vav1, SHIP-1, Cb1, ERK, p38, SHP-1, SHP-2
SLAMF5	CD84	SLAMF5	Human: 2 Mouse: 2	Human: Y^{262}, Y^{299} Mouse: Y^{265}, Y^{300}	NK, NKT, T, B, monocytes, DC, eosinophils, neutrophils, platelets	SAP, EAT-2, SHP-1, SHP-2, SHIP-1, Csk, DoK1, Cb1
SLAMF6	CD352 NTB-A (human) Ly108 (mouse)	SLAMF6	Human: 2 Mouse: 2	Human: Y^{294}, Y^{308} Mouse: Y^{294}, Y^{318}	NK, NKT, T, B, DC, eosinophils, neutrophils	Fyn, Lck, PLC-γ, PI3K, SHP-1, Cb1, Vav1
SLAMF7	CD319 CS1 CRACC	SLAMF7	Human: 2 Mouse: 2	Human: Y^{284} Mouse: Y^{302}	NK, NKT, population of T, activated B and DC, myeloma cells	Fyn, Lck, PLC-γ, Vav1, PI3K

Abbreviations: HSC: hematopoietic stem cells; T: T cells; B: B cells; NK: nature killer cells; NKT: nature killer T cells; DC: dendritic cells; SAP: SLAM-associated protein; EAT-2: Ewing's sarcomas EWS/FLI1 activated transcript-2; ERT: EAT-2-related transducer; SHIP: SH2-containing inositol polyphosphate 5-phosphatase; SHP-1/2: SH2 domain-containing phosphatase 1/2; Fyn and Lck: Src family kinases; Dok1: docking protein 1; PKC-θ: protein kinase C θ; Akt: RAC-alpha serine/threonine-protein kinase; LAT: linker for activated T cells; ERK: extracellular signal-regulated kinase; Grb2: growth factor receptor bound protein 2; PI3K: phosphatidylinositol 3-kinase; Vav-1: Vav guanine nucleotide exchange factor 1; Cb1: casitas B-lineage lymphoma; Csk: COOH-terminal Src kinase; PLC-γ: phospholipase C-γ.

Theoretically, this unique homotypic self-recognition mediated by SFRs and their ubiquitous expression on hematopoietic cells will increase the opportunity to contact-dependent cell communications, such as NKT cell selection in thymus, T-B cell contact in germinal center and NK cell recognition of hematopoietic targets.

1.2 SLAM family receptor signaling

1.2.1 SAP-family-dependent SFR signaling

SFR members contain two to four the cytoplasmic immune-tyrosine switch motifs (ITSMs) (TxYxxI/V, "x" denotes any amino acid) in their cytoplasmic domains. Akin to immune-tyrosine activation motif (ITAM) and immune-tyrosine inhibitory motif (ITIM), ITSMs are able to recruit Src homology 2 domain (SH2)-containing molecules. The homophilic engagement of SFRs transmits intracellular signaling mainly by recruiting SAP and its related adaptors EAT-2 and ERT. These three adaptors share highly amino acid similarity. All of them have only one SH2 domain that can bind to the ITSMs of SFRs.

SAP can be detected in T cells, NK cells, NKT cells, platelets, eosinophils, but not in neutrophils, monocytes, or monocyte-derived dendritic cells (Table 2). It is controversial whether SAP is expressed in B cells. SAP could be detected in a minor population of human B cells (Morra et al., 2005), but not in activated B cells (Nagy et al., 2000). Despite this, genetic study has clearly demonstrated that SAP in B cells is not essential for humoral immunity (Veillette et al., 2008).

Table 2 SAP-related adaptors.

Adaptor	Gene	Binding of SFRs	Association	Expression
SAP	Human: *SH2D1A* Mouse: *Sh2d1a*	SLAMF 1,3,4,5,6,7	Fyn, PKC-θ, Lyn, β-PIX, NCK1, Fgr	T, B (?), NK, NKT, platelets, eosinophils
EAT-2	Human: *SH2D1B* Mouse: *Sh2d1b*	SLAMF 1,3,4,5,7	Hck, Lyn, Lck, Fyn, Fgr	NK, DC, macrophages, activated mast cells, resting $CD8^+$ T cells and B cells
ERT	Mouse: *Sh2d1c*	SLAM 1,4	Hck, Lyn, Lck, Fyn, Fgr	NK, $CD8^+$ T cells (mouse)

Abbreviations: SAP: SLAM-associated protein; EAT-2: Ewing's sarcomas EWS/FLI1 activated transcript-2; ERT: EAT-2-related transducer; T: T cells; B: B cells; NK: nature killer cells; NKT: nature killer T cells; DC: dendritic cells; Fyn, Fgr, Lyn Lck and Hck: Src family tyrosine kinase; PKC-θ: protein kinase C θ; NCK1: non-catalytic region of tyrosine kinase adaptor protein 1.

The tyrosine phosphorylation of ITSMs is essential for the recruitment of SAP. Indeed, SAP can bind with high affinity to the ITSMs in many SFRs, such as SLAM, Ly9, CD84 and Ly108, whereas with low or no binding affinity to the cytoplasmic tail of CRACC. There are some patients with XLP1 carrying an arginine 55-to-leucine ($R^{55}L$) mutation in the SAP SH2 domain. Although this mutation does not affect the abundance of SAP, it prevents its binding to the tyrosine-phosphorylated ITSMs of SFRs (Cannons et al., 2010; Chan et al., 2003; Latour et al., 2003; Li et al., 2003). Given that ITSMs are not exclusively expressed in SFRs, it is debatable whether SAP is required for the signaling emanated from other ITSM-containing receptors, such as programmed cell death 1 (PD1) and Siglec-family receptors (Crocker & Varki, 2001; Sharpe & Pauken, 2018).

In addition to binding with SFRs, the SH2 domain of SAP functions as a signaling molecule that recruits many downstream Src family kinases after SAP is engaged with SFRs. In particular, SAP can recruit kinase Fyn via the interaction of its SH2 domain with the SH3 domain of Fyn. The amino acid arginine 78 (R^{78}) in SAP and aspartic acid 100 (D^{100}) in Fyn are essential for this process. Fyn-mediated phosphorylation is important for a serial of biological processes, such as T cell activation and NK cell cytotoxicity (Bloch-Queyrat et al., 2005; Davidson et al., 2004). Although SAP can bind to kinase Lck in vitro, this interaction and its physiological function remains unclear (Simarro et al., 2004). Parallel to T cells, the association between SAP and kinase Lyn was detected in B cells (Li et al., 2008), although it is controversial whether SAP is present in B cells.

In addition to the conventional insight of SAP binding to Src family kinases, SAP can also recruit protein kinase C (PKC)-θ in a R^{78}-dependent manner but independent of R^{55} or tyrosine phosphorylation (Cannons et al., 2010). SAP is able to associate with the SH3 domain of β PAK-interacting protein (PIX), a guanine nucleotide exchange factor specific for Rac/Cdc42 GTPase. Similarly, this association is R^{78}-dependent and related to the activation of nuclear factor of activated T-cells (NFAT) (Gu et al., 2006). A high affinity of SAP binding with Fgr and NCK1 was observed, whereas the ability of SH3 domains of Src, Abl and Crk to bind with SAP is relatively very weak (Li, Schibli, & Li, 2009). Collectively, the specific functions mediated by SAP may largely depend on the expression and affinity of those downstream binding protein in multiple immune cell types.

Although SAP, EAT-2 and ERT can bind to most cytoplasmic tails of SFR members and they frequently trigger positive signaling, the affinity of those binding proteins is different and thereby indicating the possible competitive roles. Although EAT-2 and ERT share sequence homology with SAP, distinct features have been observed. EAT-2 can be recruited by the ITSMs of several SFR members, such as SLAM, Ly9, CD84 and CRACC. However, the affinity of EAT-2 binding to these ITSMs are different to SAP binding. Particularly, SAP, rather than EAT-2, can bind to the non-phosphorylated ITSMs (Morra, Lu, et al., 2001). EAT-2 can bind to the ITSMs of CRACC with higher affinity comparing to SAP. ERT, a pseudo gene in human but expressed in mouse, is able to bind to cytoplasmic tail of 2B4 in mouse NK cells and $CD8^+$ T cells. ERT can also bind to SLAM and facilitate its tyrosine phosphorylation by Src kinases (Calpe et al., 2006). Unlike SAP, EAT-2 and ERT do not contain R78-based motif and are unable to recruit Fyn (Veillette, 2006). Alternatively, EAT-2, and probably ERT, exert their downstream signaling function by their C-terminal tail tyrosine phosphorylation, and it further recruits PLC-γ (Clarkson & Brown, 2009; Cruz-Munoz, Dong, Shi, Zhang, & Veillette, 2009; Roncagalli et al., 2005). The interaction of EAT-2 or ERT with Hck, Lyn, Lck and Fyn occur via their kinase domains, rather than their SH3 domain (Calpe et al., 2006).

1.2.2 SAP-family-independent signaling

Except for SAP-family adaptors, SFRs are also capable of coupling other SH2 domain phosphatases, including SH2 domain-containing phosphatase-1 (SHP-1), SH2 domain-containing phosphatase-2 (SHP-2) and SH2 domain-containing inositol polyphosphate 5-phosphatase 1 (SHIP-1) (Dong et al., 2012; Eissmann et al., 2005; Parolini et al., 2000; Tangye et al., 1999). Presumably, the diversity of those SH2 domain-containing binding partners allows SFRs to initiate different downstream signals. The recruitment of SAP-family molecules usually leads to an active signal, while the usage of SH2-domian phosphatase frequently delivers an inhibitory signal. It is largely unknown whether the net signaling mediated by SFRs is determined by a balance between the activating SAP-family adaptors and the inhibitory phosphatases. Thus, the expression profile of these binding partners will partly decide the feature of SLAM family, which may explain why the nature of same SFRs is different in various immune cells.

Biochemical studies clearly show that SAP-family adaptor molecules are preferentially bound to the ITSMs of SFRs. Thus, SAP might function as a natural blocker in a competitive way, leading to the disassociation of those inhibitory phosphatases from SFRs. Despite this, SAP itself shows short biological half-life (Morra, Simarro-Grande, et al., 2001; Okamoto et al., 2004), suggesting that the action of SAP is also dynamic and transient. This could be interpreted as an evolutionary advantage of the natural blocker functions of SAP to be more effective to maintain the balance of positive and negative processes. Indeed, the lack of SAP will result in an exacerbation of deficiency comparing to the disruption of SFRs (Chen et al., 2017;Eissmann et al., 2005; Kageyama et al., 2012; Pahima, Puzzovio, & Levi-Schaffer, 2019; Yigit, Wang, Herzog, & Terhorst, 2019).

Because the tyrosine phosphorylation of SFRs depends on SAP-mediated activating signaling. The ternary complex of SLAM-SAP-Fyn axis can promote the phosphorylation of cytoplasmic domain of SLAM and further result in the recruitment of SHIP-1 (Latour et al., 2001), implying the signaling of SFRs is very complex. Sequential recruitment of downstream SH2 domain-containing molecules will endow the signaling by SFRs more accurate spatially and temporally.

1.3 SAP-independent SLAM family signaling in the patients with XLP1

While three SAP-family adaptors are allowed to associate with the cytoplasmic tail of SFRs, only the deficiency of SAP in human leads to severe immune defects. The deficiency of EAT-2 or ERT is never reported in human. Mice lacking EAT-2 and ERT did not exhibit any XLP1-like symptoms (Roncagalli et al., 2005). These studies strongly suggest that SAP is a very critical regulator of many immune processes. There are multiple immune defects observed in the patients with XLP1 or SAP-deficient mice. In particular, SAP deficiency severely compromises the contact of follicular T helper (Tfh) cells with B cells in germinal center, which leads to long-term immune defects in humoral immunity (Qi, Cannons, Klauschen, Schwartzberg, & Germain, 2008). This defect certainly associates with the high incidence of recurrence of EBV infection. It seems to be a gain of SAP-independent SFR inhibitory signaling that suppresses the entrance of Tfh cells into germinal center at least in mice (Chen et al., 2017). It remains to investigate whether a blockage of this inhibitory signal would alleviate the defective antibody production in the patients with XLP1.

In addition, SAP deficiency impairs the cytotoxicity of $CD8^+$ T lymphocytes, a subset of T cells responsible for clearance of virally infected cells (including malignant cells) in an antigen-dependent manner. Thus, the impaired $CD8^+$ T cell function will lead to the high sensibility to EBV infection and EBV-related B-cell lymphoma in the patients with XLP1. Until now, how the loss of SAP decreases $CD8^+$ T cell function remains elusive. On the one hand, SAP deficiency will at least cause a loss of SAP-dependent SFR signaling, or SFRs become inhibitory when SAP is absent in $CD8^+$ T cells. Further study needs to investigate these two possibilities. It will be helpful for the correction of defective $CD8^+$ T cell-mediated antiviral and antitumor immunity, a major defect in the patients with XLP1. On the other hand, a new subset of cytotoxic $CD8^+$ T cells in the follicular was recently designated as follicular cytotoxic T cells (Tfc) (Yu & Ye, 2018), parallel to Tfh cells. Whether SAP deficiency dampens this particular subset of T cells in the follicular region needs further investigation.

In addition to these two defects in adaptive immunity described above, SAP deficiency also gives rise to the defective innate immunity. In the following, we will focus on how SLAM family receptors and SAP-family adaptors regulate NK cell functional acquisition.

2. Regulation of NK cell education by SLAM family receptors

NK cells have the ability to eliminate neoplastic cells and virus-infected cells. Activation of NK cells are tightly controlled by the dynamic equilibrium between the signaling of an array of germline-encoded activation and inhibitory receptors. NK cells express all SFRs except SLAM, and all SAP-family adaptors (Chen et al., 2016; Lee et al., 2004; Perez-Quintero et al., 2014; Wu et al., 2016). SLAM family-mediated homotypic interactions are critical to enhancing NK cell activation against the allogeneic hematopoietic cells and play important roles in NK cell-mediated immunosurveillance of hematopoietic malignancy (Benoit, Wang, Pabst, Dutz, & Tan, 2000; Bottino et al., 2001; Dong et al., 2009; Nakajima et al., 2000; Parolini et al., 2000). Engagement of SFRs between NK cells and hematopoietic targets trigger very complicated signaling that gives rise to distinct NK cell responses. Studies from XLP1 patients and SAP-family-deficient mice uncovered that the ability of SFRs to influence NK cell function is tightly regulated by the presence of SAP-family adaptors.

SAP-family adaptors secure SFR-mediated NK cell activation via dual mechanism. First, SAP-family proteins function as active signaling molecules that link SFRs to specific intracellular biochemical signals. SAP couples

SFRs to Fyn, by a way of a direct interaction between the arginine 78 (R^{78}) in the SH2 domain of SAP and the SH3 domain of Fyn (Chan et al., 2003; Chen et al., 2004; Latour et al., 2003). This association triggers Vav-1 phosphorylation and activation, leading to PLC-γ-mediated Ca^{2+} flux directly or indirectly, augmenting conjugate formation between NK cells and hematopoietic target cells (Chen et al., 2004; Chuang, Kumaresan, & Mathew, 2001; Dong et al., 2012). Unlike SAP, EAT-2 does not possess an R^{78}-based motif, EAT-2 associates with PLC-γ through a direct interaction between phosphorylated Tyr^{127} in the C-terminal tail of EAT-2 and the N-terminal SH2 domain of PLC-γ, which evokes calcium flux and Erk activation, leading to NK cell granule polarization (Perez-Quintero et al., 2014; Tassi & Colonna, 2005). The complementary roles of SAP-family adaptors permit SFRs to mediate a broader range of signals and effects to promote the efficiency at activating NK cells.

Except for the signaling property, SAP-family adaptors can also function as "natural blocker" to prevent the recruitment of the SH2 domain-containing inhibitory molecules, such as SHIP-1, SHP-1 and SHP-2, by either through competing with the same ITSMs or through occupancy hindrance (Dong et al., 2012; Eissmann et al., 2005; Tangye et al., 1999). In the absence of SAP-family adaptors, these inhibitory molecules, such as SHIP-1, preferentially bind to SFRs, linking SFRs to the inhibitory cascade, which strongly suppresses CD16 or natural killer group 2D (NKG2D)-mediated activating signaling to restriction of NK cell activation, as occurs in NK cells from SAP-mutated XLP1 patients (Benoit et al., 2000; Dong et al., 2012; Parolini et al., 2000).

This dual activity of SFRs in NK cell activation has extensively been elaborated in our recent review (Chen & Dong, 2019). In addition to this classical role of SFRs in NK cell activation, SFRs are involved in NK cell education in the physiological conditions (Chen et al., 2016; Meazza et al., 2017; Wu et al., 2016).

2.1 Classical MHC-I mediated NK cell education

NK cells bear potent effector mechanisms to kill target cells. To avoid inadvertent attack against self, NK cells must maintain the ability to discriminate signatures of self. The ubiquitously expressed major histocompatibility complex class I (MHC-I) molecules, termed H-2 antigens in mice and human leukocyte antigens (HLA) in humans, are recognized by NK cells as makers of self (Ljunggren & Karre, 1990). NK cell tolerance was achieved through the receptors that can sense the signature of self-MHC-I. Thus, NK cells have a serial of non-rearranged receptors for the purpose, Ly49-family receptors in mice and killer cell immunoglobulin-like receptors (KIRs) in human. In essence, if NK cells lack self-MHC-I specific inhibitory receptors, they would be uninhibited and cause auto-reactivity. However, when either those inhibitory receptors or MHC-I is absent, NK cells become hyporesponsiveness (Belanger et al., 2012). Therefore, except for induction of immune tolerance, self-MHC-I specific inhibitory receptors play an additional role for NK cell functional maturation, a process termed as education or licensing.

The basis for the concept of NK cell education comes from distinguish of the functional relationship between Ly49 inhibitory receptors and host MHC-I molecule in mice. Expression of a single MHC-I molecule selectively educates functional activity of NK cells with a cognate inhibitory receptor (Kim et al., 2005). The positive effect of both human and mouse NK cells increases quantitatively with each additional inhibitory receptor encountering to self-MHC-I molecules (Brodin, Lakshmikanth, Johansson, Karre, & Hoglund, 2009; Johansson et al., 2005; Joncker, Fernandez, Treiner, Vivier, & Raulet, 2009; Yu et al., 2007). In contrast, NK cells from MHC-deficient hosts, such as β microglobulin (β2m)-deficient mice and transporter associated with antigen processing 1 (TAP1)-deficient patients are hypofunctional in spite of bearing the inhibitory receptors (Furukawa et al., 1999; Liao, Bix, Zijlstra, Jaenisch, & Raulet, 1991). These non-educated NK cells from the MHC-I-deficient host placed in an MHC-I-sufficient setting re-attain functional competence, suggesting the non-educated NK cells can be re-educated, but the capacity is limited to the NK cells expressing an inhibitory receptor specific for a cognate host MHC-I molecule (Elliott, Wahle, & Yokoyama, 2010; Joncker, Shifrin, Delebecque, & Raulet, 2010). Furthermore, the educated NK cells lost their effector capabilities in an environment devoid of MHC-I molecules (Joncker et al., 2010). Thus, the continuous engagement of inhibitory receptors with MHC-I molecules is required to dictate NK cell responsiveness. The studies on human NK cells also show a similar observation that NK cells expressing an individual KIR specific for self-HLA display more robust cytokine production than the self-KIR-negative NK cells (Anfossi et al., 2006). The results from KIR and HLA-transgenic mice provide additional evidence supporting the concept that self-MHC-specific inhibitory receptors confer functional competence of human NK cells (Kim et al., 2008; Sola et al., 2009). Thus, NK cell education results in two types of self-tolerant NK cells, the functionally competent NK cells and the non-educated NK cells that do not express self-MHC-specific inhibitory receptors and thus are self-tolerance. The former subset will be suppressed during later effector phase by the same self-MHC-specific inhibitory receptors that originally conferred the process of education.

There is general consensus that self-MHC-I-specific inhibitory receptors deliver inhibitory signaling in the context of an effector response. These receptors exert their function by the signaling through the intracytoplasmic ITIMs. Upon the engagement with self-MHC-I, ITIMs undergo tyrosine phosphorylation, enabling them to recruit the tyrosine phosphatases SHP-1, or probably SHP-2 as well as SHIP-1 (Long, Kim, Liu, Peterson, & Rajagopalan, 2013; Nakamura et al., 1997; Wang et al., 2002). SHP-1 is the major mediator of the inhibitory function of self-MHC-I specific receptors at least in mouse NK cells. However, the inactivation of SHP-1 in mouse NK cells leads to NK cell hyporesponsiveness rather than hyperactivation (Viant et al., 2014). Thus, it is hypotheses that SHP-1 expression in NK cells is required for their functional competence. It is still difficult to reconcile the transmission of inhibitory to be a positive role in the context of education. It predicts that the signaling from an unidentified signaling motif guiding NK cell education. Recent study using the knock-in mice with a targeted loss-of-function mutation in the ITIM of Ly49A shows that both inhibition and education of NK cells require the signaling through the same ITIM (Bern et al., 2017). It is probably that ITIM can signal through distinct pathways in the setting of governing inhibition and education of NK cells. Indeed, except for the recruitment of tyrosine phosphatases that might counteract kinases activity downstream of many activation receptors, the inhibitory receptor signaling plays a key role in ensuring the self-tolerance of NK cells by the confinement of activating receptors to the plasma membrane (Guia et al., 2011). Alternatively, the inhibitory receptor signaling probably prevent NK cells from the sustained protein tyrosine kinase-dependent activation. Consistently, the absence of SHP-1 will give rise to an impairment of Ca^{2+} mobilization upon engagement of activating receptors, such as Ly49D or NKG2D, which maybe account for the desensitization of NK cells (Viant et al., 2014).

Certain inhibitory MHC-I receptors have the capacity to associate with the MHC-I molecules expressed by other cells (in *trans*) and by NK cell itself (in *cis*) (Scarpellino et al., 2007). The former plays a key role in NK cell education (Bessoles et al., 2013). Adoptive transfer of mature MHC-I-deficient

NK cells to MHC-I-sufficient WT hosts restore NK cell reactivity (Elliott et al., 2010; Joncker et al., 2010). Reciprocally, NK cells transferred from WT mice to MHC-I-deficient hosts present decreased responsiveness (Joncker et al., 2010). These findings support the critical role for *trans* interaction in shaping mouse NK cell education. Recent studies show that *cis* interaction also occurs through the same binding site as *trans* interaction of Ly49A (Doucey et al., 2004). *Cis* association sequesters the inhibitory receptors available for *trans* binding, lowering the threshold of NK cell activation, which is critical to optimal discrimination of target cells (Andersson, Williams, Davis, & Hoglund, 2007; Doucey et al., 2004). NK cells appear not to be properly educated when devoid of the *cis* interaction with MHC-I in a transgenic mouse model (Chalifour et al., 2009). Studies from a humanized mouse uncovered the contributions of HLA-I molecules presented both in *trans* from neighboring cells and in *cis* to human NK cell education, and the *cis* interaction is necessary to maintain education (Boudreau et al., 2016). Interestingly, in the context of stem cell transplantation or adoptive transfer of mature human NK cells, the uneducated donor NK cells can "acquire" cognate MHC-I molecules from host cells, leading NK cell education in *cis* to adjust NK cell reactivity (Boudreau et al., 2016).

2.2 Non-MHC-I mediated NK cell education: SFR inhibitory signaling

The inhibitory receptors specific for self-MHC-I predominantly convey the inhibitory signals guaranteeing NK cell effector inhibition and functional maturation. However, many other inhibitory receptors are also reported to be involved in NK cell education (He & Tian, 2017; Kumar & McNerney, 2005). This phenomenon is called non-MHC-I mediated NK cell education. As we have known that SFRs bear dual activity, which is largely determined by the presence of SAP-family adaptors. Therefore, in SAP family-deficient NK cells, nearly all of SFR members are inhibitory, which can substantially inhibit NK cell activation (Benoit et al., 2000; Bottino et al., 2001; Dong et al., 2009; Nakajima et al., 2000; Parolini et al., 2000; Tangye, Phillips, Lanier, & Nichols, 2000). Interestingly, similar to the MHC-I molecules that are ubiquitously expressed, SFRs as self-ligands are also widely distributed on hematopoietic cells. Thus, it was speculated that the hematopoietic cells might be qualified as NK cell educating cells via the engagement of SFR pairs.

As predicted, NK cell activation is much enhanced in mice lacking all of SAP-family adaptors when non-hematopoietic cells are used as targets.

SAP-family-deficient NK cells are also over activated when they are triggered through multiple activation receptors, including DNAM-1, NKp46, Ly49D and CD16 (Roncagalli et al., 2005; Wu et al., 2016). Thus, the SFR inhibitory signaling endows NK cell activation receptors with functional competence. Interestingly, akin to the scenario that self-MHC-I specific inhibitory receptors suppress NK cell effector function when encountering MHC-I matched self-cells, NK cells that are educated by SFRs will be inhibited when they are encountered the hematopoietic cells targets that bear SFR ligands. By contrast, it will be more responsive toward the targets that do not express SFR ligands. Indeed, although NK cells from the SAP-deficient human patients with XLP1 or SAP-deficient mice are not able to kill allogeneic hematopoietic target cells, they are more responsive to a wide range of non-hematopoietic target cells (Dong et al., 2009; Roncagalli et al., 2005; Wu et al., 2016). Hence, the SAP-independent SFR inhibitory signaling very likely set the threshold of NK cell responsiveness to non-hematopoietic cells.

It is largely undetermined whether NK cells are educated via SAP-independent SFR signaling in human. A limited clue shows that the extensive liver damage was observed in some of patients with XLP1 following EBV infection, suggesting that SAP-deficient NK cells that are unduly educated likely over-attack non-hematopoietic hepatocytes (Tangye, 2014; Veillette, Perez-Quintero, & Latour, 2013). We realize that this signal has the ability to educate NK cells only in the situation of SAP absence, it is hard to prove whether NK cell education relies on or are dedicatedly tuned by SFR inhibitory signaling in physiological condition.

The next question is which SFR members are involved in NK cell education. There are many SFR members on the NK cells. Among them, Ly108 displays a unique expression pattern. This receptor is highly expressed on the early-differentiated NK cells at least on the background of C57BL/6 mice. Especially, Ly108 is much more presented on the Ly49C/I-positive NK cells, which represent a subset of educated NK cells. In the mice devoid of SAP, Ly108 appears to be inhibitory, which endows increased NK cell responsiveness toward non-hematopoietic targets (Wu et al., 2016). In the patients with XLP1, 2B4-mediated inhibitory signaling seems to be involved in NK cell education and the effect appears even much pronounced in a proportion of NK cells lacking the self-MHC-I inhibitory KIRs (Meazza et al., 2017). As we know that all of SFRs will switch to be inhibitory in SAP-family-deficient NK cells, it is very puzzled why Ly108 and 2B4 are the only two receptors that can educate NK cells. It needs to further investigate which hematopoietic cells are the educating cells and where NK cells are educated by the engagement of SFR pairs. These answers may help to explain the specificity of Ly108 in NK cell education in mouse. It is speculated that Ly108 dictates NK cell education very likely occurring in the immature stage of NK cell development naturally when SAP is minimally expressed, whereas Ly108 is abundant.

NK cells are educated by SFRs only at SAP-deficient hosts and probably the early-differentiated NK cells, suggesting the SAP-independent signaling are involved in the process. During the effector phases, the engagement of 2B4 significantly induces the phosphorylation of SHIP-1, a lipid phosphatase that can dampen various activating signaling, such as MAPK, PI3K and Ca^{2+} flux. SHIP-1 is also involved during NK cell education (Gumbleton, Vivier, & Kerr, 2015). However, no evidence supports the notion that SHIP-1 is responsible for SFR-mediated NK cell education.

We previously revealed that simultaneous deletion of two phosphatases SHP-1 and SHP-2 could partially abolish 2B4-induced inhibitory signal. SHP-1 is also documented as a primary inhibitory molecule downstream Ly108 in T cells (Kageyama et al., 2012). Moreover, it is well-known that SHP-1 is critical to NK cell education mediated by the inhibitory receptors for self-MHC-I. SHP-1 is also identified as the downstream of Ly108 for NK cell education. Thus, Ly108 educates NK cells via SHP-1 in a mechanism analogous to that of Ly49-mediated education, leading to redistribution of positive molecules or dephosphorylation and inactivation of negative regulators, both of which result in enhanced proximal signaling of activating receptors (Wu et al., 2016). Ly108-mediated inhibitory signaling likely sets the threshold of NK cell responsiveness probably preceding the education by the inhibitory receptors for MHC-I. It also needs to test whether SFR inhibitory signaling is sufficient for NK cell education or this effect still relies on the presence of self-MHC-I educating signal. It is estimated that MHC-I-dependent signal is primary, while SFRs are second as co-receptors. We propose that SAP-independent SFR inhibitory signaling cooperates with self-MHC-I-dependent inhibitory signaling to tune the threshold of NK cell responsiveness (Fig. 1).

2.3 Self-specific activating receptor SLAM family in NK cell education

Given that MHC-dependent NK cell education occurs through the self-MHC-I specific inhibitory receptors, only the NK cells with the inhibitory receptors attain functional competence and maintain self-tolerance.

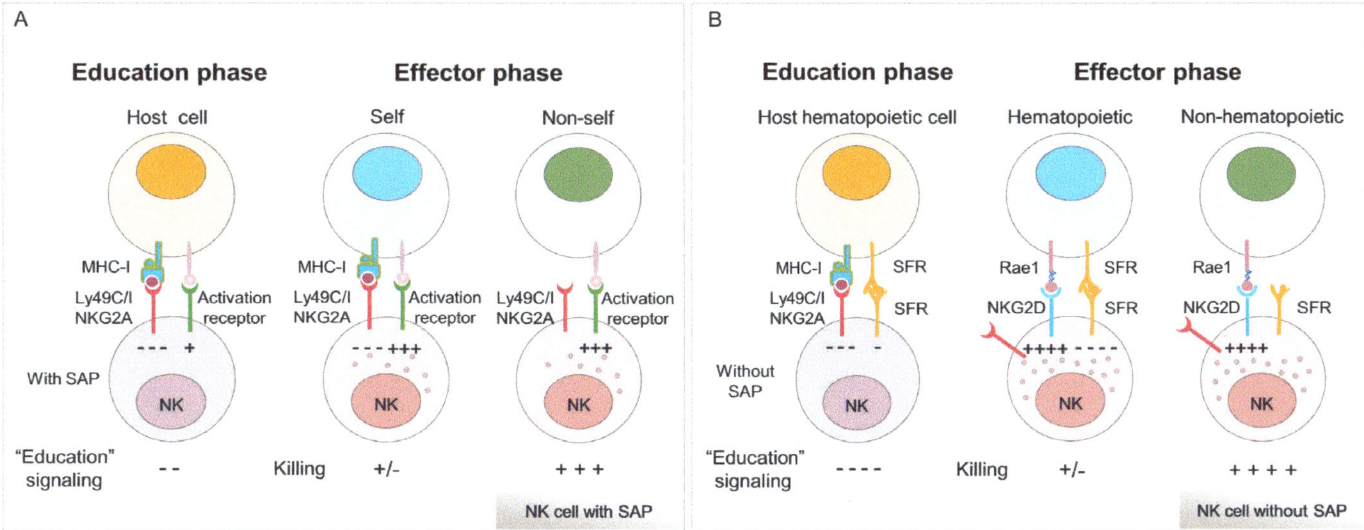

Fig. 1 Self-MHC-I-dependent inhibitory signaling and SAP-independent inhibitory SLAM family signaling in NK cell education. (A) Depicted is the physiological situation in the presence of SAP. During the education process, after engagement by the MHC class I (MHC-I) molecules on the host cells, the self-specific inhibitory receptors (such as Ly49C/I and/or NKG2A) for self-MHC-I deliver inhibitory signals that dominate NK cell education (left). During the effector phase, self-cells bearing moderate MHC-I molecules can elicit predominant inhibitory signals to prevent NK cell activation. Whereas cells display abnormal MHC-I molecules fail to engage inhibitory NK cell receptors, therefore, they are recognized as "non-self" and become susceptible to NK cell-mediated lysis through simultaneous activating signals (right). (B) Under the circumstances in the absence of SAP-family adaptors. During the education process, NK cells not only receive inhibitory signals from the self-specific inhibitory receptors, SFRs can also deliver the SAP-family-independent inhibitory signals when encounter the host hematopoietic cells, which has added effect to NK cell functional maturation (left). During the effector phase, akin to the scenario of self-MHC-specific inhibitory receptor mediated NK cell effector inhibition, when SAP-family-deficient NK cells encounter hematopoietic target cells with SLAM family ligands, the inhibitory signals from SFRs will repress the positive signaling emanates from primary activating receptors like NKG2D, leading to the suppression of NK cell activation. By contrast, non-hematopoietic cells cannot elicit SFRs-mediated inhibition, they are more susceptible to NK cell-mediated lysis due to the enhanced NK cell functional maturation (right).

However, the germline-encoded MHC-I-specific inhibitory receptors are expressed in a stochastic manner, acquisition of these receptors usually occurs after the expression of a series of NK cell activation receptors. Indeed, the NK cells lacking self-specific inhibitory receptors are detectable in MHC-sufficient hosts, but they are kept from autoreactive in spite of failing to recognize self (Anfossi et al., 2006; Fernandez et al., 2005).

It has proposed that NK cell express several activation receptors that are potentially specific for self-molecules, setting the threshold of NK cell responsiveness in the absence of the self-MHC-dependent inhibitory signaling to prevent inadvertent activation against normal tissues. NK cell desensitization can be induced by the sustained engagement of activation receptors. For examples, constitutive transgene expression of Rae1, a ligand for NKG2D, causes a reduced NK cell responsiveness to mismatched cells (Oppenheim et al., 2005). Similarly, the ability of Ly49H^{+} NK cells is reduced in mice with transgenic expression of m157, a mouse CMV (MCMV)-encoded protein specific for activation receptor Ly49H (Sun & Lanier, 2008; Tripathy et al., 2008). The responsiveness of human NK cells expressing activating KIR2DS1 is tune down when derived from the donors bearing its ligand, HLA-C2 (Fauriat, Ivarsson, Ljunggren, Malmberg, & Michaelsson, 2010). Thus, activation signaling probably induce NK cell anergy. Additional evidence comes from several mice lacking activating receptors. A loss-of-function mutation of NKp46 leads to NK cell hyperresponsiveness (Narni-Mancinelli et al., 2012). A modest increase in NK cell activity is found in NKG2D-deficient mice (Zafirova et al., 2009). In line with this finding, blockage of NKG2D by the soluble NKG2D ligands HLA class I chain-related A (MICA) results in enhanced NK cell responsiveness and tumor rejection (Deng et al., 2015). These data strongly support the speculation that the engagement of NK activating receptors, such as NKp46 and NKG2D, would lead to NK cell desensitization during NK cell functional maturation. However, the relevant ligands for NKp46 or NKG2D have not yet been discovered in healthy organisms. Thus, the limited number of NK cell receptors defined can directly recognize endogenous "self" ligands that are constitutively expressed on hematopoietic cells.

SFRs are self-ligands and widely expressed on hematopoietic cells, we proposed that these receptors very likely mediate the close contact between NK cells and other hematopoietic cells. The data from our studies show that SFR deficiency either on donor hematopoietic cells or recipient mice significantly enhanced the acceptance of transplantation, suggesting that SFRs act as the self-specific activation receptors in NK cell-mediated missing-self recognitions of allogenic hematopoietic cells, in particular hybrid resistance (Chen et al., 2016). However, SFR-deficient mice indeed exhibited an enhanced reactivity to hematopoietic cells. These data are very similar to that observed in mice lacking NKp46 or NKG2D. Thus, SFRs may be the first activating receptors that are involved in NK cell education by sensing the constitutively expressed ligands. The chronic engagement of activating signaling will tolerate NK cell activity, akin to T cell tolerance to self-antigens.

Although SFR-deficient mice exhibited the enhanced NK cell reactivity, SAP family-deficient NK cells were impaired. Due to the switch of SFR function, it is hard to test whether the downstream activating signaling by SAP-family adaptors is indeed involved in NK cell education. We know little about how SFRs regulates NK cell education.

SFR-deficient NK cells have an elevated expression of NKG2D and DNAM-1. This suggests that SFR signaling probably regulates the distribution of NK cell activation receptors to prevent the inadequate activation against normal cells (Guo et al., 2016). It is notable that an enhanced response is observed in NK cells lacking SFRs when triggered through some activation receptors, including NK1.1, Ly49D, NKG2D and CD16 (Chen et al., 2016; Guo et al., 2016). As an alternative mechanism, it could be proposed that sustained engagement of activation receptors induces cross-tolerance of multiple distinct NK cell activation pathways. It is plausible as the higher NK cell reactivity upon NK1.1 triggering is also detected in mice lacking NKp46 and NKG2D (Narni-Mancinelli et al., 2012; Zafirova et al., 2009). Along with these lines, continuous engagement of the activating Ly49H in vivo by m157 impairs NK cell activation upon stimulation with NK1.1 (Tripathy et al., 2008). The chronic exposure of NK cells to cell bound NKG2D ligands in vitro selectively dysfunction of several NK cell activation receptors, in this cases sustained NKG2D signaling seems preferentially to modulates cytoplasmic signaling downstream of Fc receptor γ (FcRγ), leading to cross-tolerance of FcRγ-dependent NK cell activation receptors, like CD16, NK1.1, and NKp46 (Coudert, Scarpellino, Gros, Vivier, & Held, 2008). In line with this notion, there is evidence for functional crosstalk in human NK cells, which is specifically occurs among certain natural cytotoxicity receptors (NCR), typically NKp46, NKp30 and NKp44 (Augugliaro et al., 2003).

2.4 An integrated education model

There are some clues that activation signaling influences the functional acquisition mediated by the self-MHC-I-specific inhibitory receptors. Notably, both the Ly49C$^+$ and Ly49C$^-$ cells from the Ly49H$^+$ subset in the m157-Tg mice are hypofunctional compared with the same NK cell subset of WT mice (Tripathy et al., 2008). Additionally, in m157-transgenic (m157-Tg) mice, Ly49H$^+$ NK cells that express self-specific inhibitory receptors for autologous MHC-I molecules exhibit comparable reactivity as their counterparts that lack an inhibitory receptor for MHC-I following activation receptor crosslinking (Tripathy et al., 2008). This has also been described in a human-based study, in which tuning down of the NK cell responsiveness by the activating receptor KIR2DS1 is apparent in cells lacking expression of inhibitory MHC-I-specific receptors, as well as those coexpressing these receptors (Fauriat et al., 2010). In line with those studies, SFRs reset NK cell responsiveness irrespective of expressing the self-MHC-I dependent inhibitory receptors. However, they differentially fine-tune NK cell subsets, the extent of which is negatively correlated with the expression levels of the self-MHC-I specific inhibitory receptors (Chen et al., 2016). Thus, the education of NK cells via self-specific activating receptors is a mechanism to secure tolerance that complements education via inhibitory self-MHC-I receptors.

In the end, we propose that NK cell education can be achieved by at least two distinct signals that are derived from self-MHC-I-specific inhibitory receptors and from self-specific activation receptors, respectively. Engagement of inhibitory receptors with cognate MHC-I molecules results in the generation of functional competence. On the contrary, the ligation of activating receptor with endogenous self-ligands leads to anergy. Both of opposite signals secure NK cell self-tolerance, whereas the fine balance between these two types of signaling will set the threshold of NK cell responsiveness, a process negatively related with the scenario of NK cell activation (Fig. 2).

3. Concluding remarks

Mutation of SAP in patients with XLP1 highlights the indispensable role of SFRs in humoral immunity and cytotoxic lymphocyte activation and NKT cell development. SFRs can transmit two different signaling,

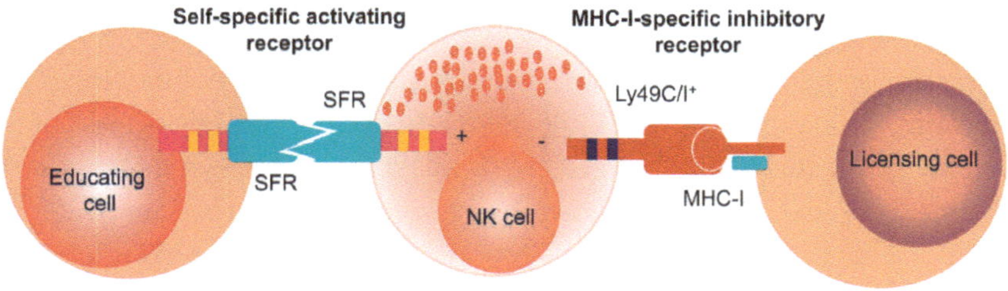

Fig. 2 Self-MHC-I-specific inhibitory receptors and self-specific activation receptors coordinately regulate NK cell education. NK cell education can be achieved by at least two distinct signals derived from self-MHC-I-specific inhibitory receptors and self-specific activation receptors (such as SFRs), engagement of inhibitory receptors by cognate MHC-I molecules result in the generation of the inhibitory signaling, on the contrary, activating receptor ligation by self-ligands leading to the generation of activation signaling, the fine balance between these two types of signaling will set the threshold of NK cell education.

SAP-dependent and SAP-independent. These two signals play the opposite roles at least in NK cell activation. Recent studies also reveal that SFRs are involved in NK cell education. SAP-independent SFR signaling seems to promote NK cell functional competence, while SFRs as self-specific activation receptors can desensitize NK cell responsiveness, a process akin to NK cell education. Further studies need to focus on how SFRs cooperate with self-specific inhibitory receptors during NK cell education. In particular, it remains elusive how the net signaling for NK cell education is balanced among self-MHC-I specific inhibitory signaling, SAP-dependent SLAM signaling and SAP-independent inhibitory signaling. These further investigations will expand our insight into MHC-I-independent NK cell education.

Acknowledgments

Work in the Dong's lab is supported by National Key Research & Developmental Program of China (to Z.D., 2018YFC1003900), Natural Science Foundation of China (to Z.D., 81725007, 31830027 and 31821003), Beijing Natural Science Foundation (to Z.D., 5172018) and Natural Science Foundation of China (to S.C., 81901671).

Competing financial interests

The authors declare no competing financial interests.

References

Ames, J. B., Vyas, V., Lusin, J. D., & Mariuzza, R. (2005). NMR structure of the natural killer cell receptor 2B4 (CD244): Implications for ligand recognition. *Biochemistry*, *44*, 6416–6423.

Andersson, K. E., Williams, G. S., Davis, D. M., & Hoglund, P. (2007). Quantifying the reduction in accessibility of the inhibitory NK cell receptor Ly49A caused by binding MHC class I proteins in cis. *European Journal of Immunology*, *37*, 516–527.

Anfossi, N., Andre, P., Guia, S., Falk, C. S., Roetynck, S., Stewart, C. A., et al. (2006). Human NK cell education by inhibitory receptors for MHC class I. *Immunity*, *25*, 331–342.

Angulo, A., Cuenca, M., Martinez-Vicente, P., & Engel, P. (2019). Viral CD229 (Ly9) homologs as new manipulators of host immunity. *Journal of Leukocyte Biology*, *105*, 947–954.

Arulanandam, A. R., Moingeon, P., Concino, M. F., Recny, M. A., Kato, K., Yagita, H., et al. (1993). A soluble multimeric recombinant CD2 protein identifies CD48 as a low affinity ligand for human CD2: Divergence of CD2 ligands during the evolution of humans and mice. *The Journal of Experimental Medicine*, *177*, 1439–1450.

Augugliaro, R., Parolini, S., Castriconi, R., Marcenaro, E., Cantoni, C., Nanni, M., et al. (2003). Selective cross-talk among natural cytotoxicity receptors in human natural killer cells. *European Journal of Immunology*, *33*, 1235–1241.

Belanger, S., Tu, M. M., Rahim, M. M., Mahmoud, A. B., Patel, R., Tai, L. H., et al. (2012). Impaired natural killer cell self-education and "missing-self" responses in Ly49-deficient mice. *Blood*, *120*, 592–602.

Benoit, L., Wang, X., Pabst, H. F., Dutz, J., & Tan, R. (2000). Defective NK cell activation in X-linked lymphoproliferative disease. *Journal of Immunology*, *165*, 3549–3553.

Bern, M. D., Beckman, D. L., Ebihara, T., Taffner, S. M., Poursine-Laurent, J., White, J. M., et al. (2017). Immunoreceptor tyrosine-based inhibitory motif-dependent functions of an MHC class I-specific NK cell receptor. *Proceedings of the National Academy of Sciences of the United States of America*, *114*, E8440–E8447.

Bessoles, S., Angelov, G. S., Back, J., Leclercq, G., Vivier, E., & Held, W. (2013). Education of murine NK cells requires both cis and trans recognition of MHC class I molecules. *Journal of Immunology*, *191*, 5044–5051.

Bloch-Queyrat, C., Fondaneche, M. C., Chen, R., Yin, L., Relouzat, F., Veillette, A., et al. (2005). Regulation of natural cytotoxicity by the adaptor SAP and the Src-related kinase Fyn. *The Journal of Experimental Medicine*, *202*, 181–192.

Bottino, C., Falco, M., Parolini, S., Marcenaro, E., Augugliaro, R., Sivori, S., et al. (2001). NTB-A [correction of GNTB-A], a novel SH2D1A-associated surface molecule contributing to the inability of natural killer cells to kill Epstein-Barr virus-infected B cells in X-linked lymphoproliferative disease. *The Journal of Experimental Medicine*, *194*, 235–246.

Boudreau, J. E., Liu, X. R., Zhao, Z., Zhang, A., Shultz, L. D., Greiner, D. L., et al. (2016). Cell-extrinsic MHC class I molecule engagement augments human NK cell education programmed by cell-intrinsic MHC class I. *Immunity*, *45*, 280–291.

Brodin, P., Lakshmikanth, T., Johansson, S., Karre, K., & Hoglund, P. (2009). The strength of inhibitory input during education quantitatively tunes the functional responsiveness of individual natural killer cells. *Blood*, *113*, 2434–2441.

Brown, M. H., Boles, K., van der Merwe, P. A., Kumar, V., Mathew, P. A., & Barclay, A. N. (1998). 2B4, the natural killer and T cell immunoglobulin superfamily surface protein, is a ligand for CD48. *The Journal of Experimental Medicine*, *188*, 2083–2090.

Cabrero, J. G., Freeman, G. J., Lane, W. S., & Reiser, H. (1993). Identification, by protein sequencing and gene transfection, of sgp-60 as the murine homologue of CD48. *Proceedings of the National Academy of Sciences of the United States of America*, *90*, 3418–3422.

Calpe, S., Erdos, E., Liao, G., Wang, N., Rietdijk, S., Simarro, M., et al. (2006). Identification and characterization of two related murine genes, Eat2a and Eat2b, encoding single SH2-domain adapters. *Immunogenetics*, *58*, 15–25.

Calpe, S., Wang, N., Romero, X., Berger, S. B., Lanyi, A., Engel, P., et al. (2008). The SLAM and SAP gene families control innate and adaptive immune responses. *Advances in Immunology*, *97*, 177–250.

Cannons, J. L., Tangye, S. G., & Schwartzberg, P. L. (2011). SLAM family receptors and SAP adaptors in immunity. *Annual Review of Immunology*, *29*, 665–705.

Cannons, J. L., Wu, J. Z., Gomez-Rodriguez, J., Zhang, J., Dong, B., Liu, Y., et al. (2010). Biochemical and genetic evidence for a SAP-PKC-theta interaction contributing to IL-4 regulation. *Journal of Immunology*, *185*, 2819–2827.

Chalifour, A., Scarpellino, L., Back, J., Brodin, P., Devevre, E., Gros, F., et al. (2009). A role for cis interaction between the inhibitory Ly49A receptor and MHC class I for natural killer cell education. *Immunity*, *30*, 337–347.

Chan, B., Lanyi, A., Song, H. K., Griesbach, J., Simarro-Grande, M., Poy, F., et al. (2003). SAP couples Fyn to SLAM immune receptors. *Nature Cell Biology*, *5*, 155–160.

Chen, S., Cai, C., Li, Z., Liu, G., Wang, Y., Blonska, M., et al. (2017). Dissection of SAP-dependent and SAP-independent SLAM family signaling in NKT cell development and humoral immunity. *The Journal of Experimental Medicine*, *214*, 475–489.

Chen, S., & Dong, Z. (2019). NK cell recognition of hematopoietic cells by SLAM-SAP families. *Cellular & Molecular Immunology*, *16*, 452–459.

Chen, R., Relouzat, F., Roncagalli, R., Aoukaty, A., Tan, R., Latour, S., et al. (2004). Molecular dissection of 2B4 signaling: Implications for signal transduction by SLAM-related receptors. *Molecular and Cellular Biology*, *24*, 5144–5156.

Chen, S., Yang, M., Du, J., Li, D., Li, Z., Cai, C., et al. (2016). The self-specific activation receptor SLAM family is critical for NK cell education. *Immunity*, *45*, 292–304.

Chuang, S. S., Kumaresan, P. R., & Mathew, P. A. (2001). 2B4 (CD244)-mediated activation of cytotoxicity and IFN-gamma release in human NK cells involves distinct pathways. *Journal of Immunology*, *167*, 6210–6216.

Clarkson, N. G., & Brown, M. H. (2009). Inhibition and activation by CD244 depends on CD2 and phospholipase C-gamma1. *The Journal of Biological Chemistry*, *284*, 24725–24734.

Coudert, J. D., Scarpellino, L., Gros, F., Vivier, E., & Held, W. (2008). Sustained NKG2D engagement induces cross-tolerance of multiple distinct NK cell activation pathways. *Blood*, *111*, 3571–3578.

Crocker, P. R., & Varki, A. (2001). Siglecs, sialic acids and innate immunity. *Trends in Immunology*, *22*, 337–342.

Cruz-Munoz, M. E., Dong, Z., Shi, X., Zhang, S., & Veillette, A. (2009). Influence of CRACC, a SLAM family receptor coupled to the adaptor EAT-2, on natural killer cell function. *Nature Immunology*, *10*, 297–305.

Davidson, D., Shi, X., Zhang, S., Wang, H., Nemer, M., Ono, N., et al. (2004). Genetic evidence linking SAP, the X-linked lymphoproliferative gene product, to Src-related kinase FynT in T(H)2 cytokine regulation. *Immunity*, *21*, 707–717.

Davis, S. J., & van der Merwe, P. A. (1996). The structure and ligand interactions of CD2: Implications for T-cell function. *Immunology Today*, *17*, 177–187.

de la Fuente, M. A., Tovar, V., Villamor, N., Zapater, N., Pizcueta, P., Campo, E., et al. (2001). Molecular characterization and expression of a novel human leukocyte cell-surface marker homologous to mouse Ly-9. *Blood*, *97*, 3513–3520.

Deng, W., Gowen, B. G., Zhang, L., Wang, L., Lau, S., Iannello, A., et al. (2015). Antitumor immunity. A shed NKG2D ligand that promotes natural killer cell activation and tumor rejection. *Science, 348*, 136–139.

Dong, Z., Cruz-Munoz, M. E., Zhong, M. C., Chen, R., Latour, S., & Veillette, A. (2009). Essential function for SAP family adaptors in the surveillance of hematopoietic cells by natural killer cells. *Nature Immunology, 10*, 973–980.

Dong, Z., Davidson, D., Perez-Quintero, L. A., Kurosaki, T., Swat, W., & Veillette, A. (2012). The adaptor SAP controls NK cell activation by regulating the enzymes Vav-1 and SHIP-1 and by enhancing conjugates with target cells. *Immunity, 36*, 974–985.

Doucey, M. A., Scarpellino, L., Zimmer, J., Guillaume, P., Luescher, I. F., Bron, C., et al. (2004). Cis association of Ly49A with MHC class I restricts natural killer cell inhibition. *Nature Immunology, 5*, 328–336.

Dustin, M. L., Sanders, M. E., Shaw, S., & Springer, T. A. (1987). Purified lymphocyte function-associated antigen 3 binds to CD2 and mediates T lymphocyte adhesion. *The Journal of Experimental Medicine, 165*, 677–692.

Eissmann, P., Beauchamp, L., Wooters, J., Tilton, J. C., Long, E. O., & Watzl, C. (2005). Molecular basis for positive and negative signaling by the natural killer cell receptor 2B4 (CD244). *Blood, 105*, 4722–4729.

Elliott, J. M., Wahle, J. A., & Yokoyama, W. M. (2010). MHC class I-deficient natural killer cells acquire a licensed phenotype after transfer into an MHC class I-sufficient environment. *The Journal of Experimental Medicine, 207*, 2073–2079.

Fauriat, C., Ivarsson, M. A., Ljunggren, H. G., Malmberg, K. J., & Michaelsson, J. (2010). Education of human natural killer cells by activating killer cell immunoglobulin-like receptors. *Blood, 115*, 1166–1174.

Fernandez, N. C., Treiner, E., Vance, R. E., Jamieson, A. M., Lemieux, S., & Raulet, D. H. (2005). A subset of natural killer cells achieves self-tolerance without expressing inhibitory receptors specific for self-MHC molecules. *Blood, 105*, 4416–4423.

Furukawa, H., Yabe, T., Watanabe, K., Miyamoto, R., Miki, A., Akaza, T., et al. (1999). Tolerance of NK and LAK activity for HLA class I-deficient targets in a TAP1-deficient patient (bare lymphocyte syndrome type I). *Human Immunology, 60*, 32–40.

Gu, C., Tangye, S. G., Sun, X., Luo, Y., Lin, Z., & Wu, J. (2006). The X-linked lymphoproliferative disease gene product SAP associates with PAK-interacting exchange factor and participates in T cell activation. *Proceedings of the National Academy of Sciences of the United States of America, 103*, 14447–14452.

Guia, S., Jaeger, B. N., Piatek, S., Mailfert, S., Trombik, T., Fenis, A., et al. (2011). Confinement of activating receptors at the plasma membrane controls natural killer cell tolerance. *Science Signaling, 4*, ra21.

Gumbleton, M., Vivier, E., & Kerr, W. G. (2015). SHIP1 intrinsically regulates NK cell signaling and education, resulting in tolerance of an MHC class I-mismatched bone marrow graft in mice. *Journal of Immunology, 194*, 2847–2854.

Guo, H., Cranert, S. A., Lu, Y., Zhong, M. C., Zhang, S., Chen, J., et al. (2016). Deletion of slam locus in mice reveals inhibitory role of SLAM family in NK cell responses regulated by cytokines and LFA-1. *The Journal of Experimental Medicine, 213*, 2187–2207.

Hagberg, N., Theorell, J., Schlums, H., Eloranta, M. L., Bryceson, Y. T., & Ronnblom, L. (2013). Systemic lupus erythematosus immune complexes increase the expression of SLAM family members CD319 (CRACC) and CD229 (LY-9) on plasmacytoid dendritic cells and CD319 on CD56(dim) NK cells. *Journal of Immunology, 191*, 2989–2998.

He, Y., & Tian, Z. (2017). NK cell education via nonclassical MHC and non-MHC ligands. *Cellular & Molecular Immunology, 14*, 321–330.

Ishibashi, M., Soeda, S., Sasaki, M., Handa, H., Imai, Y., Tanaka, N., et al. (2018). Clinical impact of serum soluble SLAMF7 in multiple myeloma. *Oncotarget*, *9*, 34784–34793.
Johansson, S., Johansson, M., Rosmaraki, E., Vahlne, G., Mehr, R., Salmon-Divon, M., et al. (2005). Natural killer cell education in mice with single or multiple major histocompatibility complex class I molecules. *The Journal of Experimental Medicine*, *201*, 1145–1155.
Joncker, N. T., Fernandez, N. C., Treiner, E., Vivier, E., & Raulet, D. H. (2009). NK cell responsiveness is tuned commensurate with the number of inhibitory receptors for self-MHC class I: The rheostat model. *Journal of Immunology*, *182*, 4572–4580.
Joncker, N. T., Shifrin, N., Delebecque, F., & Raulet, D. H. (2010). Mature natural killer cells reset their responsiveness when exposed to an altered MHC environment. *The Journal of Experimental Medicine*, *207*, 2065–2072.
Kageyama, R., Cannons, J. L., Zhao, F., Yusuf, I., Lao, C., Locci, M., et al. (2012). The receptor Ly108 functions as a SAP adaptor-dependent on-off switch for T cell help to B cells and NKT cell development. *Immunity*, *36*, 986–1002.
Kiel, M. J., Yilmaz, O. H., Iwashita, T., Yilmaz, O. H., Terhorst, C., & Morrison, S. J. (2005). SLAM family receptors distinguish hematopoietic stem and progenitor cells and reveal endothelial niches for stem cells. *Cell*, *121*, 1109–1121.
Kim, S., Poursine-Laurent, J., Truscott, S. M., Lybarger, L., Song, Y. J., Yang, L., et al. (2005). Licensing of natural killer cells by host major histocompatibility complex class I molecules. *Nature*, *436*, 709–713.
Kim, S., Sunwoo, J. B., Yang, L., Choi, T., Song, Y. J., French, A. R., et al. (2008). HLA alleles determine differences in human natural killer cell responsiveness and potency. *Proceedings of the National Academy of Sciences of the United States of America*, *105*, 3053–3058.
Kumar, V., & McNerney, M. E. (2005). A new self: MHC-class-I-independent natural-killer-cell self-tolerance. *Nature Reviews. Immunology*, *5*, 363–374.
Latour, S., Gish, G., Helgason, C. D., Humphries, R. K., Pawson, T., & Veillette, A. (2001). Regulation of SLAM-mediated signal transduction by SAP, the X-linked lymphoproliferative gene product. *Nature Immunology*, *2*, 681–690.
Latour, S., Roncagalli, R., Chen, R., Bakinowski, M., Shi, X., Schwartzberg, P. L., et al. (2003). Binding of SAP SH2 domain to FynT SH3 domain reveals a novel mechanism of receptor signalling in immune regulation. *Nature Cell Biology*, *5*, 149–154.
Lee, K. M., McNerney, M. E., Stepp, S. E., Mathew, P. A., Schatzle, J. D., Bennett, M., et al. (2004). 2B4 acts as a non-major histocompatibility complex binding inhibitory receptor on mouse natural killer cells. *The Journal of Experimental Medicine*, *199*, 1245–1254.
Li, C., Chung, B., Tao, J., Iosef, C., Aoukaty, A., Wang, Y., et al. (2008). The X-linked lymphoproliferative syndrome gene product SAP regulates B cell function through the FcgammaRIIB receptor. *Cellular Signalling*, *20*, 1960–1967.
Li, C., Iosef, C., Jia, C. Y., Gkourasas, T., Han, V. K., & Shun-Cheng Li, S. (2003). Disease-causing SAP mutants are defective in ligand binding and protein folding. *Biochemistry*, *42*, 14885–14892.
Li, C., Schibli, D., & Li, S. S. (2009). The XLP syndrome protein SAP interacts with SH3 proteins to regulate T cell signaling and proliferation. *Cellular Signalling*, *21*, 111–119.
Liao, N. S., Bix, M., Zijlstra, M., Jaenisch, R., & Raulet, D. (1991). MHC class I deficiency: Susceptibility to natural killer (NK) cells and impaired NK activity. *Science*, *253*, 199–202.
Limaye, N., Belobrajdic, K. A., Wandstrat, A. E., Bonhomme, F., Edwards, S. V., & Wakeland, E. K. (2008). Prevalence and evolutionary origins of autoimmune susceptibility alleles in natural mouse populations. *Genes and Immunity*, *9*, 61–68.
Ljunggren, H. G., & Karre, K. (1990). In search of the 'missing self': MHC molecules and NK cell recognition. *Immunology Today*, *11*, 237–244.

Long, E. O., Kim, H. S., Liu, D., Peterson, M. E., & Rajagopalan, S. (2013). Controlling natural killer cell responses: Integration of signals for activation and inhibition. *Annual Review of Immunology, 31*, 227–258.
McArdel, S. L., Terhorst, C., & Sharpe, A. H. (2016). Roles of CD48 in regulating immunity and tolerance. *Clinical Immunology, 164*, 10–20.
Meazza, R., Falco, M., Marcenaro, S., Loiacono, F., Canevali, P., Bellora, F., et al. (2017). Inhibitory 2B4 contributes to NK cell education and immunological derangements in XLP1 patients. *European Journal of Immunology, 47*, 1051–1061.
Morra, M., Barrington, R. A., Abadia-Molina, A. C., Okamoto, S., Julien, A., Gullo, C., et al. (2005). Defective B cell responses in the absence of SH2D1A. *Proceedings of the National Academy of Sciences of the United States of America, 102*, 4819–4823.
Morra, M., Lu, J., Poy, F., Martin, M., Sayos, J., Calpe, S., et al. (2001). Structural basis for the interaction of the free SH2 domain EAT-2 with SLAM receptors in hematopoietic cells. *The EMBO Journal, 20*, 5840–5852.
Morra, M., Simarro-Grande, M., Martin, M., Chen, A. S., Lanyi, A., Silander, O., et al. (2001). Characterization of SH2D1A missense mutations identified in X-linked lymphoproliferative disease patients. *The Journal of Biological Chemistry, 276*, 36809–36816.
Nagy, N., Cerboni, C., Mattsson, K., Maeda, A., Gogolak, P., Sumegi, J., et al. (2000). SH2D1A and SLAM protein expression in human lymphocytes and derived cell lines. *International Journal of Cancer, 88*, 439–447.
Nakajima, H., Cella, M., Bouchon, A., Grierson, H. L., Lewis, J., Duckett, C. S., et al. (2000). Patients with X-linked lymphoproliferative disease have a defect in 2B4 receptor-mediated NK cell cytotoxicity. *European Journal of Immunology, 30*, 3309–3318.
Nakamura, M. C., Niemi, E. C., Fisher, M. J., Shultz, L. D., Seaman, W. E., & Ryan, J. C. (1997). Mouse Ly-49A interrupts early signaling events in natural killer cell cytotoxicity and functionally associates with the SHP-1 tyrosine phosphatase. *The Journal of Experimental Medicine, 185*, 673–684.
Narni-Mancinelli, E., Jaeger, B. N., Bernat, C., Fenis, A., Kung, S., De Gassart, A., et al. (2012). Tuning of natural killer cell reactivity by NKp46 and Helios calibrates T cell responses. *Science, 335*, 344–348.
Oguro, H., Ding, L., & Morrison, S. J. (2013). SLAM family markers resolve functionally distinct subpopulations of hematopoietic stem cells and multipotent progenitors. *Cell Stem Cell, 13*, 102–116.
Okamoto, S., Ji, H., Howie, D., Clarke, K., Gullo, C., Manning, S., et al. (2004). Expression of the SH2D1A gene is regulated by a combination of transcriptional and post-transcriptional mechanisms. *European Journal of Immunology, 34*, 3176–3186.
Oppenheim, D. E., Roberts, S. J., Clarke, S. L., Filler, R., Lewis, J. M., Tigelaar, R. E., et al. (2005). Sustained localized expression of ligand for the activating NKG2D receptor impairs natural cytotoxicity in vivo and reduces tumor immunosurveillance. *Nature Immunology, 6*, 928–937.
Pahima, H., Puzzovio, P. G., & Levi-Schaffer, F. (2019). 2B4 and CD48: A powerful couple of the immune system. *Clinical Immunology, 204*, 64–68.
Parolini, S., Bottino, C., Falco, M., Augugliaro, R., Giliani, S., Franceschini, R., et al. (2000). X-linked lymphoproliferative disease. 2B4 molecules displaying inhibitory rather than activating function are responsible for the inability of natural killer cells to kill Epstein-Barr virus-infected cells. *The Journal of Experimental Medicine, 192*, 337–346.
Perez-Quintero, L. A., Roncagalli, R., Guo, H., Latour, S., Davidson, D., & Veillette, A. (2014). EAT-2, a SAP-like adaptor, controls NK cell activation through phospholipase Cgamma, Ca++, and Erk, leading to granule polarization. *The Journal of Experimental Medicine, 211*, 727–742.

Postelnek, J., Neely, R. J., Robbins, M. D., Gleason, C. R., Peterson, J. E., & Piccoli, S. P. (2016). Development and validation of electrochemiluminescence assays to measure free and total sSLAMF7 in human serum in the absence and presence of elotuzumab. *The AAPS Journal*, *18*, 989–999.

Qi, H., Cannons, J. L., Klauschen, F., Schwartzberg, P. L., & Germain, R. N. (2008). SAP-controlled T-B cell interactions underlie germinal centre formation. *Nature*, *455*, 764–769.

Romero, X., Benitez, D., March, S., Vilella, R., Miralpeix, M., & Engel, P. (2004). Differential expression of SAP and EAT-2-binding leukocyte cell-surface molecules CD84, CD150 (SLAM), CD229 (Ly9) and CD244 (2B4). *Tissue Antigens*, *64*, 132–144.

Romero, X., Sintes, J., & Engel, P. (2014). Role of SLAM family receptors and specific adapter SAP in innate-like lymphocytes. *Critical Reviews in Immunology*, *34*, 263–299.

Romero, X., Zapater, N., Calvo, M., Kalko, S. G., de la Fuente, M. A., Tovar, V., et al. (2005). CD229 (Ly9) lymphocyte cell surface receptor interacts homophilically through its N-terminal domain and relocalizes to the immunological synapse. *Journal of Immunology*, *174*, 7033–7042.

Roncagalli, R., Taylor, J. E., Zhang, S., Shi, X., Chen, R., Cruz-Munoz, M. E., et al. (2005). Negative regulation of natural killer cell function by EAT-2, a SAP-related adaptor. *Nature Immunology*, *6*, 1002–1010.

Sandrin, M. S., Mouhtouris, E., Vaughan, H. A., Warren, H. S., & Parish, C. R. (1993). CD48 is a low affinity ligand for human CD2. *Journal of Immunology*, *151*, 4606–4613.

Scarpellino, L., Oeschger, F., Guillaume, P., Coudert, J. D., Levy, F., Leclercq, G., et al. (2007). Interactions of Ly49 family receptors with MHC class I ligands in trans and cis. *Journal of Immunology*, *178*, 1277–1284.

Sharpe, A. H., & Pauken, K. E. (2018). The diverse functions of the PD1 inhibitory pathway. *Nature Reviews. Immunology*, *18*, 153–167.

Simarro, M., Lanyi, A., Howie, D., Poy, F., Bruggeman, J., Choi, M., et al. (2004). SAP increases FynT kinase activity and is required for phosphorylation of SLAM and Ly9. *International Immunology*, *16*, 727–736.

Smith, G. M., Biggs, J., Norris, B., Anderson-Stewart, P., & Ward, R. (1997). Detection of a soluble form of the leukocyte surface antigen CD48 in plasma and its elevation in patients with lymphoid leukemias and arthritis. *Journal of Clinical Immunology*, *17*, 502–509.

Sola, C., Andre, P., Lemmers, C., Fuseri, N., Bonnafous, C., Blery, M., et al. (2009). Genetic and antibody-mediated reprogramming of natural killer cell missing-self recognition in vivo. *Proceedings of the National Academy of Sciences of the United States of America*, *106*, 12879–12884.

Sun, J. C., & Lanier, L. L. (2008). Tolerance of NK cells encountering their viral ligand during development. *The Journal of Experimental Medicine*, *205*, 1819–1828.

Tangye, S. G. (2014). XLP: Clinical features and molecular etiology due to mutations in SH2D1A encoding SAP. *Journal of Clinical Immunology*, *34*, 772–779.

Tangye, S. G., Lazetic, S., Woollatt, E., Sutherland, G. R., Lanier, L. L., & Phillips, J. H. (1999). Cutting edge: Human 2B4, an activating NK cell receptor, recruits the protein tyrosine phosphatase SHP-2 and the adaptor signaling protein SAP. *Journal of Immunology*, *162*, 6981–6985.

Tangye, S. G., Phillips, J. H., Lanier, L. L., & Nichols, K. E. (2000). Functional requirement for SAP in 2B4-mediated activation of human natural killer cells as revealed by the X-linked lymphoproliferative syndrome. *Journal of Immunology*, *165*, 2932–2936.

Tassi, I., & Colonna, M. (2005). The cytotoxicity receptor CRACC (CS-1) recruits EAT-2 and activates the PI3K and phospholipase Cgamma signaling pathways in human NK cells. *Journal of Immunology*, *175*, 7996–8002.

Tripathy, S. K., Keyel, P. A., Yang, L., Pingel, J. T., Cheng, T. P., Schneeberger, A., et al. (2008). Continuous engagement of a self-specific activation receptor induces NK cell tolerance. *The Journal of Experimental Medicine*, *205*, 1829–1841.

van der Merwe, P. A., Barclay, A. N., Mason, D. W., Davies, E. A., Morgan, B. P., Tone, M., et al. (1994). Human cell-adhesion molecule CD2 binds CD58 (LFA-3) with a very low affinity and an extremely fast dissociation rate but does not bind CD48 or CD59. *Biochemistry, 33*, 10149–10160.

Veillette, A. (2006). Immune regulation by SLAM family receptors and SAP-related adaptors. *Nature Reviews. Immunology, 6*, 56–66.

Veillette, A., Perez-Quintero, L. A., & Latour, S. (2013). X-linked lymphoproliferative syndromes and related autosomal recessive disorders. *Current Opinion in Allergy and Clinical Immunology, 13*, 614–622.

Veillette, A., Zhang, S., Shi, X., Dong, Z., Davidson, D., & Zhong, M. C. (2008). SAP expression in T cells, not in B cells, is required for humoral immunity. *Proceedings of the National Academy of Sciences of the United States of America, 105*, 1273–1278.

Viant, C., Fenis, A., Chicanne, G., Payrastre, B., Ugolini, S., & Vivier, E. (2014). SHP-1-mediated inhibitory signals promote responsiveness and anti-tumour functions of natural killer cells. *Nature Communications, 5*, 5108.

Wang, J. W., Howson, J. M., Ghansah, T., Desponts, C., Ninos, J. M., May, S. L., et al. (2002). Influence of SHIP on the NK repertoire and allogeneic bone marrow transplantation. *Science, 295*, 2094–2097.

Wang, J. H., Smolyar, A., Tan, K., Liu, J. H., Kim, M., Sun, Z. Y., et al. (1999). Structure of a heterophilic adhesion complex between the human CD2 and CD58 (LFA-3) counterreceptors. *Cell, 97*, 791–803.

Wu, N., Zhong, M. C., Roncagalli, R., Perez-Quintero, L. A., Guo, H., Zhang, Z., et al. (2016). A hematopoietic cell-driven mechanism involving SLAMF6 receptor, SAP adaptors and SHP-1 phosphatase regulates NK cell education. *Nature Immunology, 17*, 387–396.

Yigit, B., Wang, N., Herzog, R. W., & Terhorst, C. (2019). SLAMF6 in health and disease: Implications for therapeutic targeting. *Clinical Immunology, 204*, 3–13.

Yu, J., Heller, G., Chewning, J., Kim, S., Yokoyama, W. M., & Hsu, K. C. (2007). Hierarchy of the human natural killer cell response is determined by class and quantity of inhibitory receptors for self-HLA-B and HLA-C ligands. *Journal of Immunology, 179*, 5977–5989.

Yu, D., & Ye, L. (2018). A portrait of CXCR5(+) follicular cytotoxic CD8(+) T cells. *Trends in Immunology, 39*, 965–979.

Zafirova, B., Mandaric, S., Antulov, R., Krmpotic, A., Jonsson, H., Yokoyama, W. M., et al. (2009). Altered NK cell development and enhanced NK cell-mediated resistance to mouse cytomegalovirus in NKG2D-deficient mice. *Immunity, 31*, 270–282.

CHAPTER SEVEN

Metalloimmunology: The metal ion-controlled immunity

Chenguang Wang[a,b], Rui Zhang[a,b], Xiaoming Wei[a,b], Mengze Lv[a,b], Zhengfan Jiang[a,b,*]

[a]Key Laboratory of Cell Proliferation and Differentiation of the Ministry of Education, School of Life Sciences, Peking University, Beijing, China
[b]Peking-Tsinghua Center for Life Sciences, Peking University, Beijing, China
*Corresponding author: e-mail address: jiangzf@pku.edu.cn

Contents

Abstract

Metals are essential components in all forms of life required for the function of nearly half of all enzymes and are critically involved in virtually all fundamental biological processes. Especially, the transition metals iron (Fe), zinc (Zn), manganese (Mn), nickel (Ni), copper (Cu) and cobalt (Co) are crucial micronutrients known to play vital roles in metabolism as well due to their unique redox properties. Metals carry out three major functions within metalloproteins: to provide structural support, to serve as enzymatic cofactors, and to mediate electron transportation. Metal ions are also involved in the immune system from metal allergies to nutritional immunity. Within the past decade,

Advances in Immunology, Volume 145
ISSN 0065-2776
https://doi.org/10.1016/bs.ai.2019.11.007

much attention has been drawn to the roles of metal ions in the immune system, since increasing evidence has mounted to suggest that metals are critically implicated in regulating both the innate immune sensing of and the host defense against invading pathogens. The importance of ions in immunity is also evidenced by the identification of various immunodeficiencies in patients with mutations in ion channels and transporters. In addition, cancer immunotherapy has recently been conclusively demonstrated to be effective and important for future tumor treatment, although only a small percentage of cancer patients respond to immunotherapy because of inadequate immune activation. Importantly, metal ion-activated immunotherapy is becoming an effective and potential way in tumor therapy for better clinical application. Nevertheless, we are still in a primary stage of discovering the diverse immunological functions of ions and mechanistically understanding the roles of these ions in immune regulation. This review summarizes recent advances in the understanding of metal-controlled immunity. Particular emphasis is put on the mechanisms of innate immune stimulation and T cell activation by the essential metal ions like calcium (Ca^{2+}), zinc (Zn^{2+}), manganese (Mn^{2+}), iron (Fe^{2+}/Fe^{3+}), and potassium (K^{+}), followed by a few unessential metals, in order to draw a general diagram of metalloimmunology.

1. Introduction

The cellular membrane system, including plasma membranes (PM) and membranes of various intracellular organelles such as mitochondria, the endoplasmic reticulum (ER) and vacuoles, is composed of impermeable hydrophobic lipid layers which restrict free penetration of the charged metal ions. The active transportation of ions thus creates concentration and electric gradients across the membranes via many integral pore-forming membrane proteins, such as ion channels, transporters and pumps, which allow the influx and efflux of ions across membranes to transform different signals by simple changes of ion permeability. Cellular ion signals play crucial roles in various physiological processes including nerve impulse transmission, muscle contraction, gene expression, cell fate decision, development and migration. Therefore, various ion signals act as the fundamental vowel phonemes in the sophisticated cellular language, and are even more precious in the context of immune responses against infections under which the cellular emergency communications determine a matter of life or death.

Ion signals have been widely studied in excitable cells, but they also function in non-excitable cells in the immune system which express various ion channels and ion transporters. From the initial recognition of pathogen/damage-associated molecular patterns (PAMPs/DAMPs) to the terminal generation of protective immunity and immunological memories, successful immune responses against infections or neoplastic transformations are orchestrated by a series of transcellular and intracellular signaling cascades with no exception, in which different metal cations including Ca^{2+}, Zn^{2+}, Mn^{2+}, $Fe^{2+/3+}$ and K^{+}, play important roles in transmitting various signals. Given the fact that the immune system usually responds to sudden changes like microbial infection, and is rendered tolerance by slow or continuous stimulations (Pradeu & Vivier, 2016), these metal cations are naturally fit for the abrupt immune responses by rapidly changing their concentrations in several orders of magnitude.

Moreover, some unessential metal cations and the corresponding metallic compounds have been used therapeutically to regulate the immune responses, among which the anti-cancer drug cis-platinum, arsenic compounds and aluminum adjuvants are the most famous examples. Herein, we summarize recent advances in our understanding of the metal-regulated immune activation. This review intends to clarify and emphasize the scientific value and future directions in metalloimmunology (Li, Zheng, Zhao, Chen, & Guo, 2019). Of note, the nutritional immunity and metal allergies are not included due to space limitation, which have been extensively discussed elsewhere (Hood & Skaar, 2012; Thyssen & Menne, 2010).

2. Calcium (Ca)

The concentration gradient of Ca^{2+} is the largest among all the metal ions discussed, and the subcellular distribution of calcium is highly heterogeneous. Most of the cellular Ca^{2+} is stored in the extracellular space and the endoplasmic reticulum, where the concentration of Ca^{2+} varies from 0.3 to 2 mM. In the resting state, the intracellular concentration of Ca^{2+} is about 0.1 μM, but it significantly increases nearly 10-fold when cells are activated. The Ca^{2+} influx is particularly important at each step of the cell cycle progression and the proliferation of the immune cells (Bose, Cieslar-Pobuda, & Wiechec, 2015). So far, Ca^{2+} is the most well-studied and widely accepted ionic second messenger in regulating various immune responses, including the calcium–NFAT (Nuclear factor of activated T cells) pathway, the NLRP3 (Nod-like receptor 3) inflammasome and the cGAS (cyclic GMP-AMP (cGAMP) synthase)-STING (stimulator of IFN genes, also named MITA or ERIS) (Ishikawa & Barber, 2008; Sun et al., 2009; Sun, Wu, Du, Chen, & Chen, 2013; Zhong et al., 2008) pathway.

2.1 Calcium and the NFAT pathway

The general aspects of the calcium–NFAT signaling have been thoroughly reviewed (Hogan, Chen, Nardone, & Rao, 2003; Macian, 2005) and are briefly summarized here. The calcium mobilization is coupled with the engagement of immune-receptors and the subsequent activation of the phospholipase Cγ (PLCγ) which hydrolyses phosphatidylinositol-4, 5-bisphosphate to produce inositol 1,4,5-trisphosphate ($InsP_3$) and diacylglycerol. The $InsP_3$-operated channels then release Ca^{2+} from the intracellular calcium stores. The consequent decrease of Ca^{2+} concentration in the endoplasmic reticulum activates the stromal interaction molecules (STIM1/2) which subsequently bind to and open the Ca^{2+} release-activated Ca^{2+} (CRAC) channels formed by ORAI1 and ORAI2 on the plasma membrane. The resultant influx of extracellular Ca^{2+} is called store-operated Ca^{2+} entry (SOCE). The maintained increased levels of intracellular Ca^{2+} activates the Ca^{2+} sensor calmodulin and diverse calmodulin-dependent enzymes including calcineurin (Vaeth & Feske, 2018b). Calcineurin then dephosphorylates multiple phosphoserines in the regulatory domain of the transcription factor NFAT (Nuclear factor of activated T cells), leading to its nuclear translocation. Cooperating with several transcriptional partners like AP1, EGR1/4, GATA3, and IRF4, etc., the translocated NFAT initiates the expression of a cluster of NFAT-regulated genes, such as cytokines, transcription factors, glycolytic enzymes and mitochondrial genes which regulate a variety of cellular processes (Vaeth & Feske, 2018a) (Fig. 1).

The most direct and convincing evidence manifesting the role of calcium signaling in the immune defenses is underscored by a bundle of human genetic data. Loss-of-function mutations in *ORAI1* (Feske et al., 2006; Lian et al., 2018; McCarl et al., 2009; Vig et al., 2006) or *STIM1* (Byun et al., 2010; Fuchs et al., 2012; Maus et al., 2015; Picard et al., 2009) abolish the SOCE mediated Ca^{2+} signal, which result in a unique disease syndrome named CRAC channelopathy. Patients with this syndrome are characterized by combined immunodeficiency and are life-threatened by the uncontrolled common-pathogen infections including cytomegalovirus (CMV), herpes simplex virus (HSV), Epstein-Barr virus (EBV), *Candida albicans* and *Streptococcus pneumoniae* (Byun et al., 2010; McCarl et al., 2009). Without Ca^{2+} signaling, T cells from these patients fail to express the growth cytokine IL-2 (Feske, Draeger, Peter, Eichmann, & Rao, 2000; Feske, Giltnane, Dolmetsch, Staudt, & Rao, 2001), with impaired aerobic glycolysis and lipid metabolism, and can hardly proliferate and differentiate

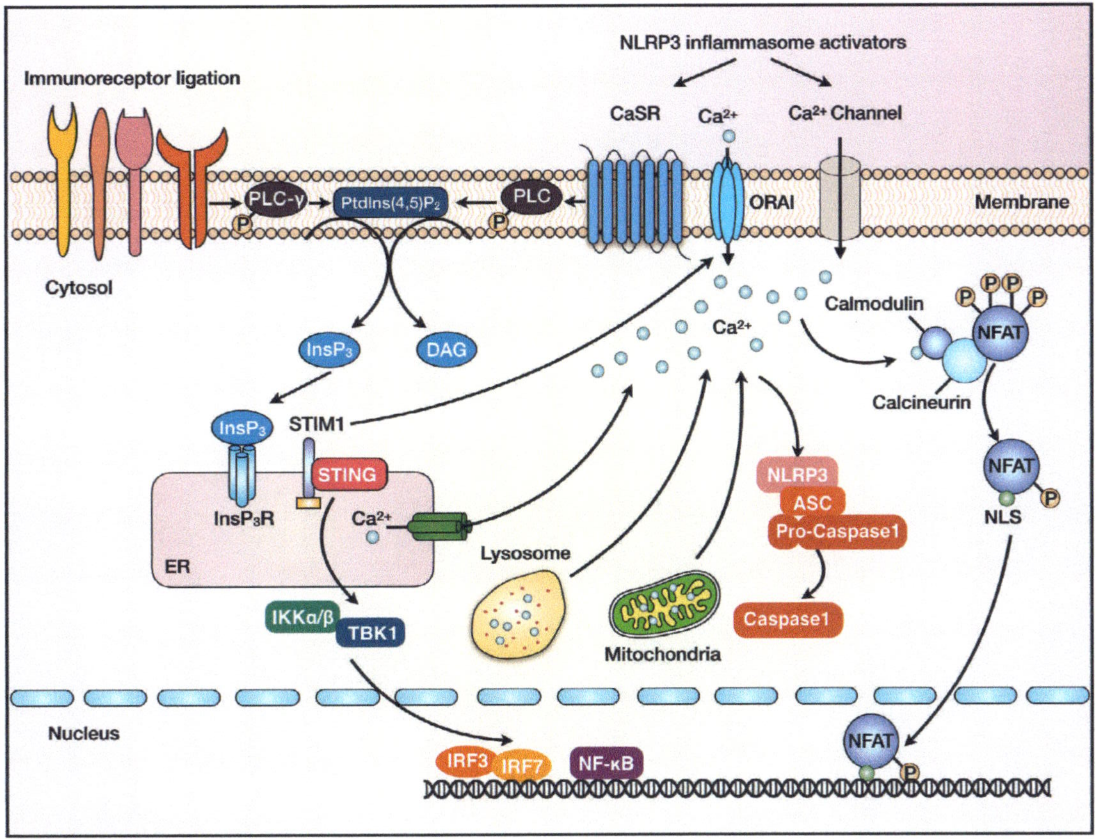

Fig. 1 See legend on next page.

(Maus et al., 2017; Vaeth et al., 2017). What is more, the attenuated function of follicular T helper cells impairs antibody affinity maturation, thus exacerbating the immunodeficiency (Vaeth et al., 2016). Meanwhile, the successful medical application of calcineurin inhibitors (Liu et al., 1991), namely sirolimus (rapamycin), cyclosporine A (CsA) and tacrolimus (FK506), as immunosuppressive drugs to reduce the risk of rejection after allogeneic organ transplantation (Mukherjee & Mukherjee, 2009; O'Grady et al., 2002) and to treat T cell-mediated autoimmune diseases (Baumgart, Macdonald, & Feagan, 2008; Baumgart, Pintoffl, Sturm, Wiedenmann, & Dignass, 2006; Gremese & Ferraccioli, 2004; Griffiths & Emery, 2001), equally highlights the importance of Ca^{2+} signaling in the adaptive immune responses.

As one of the direct responders in the intracellular Ca^{2+} signaling, the transcription factor NFAT is critically involved in the entire lifespan of T lymphocytes. In the thymus, T-cell progenitors successively undergo positive and negative selections, thus generating a mature conventional T-cell repertoire that is both MHC-restricted and self-tolerant. Considering that the strength of the Ca^{2+} signaling represents the binding affinity of pre-TCR on thymocytes to the peptide-MHC complexes on thymic epithelia (Aifantis, Gounari, Scorrano, Borowski, & von Boehmer, 2001; Bhakta, Oh, & Lewis, 2005; Daniels et al., 2006), it is not surprising that the calcium–NFAT signals are involved in the regulation of thymocyte proliferation and the development of immature CD4/CD8 double negative (DN) thymocytes into mature $CD8^+$ or $CD4^+$ single positive (SP) cells. The

Fig. 1 Ca^{2+} is a second messenger in various immune responses. Ca^{2+} is the most well accepted ionic second messenger that regulates various immune responses, including the Ca^{2+}–NFAT pathway, the NLRP3 inflammasome and the cGAS-STING pathway. For the Ca^{2+}–NFAT activation, the ligation of immune-receptor by its ligands activates PLC-γ which in turn hydrolyzes PtdIns (4, 5) P_2 into $InsP_3$ and DAG. $InsP_3$ binds to its receptor on the ER, then drives Ca^{2+} release into the cytoplasm from the ER. Decrease of ER-stored Ca^{2+} level triggers STIM1/2-mediated opening of the plasma membrane channels ORAI1/2 to induce the Ca^{2+} influx. Increased cytoplasmic Ca^{2+} activates calmodulin, calcineurin and NFAT. NFAT then translocates into the nucleus and regulates gene expression. For the Ca^{2+}-NLRP3 inflammasome activation, Ca^{2+} signaling is triggered by the NLRP3 inflammasome activators. G protein-coupled calcium-sensing receptor (CaSR) induces Ca^{2+} signaling via the PLC-$InsP_3$ pathway. Organelle destabilization also leads to the leakage of Ca^{2+} into the cytoplasm during NLRP3 inflammasome activation. For the cGAS-STING pathway, the Ca^{2+} sensor STIM1 retains STING in the ER, preventing the aberrant activation of cGAS-STING and inhibiting the production of type I-IFNs and other proinflammatory cytokines in the resting state.

inhibition of calcineurin activity with CsA led to defects in negative selection featured by the impaired DP-to-SP transition (Gao, Lo, Cheney, Kanagawa, & Sprent, 1988; Hiramine, Hojo, & Matsumoto, 1988; Jenkins, Schwartz, & Pardoll, 1988). Moreover, gene knockout mice deleting the catalytic or regulatory subunit of calcineurin were reported to have a decreased amount of SP thymocytes, suggesting the involvement of calcium signaling in positive selection (Bueno, Brandt, Rothenberg, & Molkentin, 2002; Neilson, Winslow, Hur, & Crabtree, 2004). In the periphery where T cells encounter various antigens, the calcium–NFAT signal seems to be indispensable for the expression of the lineage-signature cytokines in all T-helper cell subsets, including T helper 1 (TH_1) (Ma, McCarl, Khalil, Luthy, & Feske, 2010; Yu, Wang, et al., 2011), T helper 2 (TH_2) (Cabral et al., 2010; Fanger, Neben, & Cahalan, 2000; Robert et al., 2014; Weber, Hildner, Murphy, & Allen, 2010), T helper 17 (TH_{17}) (Ghosh et al., 2010; Gomez-Rodriguez et al., 2009; Kim et al., 2014) and T follicular helper (T_{FH}) cells (Bauquet et al., 2009; Vaeth et al., 2016). Besides, the fact that STIM1/2 double-deficient regulatory T (T_{Reg}) cells fail to inhibit the proliferation of $CD4^+$ T cells in vitro provides new roles of Ca^{2+} signaling in T-cell tolerance, which include not only the cell-intrinsic mechanisms of T cell anergy (Heissmeyer et al., 2004; Hsiao et al., 2009) but also the proper functions of T_{Reg} cells (Bopp et al., 2005; Jin et al., 2013; Oh-Hora et al., 2008; Schenk et al., 2011; Tone et al., 2008). Besides, Ca^{2+} signaling also plays a pivotal role in the activation of $CD8^+$ cytotoxic T lymphocytes (CTLs). For example, the full activation of the adhesion molecule LFA-1 is dependent on the cytoplasmic Ca^{2+} signaling, which is required for the lytic immune synapsis formation between CTLs and their target cells (Franciszkiewicz et al., 2013; Zweifach, 2000). After that, the Ca^{2+} signal at the immune synapse precisely controls the polarization of perforin and granzyme containing cytotoxic granules to the target cells (MacLennan, Gotch, & Golstein, 1980; Pores-Fernando & Zweifach, 2009; Quintana et al., 2011; Schwarz, Qu, & Hoth, 2013; Takayama & Sitkovsky, 1987). Thereby, the inhibition of Ca^{2+} signaling in the $CD8^+$ CTLs almost completely abolishes the lytic granule exocytosis of those tumor cells and virus-infected cells (Maul-Pavicic et al., 2011; Shaw et al., 2014; Weidinger, Shaw, & Feske, 2013).

The Ca^{2+}–NFAT signaling is not limited to T cells only. In fact, at least one NFAT family member is expressed by almost all the cell types that have been examined (Crabtree & Olson, 2002; Hogan et al., 2003). The calcium/NFAT-regulated genes have subsequently been shown to modulate the functions of a broad range of myeloid cells. In the dendritic cells (DCs), the Ca^{2+} signaling is reported to couple with the toll-like receptors (TLRs) pathway, where the engagement of the endotoxin lipopolysaccharide (LPS) by TLR4/CD14 is mediated by lipid rafts and leads to the activation of the Src-family kinase PLCγ2. The resultant Ca^{2+} influx is followed by the nuclear translocation of NFAT and the increased production of IL-2 (Zanoni et al., 2009). Likewise, the detection of the fungal zymosan by the C-type lectin receptor Dectin-1 will result in Ca^{2+} mobilization and NFAT-regulated expressions of IL-2, IL-10 and IL-12 (Goodridge, Simmons, & Underhill, 2007; Rogers et al., 2005). A similar mechanism for Ca^{2+} signaling has also been suggested in B cells on BCR stimulation, resulting in the production of IL-10 (Matsumoto et al., 2011). In the meantime, a kind of Ca^{2+}-flux oscillation is observed only in the immature DCs rather than the mature ones, which has been speculated to contribute to the maintenance of an immature DC phenotype and immune homeostasis (Vukcevic, Zorzato, Spagnoli, & Treves, 2010). Additionally, the Ca^{2+} signaling-dependent gene expression also modulates the life cycles of DCs in response to LPS, leading to the apoptosis of terminally differentiated DCs, a process that is important for maintaining self-tolerance and preventing autoimmunity (Granucci & Zanoni, 2009). In macrophages, the Ca^{2+} influx is triggered by the engagement of antibodies to the Fcγ receptors, which regulates the basic physiological functions like phagocytosis, phagosome-lysosome fusion and the production of nitric oxide (NO) (Chen, Chou, & Lin, 1998; Chen, Ji, et al., 2015; Watanabe, Suzuki, & Kobayashi, 1996). In mast cells, high-affinity Fc receptor for IgE (FcεRI) crosslinking is responsible for the Ca^{2+} flux and NFAT translocation, which governs mast cell functions, including degranulation, the release of leukotriene C4 (Baba et al., 2008; Suzuki, Inoue, & Ra, 2012) and survival related expression of inflammatory cytokines IL-13, TNF-α, anti-hypoxia transcription factor HIF1α and the prosurvival protein A1 (Klein et al., 2006; Ulleras et al., 2008; Walczak-Drzewiecka, Ratajewski, Wagner, & Dastych, 2008). For the neutrophils, the Ca^{2+} signaling is critical for the maintenance of the antifungal and antibacterial activities by recruiting phagosomes to the ER and promoting high-efficiency phagocytosis (Greenblatt, Aliprantis, Hu, & Glimcher, 2010; Salmon & Ahluwalia, 2011; Schaff et al., 2010; Steinckwich, Schenten, Melchior, Brechard, & Tschirhart, 2011; Zhang et al., 2014). Moreover, the expression of IL-28 and GM-CSF and the degranulation in the eosinophils are dependent on the Ca^{2+} signaling (Bosse et al., 1996; Kunsleben et al., 2015;

Meng et al., 1997). A similar indispensable role of the Ca^{2+} signaling has also been observed in IL-4 synthesis in basophils, in which Ca^{2+} motivation is triggered by the crosslinking of FcRI receptors (MacGlashan & Guo, 1991; Qi, Nishida, Chaves, Ohmori, & Huang, 2011). The Ca^{2+} flux is detected in the natural killer (NK) cells interacting with their target cells, leading to the transcription of NFAT-dependent cytokines including TNF-α, GM-CSF and interferons (Hess, Oortgiesen, & Cahalan, 1993; Tassi et al., 2008; Wang et al., 2007).

2.2 Calcium and the NLRP3 inflammasome

Ca^{2+} mobilization has been reported as a physiological or pathological stimulation in the activation of the NLRP3 inflammasome, leading to caspase-1 activation, IL-1β/IL-18 maturation and the consequent proinflammatory cell death named pyroptosis, which has been considered as the central biomolecular event during infection and metabolic diseases in various clinically important settings (Agostini et al., 2004). Based on the Ca^{2+} chelator BAPTA-AM treatment or incubation in the calcium-free media, several studies report a linkage between Ca^{2+} mobilization and NLRP3 inflammasome activation (Brough et al., 2003; Chu et al., 2009; Feldmeyer et al., 2007). Further, detailed pharmacological inhibitors and genetic models of Ca^{2+} signaling are used to reveal the general requirement for Ca^{2+} in the proximal steps upstream of NLRP3 inflammasome activation (Ferrari et al., 2006; Lee et al., 2012; Murakami et al., 2012; Solle et al., 2001). Of note, the NLRP3 inflammasome can be activated by multiple chemically and structurally distinct inducers. Ca^{2+} mobilization from the extracellular space as well as the intracellular stores seems able to explain the better part of the underlying mechanisms of NLRP3 inflammasome activation in a context-dependent manner (Horng, 2014). For the extracellular influx of Ca^{2+}, the G protein-coupled calcium-sensing receptor GPRC6A is reported to transport Ca^{2+} and to activate the NLRP3 inflammasome during the extracellular Ca^{2+} treatment (Rossol et al., 2012). Alternatively, Ca^{2+} can enter the cells via Ca^{2+}-specific channels such as the P2X7 receptor upon ATP stimulation (Lopez-Castejon et al., 2010; Lupfer et al., 2013; Shimada et al., 2012) and the TRPM2 for lysosomal destabilization crystals stimulation (Zhong et al., 2013). The formation of complement membrane attack complex also triggers Ca^{2+} influx, which then leads to NLRP3 inflammasome activation (Laudisi et al., 2013; Triantafilou, Hughes, Triantafilou, & Morgan, 2013). PLC-mediated Ca^{2+} release from ER and

Ca^{2+} leakage by lysosomal destabilization (Allam et al., 2014; Camello-Almaraz, Gomez-Pinilla, Pozo, & Camello, 2006; Orrenius, Gogvadze, & Zhivotovsky, 2015) are reported to activate the NLRP3 inflammasome. Thus, Ca^{2+} is considered as a common danger signal that can activate the inflammasomes against infection.

2.3 Calcium and the cGAS-STING pathway

The Ca^{2+} signaling has recently been discovered as a regulatory factor in the cGAS-STING pathway. The cyclic GMP-AMP synthase (cGAS) is a DNA-sensing enzyme that catalyzes the conversion of GTP and ATP to cyclic GAMP (cGAMP) (Sun et al., 2013; Wu et al., 2013) which activates the adaptor STING. This, in turn, induces the recruitment of the kinase TBK1/IKKε, the phosphorylation of IRF3 and STAT6 and the expression of type I interferons and other cytokines (Chen et al., 2011; Fang et al., 2017). The Ca^{2+} leak or dysregulation can be detected as a result of virus infection, for example, HSV-1 and hepatitis C virus (HCV) (Casciano, Duchemin, Lamontagne, Steel, & Bouchard, 2017; Cheshenko et al., 2003; Hare et al., 2015; Robinson & Marchant, 2008), which is essential for virus entry. Besides, the Ca^{2+}-mobilizing ER stress induced by the pharmacologic unfolded protein response or the oxygen-glucose deprivation is reported to activate STING-dependent IRF3 phosphorylation and the expression of the antiviral genes (Liu et al., 2012). More recently, the Ca^{2+} sensor STIM1 has been demonstrated to hold the N-terminal tail of STING for its retention at the ER, suppressing the sensitivity of the cGAS-STING pathway. The disruption of Ca^{2+} homeostasis induced by STIM1-deletion can prime the STING-dependent antiviral activity, which is consistent with the phenotypes that both STIM1-KO mouse models and patients with STIM1 mutations showed mild immunodeficiency but enhanced production of interferons and cytokines (Srikanth et al., 2019). Taken together, these studies raise the possibility that the Ca^{2+} homeostasis might serve as the stabilizer in the cGAS-STING pathway, which is featured by its unique immune surveillance activity in tumor progression (Ablasser & Chen, 2019). The assumption is reminiscent of the observations that the Ca^{2+} channels hyperpolarize the cancer cells and influence their proliferation and metastasis (Bose et al., 2015), indicating that the Ca^{2+} signaling serves as a druggable target for cancer immunotherapy under which the tumor suppression and anticancer-immunity enhancement can be simultaneously achieved.

3. Zinc (Zn)

3.1 Zinc homeostasis and Zn-related immunodeficiency

Altogether the human body contains 2–3 g of zinc, 0.1% of which is exchanged daily (Maret & Sandstead, 2006), and nearly 90% is found in muscles and bones (Wastney, Aamodt, Rumble, & Henkin, 1986). In the serum, zinc is predominantly bound to albumin (60%, low-affinity), α2-macroglobulin (30%, high-affinity) and transferrin (10%) (Rink & Gabriel, 2000; Scott & Bradwell, 1983). Zinc is referred to as a trace element, as its plasma concentration is only 10–20 μM. However, the Zn^{2+} gradient across the PM is obvious, as the intracellular free Zn^{2+} is no more than 1 nM (Haase, Hebel, Engelhardt, & Rink, 2006; Rukgauer, Klein, & Kruse-Jarres, 1997). Zn^{2+} serves as the catalytic core or structural stabilizer in over 300 enzymes, and is a component of an even larger number of additional metalloproteins (Vallee & Falchuk, 1993). According to bioinformatics searches, about 15% enzymes and a comparable number of transcription factors in the human proteome contain zinc binding motif(s) (Andreini, Bertini, & Rosato, 2009; Brylinski & Skolnick, 2011; Rink & Haase, 2007). The cellular Zn^{2+} is distributed among the nucleus (30–40%), membranes (10%) and the cytoplasm (50%) (Vallee & Falchuk, 1993), and its homeostasis is achieved by four main mechanisms (Plum, Rink, & Haase, 2010). Firstly, the tissue specific expression profiles and distinct subcellular localization of specialized Zn^{2+} transporters precisely control the Zn^{2+} homeostasis. Zn^{2+} transporters include importers like the Zrt/Irt-like protein (ZIP) family consisting of 14 genes (solute carrier family 39 from *SLC39A1* to *SLC39A14*) and exporters like the zinc transporter (ZnT) family of 10 genes (*SLC30A1* to *SLC30A10*) (Cousins, Liuzzi, & Lichten, 2006; Eide, 2006). Secondly, the cytosolic free Zn^{2+} is regulated by the zinc-buffer proteins. About 20% of the intracellular zinc is clamped by those ubiquitously expressed proteins known as metallothioneins (MTs). These 6–7 kDa small proteins each contains 20 conserved cysteines and is able to complex up to seven zinc ions through its zinc-sulfur clusters (Chimienti, Aouffen, Favier, & Seve, 2003; Kambe, Weaver, & Andrews, 2008; Tapiero & Tew, 2003). Thereby, the MTs buffer the cellular zinc over several orders of magnitude (Krezel & Maret, 2007), a process that is regulated not only by the quantity of zinc but also by the oxidation of cysteine residues of the MT proteins (Maret, 2003). Thirdly, the organelle sequestration and controlled release of Zn^{2+} allow adaptation to altered environmental or physiological requirements (Fukada & Kambe, 2011; Lichten & Cousins, 2009). Surplus Zn^{2+} is sequestrated into intracellular organelles, such as ER, Golgi, lysosomes and even high amounts of zinc-containing membrane-bound vesicular structures, so-called zincosomes (Haase & Maret, 2003; Taylor et al., 2008), which are reported to release free Zn^{2+} upon the stimulation of growth factors. Finally, the metal-response-element-binding transcription factor (MTF)-1 is able to sense free Zn^{2+} through its six zinc finger domains, stabilizing the level of Zn^{2+} through the feedback-regulation of MT and Zn^{2+} transporter transcriptions. Additionally, the dynamic regulations of zinc transporter expression profiles are responsible for the Zn^{2+} mobilization upon cytokines and hormones stimulation (Laity & Andrews, 2007; Lichten, Ryu, Guo, Embury, & Cousins, 2011).

For more than 50 years, it is known that the immune system is regulated delicately by zinc homeostasis (Ibs & Rink, 2003; Rink & Kirchner, 2000; Wellinghausen, Kirchner, & Rink, 1997). Zinc malnutrition results in complex immune deficiencies, including impaired clearance of pathogens, augmented initial inflammatory response and collateral damage to host tissues (Fraker & King, 2004; Knoell & Liu, 2010; Prasad, 2012; Wellinghausen et al., 1997). The most convincing genetic example is the zinc malabsorption syndrome called acrodermatitis enteropathica, a kind of autosomal recessive disease that is caused by the loss-of-function mutations in the intestinal zinc uptake transporter ZIP4 (Ackland & Michalczyk, 2006; Geiser, Venken, De Lisle, & Andrews, 2012; Kambe, Fukue, Ishida, & Miyazaki, 2015; Kury et al., 2002). The impaired immune function is the most common symptom in this kind of disease, including severe lymphopenia (Fraker & King, 2004; Prasad, 2012) and increased susceptibility to bacterial, viral, and fungal infections (Wellinghausen & Rink, 1998). In addition, the heterozygous mutations of lysosomal zinc transporter ZnT2 in the lactation mother can cause neonatal zinc deficiency due to the production of zinc-deficient milk. Without zinc replacement therapy, the zinc-deficient milk can be lethal to the newborns who usually suffer from immunodeficiency and antibiotics-unresponsive infections (Chowanadisai, Lonnerdal, & Kelleher, 2006; Huang & Gitschier, 1997; Itsumura et al., 2013; Lasry et al., 2012). What is more, the autosomal recessive mutations in the *TMC6/8* genes, which encode the channel-like zinc transportation partner of ZnT1, are reported to associate with abnormal susceptibility to human papillomaviruses (HPVs) (Lazarczyk et al., 2008, 2012). Nutritional zinc deficiency is a leading cause of immunodeficiency especially in developing countries (Hojyo & Fukada, 2016; Kambe et al., 2015; Moynahan, 1975).

Zinc malnutrition patients have been reported with an elevated clinical risk for the high incidence of and poor outcome of sepsis (Besecker et al., 2011; Heyland, Jones, Cvijanovich, & Wong, 2008). This is consistent with the observations in the zinc-deficient sepsis mouse model which suffered from aggravated inflammation, increased bacterial burden, organ damage and mortality (Bao et al., 2010; Haase & Rink, 2014a; Knoell et al., 2009). All these observations underscore the paramount significance of zinc homeostasis in immunity.

3.2 Zinc in innate immunity

Similar to Ca^{2+}, Zn^{2+} functions as a second messenger in innate immunity. In monocytes, Zn^{2+} treatment could induce adhesion of myelomonocytic cells to the endothelium, and Zn^{2+} chelation could diminish such monocytic recruitment (Chavakis, May, Preissner, & Kanse, 1999; Dubben, Honscheid, Winkler, Rink, & Haase, 2010). Correspondingly, stimulation of monocytes with monocyte chemoattractant protein-1 (MCP-1) or phorbol myristate acetate (PMA) induces an intracellular Zn^{2+} signaling which promotes monocytic migration and differentiation in the inflamed tissues (Kojima, Kawakami, Takei, Nitta, & Yoshida, 2007). For macrophages, the phagocytosis of pathogens and the activation of respiratory burst for pathogen-killing are positively influenced by the level of Zn^{2+}. The MTs gene knockout macrophages display Zn^{2+}-dependent immune-depression that is characterized by reduced production of inflammatory cytokines, decreased inducible nitric oxide synthase (iNOS) activity (Itoh et al., 2005) and impaired phagocytosis and the antigen presentation process (Sugiura, Kuroda, & Yamashita, 2004). Upon LPS stimulation, a rapid Zn^{2+} influx was observed through the upregulation of ZIP8 (Liu et al., 2013), which inhibited the protein tyrosine phosphatases (PTP), thereby converting TLR4-induced phosphorylation signals (Haase et al., 2008). The production of proinflammatory cytokines such as IL-1β, IL-6, TNF-α (Brazao et al., 2008; Haase et al., 2008; Nowak, Harmon, Caldwell, & Wong, 2012; Ryu, Langkamp-Henken, Chang, Shankar, & Cousins, 2011), soluble IL-2 receptor and interferon-γ in human peripheral blood mononuclear cells (PBMCs) (Driessen, Hirv, Rink, & Kirchner, 1994; Salas & Kirchner, 1987; Scuderi, 1990) required Zn^{2+} signaling, and could also be induced by incubation with supraphysiological concentrations of extracellular Zn^{2+} (Haase & Rink, 2014b; Wellinghausen et al., 1997; Wellinghausen & Rink, 1998). More recently, Zn^{2+} was reported to facilitate the cGAS-DNA condensation, a phenomenon known as phase separation, that could increase the enzymatic activity of cGAS (Du & Chen, 2018). However, it is noteworthy that the high-level phosphate buffer used in this research might precipitate other tested ions which could otherwise support or enhance the activity of cGAS. In dendritic cells, paradoxically, efflux rather than influx of the intracellular Zn^{2+} was detected during the LPS induced dendritic cell maturation. Activation of DCs led to reduced expression of the importer ZIP6/10 and upregulation of the exporters ZnT1/4/6 and MTs (Kitamura et al., 2006), thereby reducing the level of free intracellular Zn^{2+} (Leibbrandt & Koropatnick, 1994). The Zn^{2+} efflux is indispensably required for DCs maturation (Kitamura et al., 2006; Liu et al., 2013; Sayadi, Nguyen, Bard, & Bard-Chapeau, 2013), compared with the Zn^{2+} influx in macrophage activation. The different requirement for Zn^{2+} signal might be distinguished by the TLR adaptor proteins MyD88 and TRIF, which were differentially regulated by zinc (Haase & Rink, 2014a). An early Zn^{2+} signaling was required for the inhibition of the phosphodiesterase (PDE) activity, the IL-1 receptor-associated kinase (IRAK) phosphorylation (von Bulow, Rink, & Haase, 2005) and the production of inflammatory cytokines by the MyD88 signaling pathway. In contrast, the basal level of Zn^{2+} at a later time point negatively regulated the TRIF-dependent production of interferons and the expression of the costimulatory molecules CD80 and CD86, which contributed to antigen presentation and the existence of the matured DC phenotypes (Brieger, Rink, & Haase, 2013; Haase & Rink, 2014a). For neutrophils, zinc deficiency inhibited both the recruitment of neutrophils and its chemotaxis (Shankar & Prasad, 1998). At the site of infection, neutrophil phagocytosis was decreased during zinc deficiency while augmented by Zn^{2+} supplementation (Sheikh et al., 2010). The release of zinc was an essential process of the ROS-dependent signal transduction leading to the formation of neutrophil extracellular traps (NETs) in vitro, a matrix of composed DNA in which extracellular pathogens were captured (Hasan, Rink, & Haase, 2013; Kehl-Fie & Skaar, 2010). In mast cells, ZnT5-mediated Zn^{2+} influx has been described to regulate immune functions, which was associated with the FcεRI-mediated PKC recruitment to the PM, NF-κB activation, degranulation and type IV (delayed or cell-mediated) hypersensitivity (Kabu et al., 2006; Nishida et al., 2009; Yamasaki et al., 2007). In NK cells, extracellular Zn^{2+} was involved in the recognition of the MHC-I complexes on target cells (Rajagopalan & Long, 1998; Rajagopalan, Winter, Wagtmann, & Long, 1995). The lytic activity of NK cells was decreased by zinc deficiency, and moderating zinc supplementation could increase NK differentiation and their cytotoxic activity (Muzzioli, Stecconi, Donnini, Re, & Provinciali, 2007).

3.3 Zinc in adaptive immunity

In the adaptive immune system, pre-T cells are most susceptible by zinc deficiency. The increased apoptosis rate leads to a 50% loss of mature T cells during zinc malnutrition (King, Frentzel, Mann, & Fraker, 2005), consistent with the common clinical spectrum in the zinc deficiency like thymus atrophy and lymphopenia (Ackland & Michalczyk, 2006; Kury et al., 2002; Wang, Zhou, Kuo, Zemansky, & Gitschier, 2002). One of the explanations is the decreased activity of the hormone thymulin, which uses Zn^{2+} as a cofactor that is critical for the pre-T cell differentiation (Marchan, Cadenas, & Bolt, 2012; Prasad et al., 1988). More likely, the zinc deficiency-induced disruption of the T cell differentiation might be explained by the Zn^{2+}-dependent endonuclease activity of the RAG protein complex, which is involved in the indispensable enzymatic steps in the RAG-dependent V(D)J rearrangements of the TCR genes (Jung, Giallourakis, Mostoslavsky, & Alt, 2006). When T cells are primed, the accompanying Zn^{2+} influx is initiated through the Zn^{2+} transporters ZIP3/6/8, which benefits the TCR signal transduction in multiple levels (Aydemir, Liuzzi, McClellan, & Cousins, 2009; Dufner-Beattie, Huang, Geiser, Xu, & Andrews, 2005; Yu, Lee, et al., 2011). Taking two things into consideration, one is that the TCR signal is critically regulated by the equilibrium between kinases and phosphatases, and the other is that Zn^{2+} is a well-known negative regulator of the Cys-containing phosphatases, it is not surprising that the Zn^{2+} influx augments the TCR signal cascades through inhibiting the recruitment of the inhibitory phosphatase SHP-1 and increasing the activation of the kinase ZAP-70 (Kaltenberg et al., 2010). Moreover, a unique "zinc clasp" motif with two cysteine residues in the cytoplasmic domain of CD4 or CD8 binds a Zn^{2+} which is also constitutively associated with a similar motif in the Src family protein tyrosine kinase Lck. When CD4 or CD8 is recruited to the immunological synapse as a result of TCR-antigen recognition, Zn^{2+} acts as a prominent bridging ligand that brings the kinase Lck into spatial proximity of its substrates, the immune-receptor tyrosine-based activation motifs (ITAMs) of the engaged TCRs, thus leading to more efficient signaling transduction (Huse, Eck, & Harrison, 1998; Iwashima, Irving, van Oers, Chan, &

Weiss, 2014; Lin, Rodriguez, Veillette, & Lodish, 1998; Maret & Li, 2009). The involvement of the Zn^{2+} influx in the TCR signal amplification might explain the observations that the addition of Zn^{2+} alone could induce the expression of the high-affinity IL-2 receptor and the proliferation of activated T cells (Dowd, Kelleher, & Guillou, 1986; Kaltenberg et al., 2010; Tanaka, Shiozawa, Morimoto, & Fujita, 1989). For T helper cell differentiation, Zn^{2+} signal shifts the TH_1/TH_2 balance to favor cell-mediated TH_1 development, and zinc deficiency reduces the expression of IFNγ and the transcription factor T-bet in the TH_1 (Bao et al., 2011; Beck, Prasad, Kaplan, Fitzgerald, & Brewer, 1997; Prasad, 2000). Furthermore, the zinc supplement seems to promote the formation of T_{Reg} cells and inhibit the development of TH_{17} subpopulation. Thus, Zn^{2+} treatment remits the T cell-mediated allogeneic immune responses in the human mixed lymphocyte reaction (Faber, Gabriel, Ibs, & Rink, 2004) and reduces the severity of experimental autoimmune encephalomyelitis, a model of multiple sclerosis (Stoye et al., 2012). In B lymphocytes, nutritional zinc deprivation causes a significant loss of premature and immature B cells (Fraker & King, 2004; Stefanidou, Maravelias, Dona, & Spiliopoulou, 2006) and decreases the antibody production (DePasquale-Jardieu & Fraker, 1984; Fraker, DePasquale-Jardieu, Zwickl, & Luecke, 1978). Loss of the plasma Zn^{2+}-transporter ZIP10 leads to a defective humoral immune response that arises from reduced mature B cell numbers and perturbed BCR signaling (Hojyo et al., 2014; Miyai et al., 2014). Recently, the identification of ZIP7 as the causative gene of a novel immunodeficiency syndrome characterized as the absence of circulating B cells and agammaglobulinemia revealed the underlying mechanism that the diminished free cytoplasmic Zn^{2+} increases the phosphatase activity, thus suppressing the BCR signaling cascade (Anzilotti et al., 2019; Woodruff et al., 2018). These findings highlight the specific sensitivity of human B cell development to the Zn^{2+} signal perturbations at the positive selection checkpoints (Fig. 2).

4. Manganese (Mn)

4.1 Manganese homeostasis

Manganese is an essential metal for human health, as it is required for the proper immune function, the regulation of blood sugar and cellular energy, reproduction, digestion, bone growth, blood coagulation and hemostasis, and the defense against reactive oxygen species (ROS). The mammalian cells contain an average range of 0.3–2.9 ppm of Mn (Aschner & Aschner, 2005;

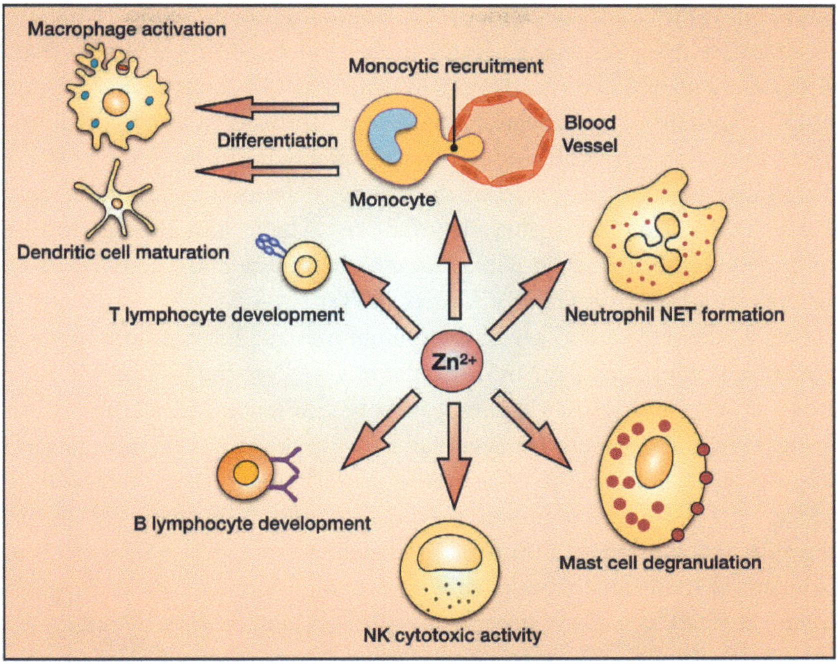

Fig. 2 Zn^{2+} is essential for the innate and adaptive immune activation. Zn^{2+} is indispensable for the proper function of the innate and adaptive immune cells. Zn^{2+} signaling promotes the recruitment of monocytes and their subsequent differentiation. Zn^{2+} positively regulates macrophage activation and dendritic cell (DC) maturation. Zn^{2+} signaling is also essential for neutrophil NET formation, mast cell degranulation and the cytotoxic activity of NK cells. Zn^{2+} augments the TCR-BCR signaling cascade, and is thus important for the development of T/B cells.

Horning, Caito, Tipps, Bowman, & Aschner, 2015), making manganese one of the most common metal ions found in tissues. The estimated safe and adequate dietary intake is an average of around 5 mg Mn/day (Greger, 1998; Trumbo, Yates, Schlicker, & Poos, 2001). The adults absorb approximately 3–5% of the ingested Mn (Davis, Zech, & Greger, 1993; Finley, Johnson, & Johnson, 1994). The absorbed Mn is transported and distributed in the plasma by gamma globulin, albumin and Mn-transferrin complex with the normal concentrations ranging from 72 to 270 μM (Aschner & Aschner, 2005; Harris & Chen, 1994; Nischwitz, Berthele, & Michalke, 2008). The circulatory Mn is largely taken up in the hepatocytes and sequestered in the mitochondria. The excess Mn is then conjugated to bile and passed to the intestine for fecal excretion (Davis et al., 1993; Schroeder, Balassa, & Tipton, 1966). Manganese exerts its function by regulating various Mn-dependent enzymes, including oxido-reductases, isomerases, transferases, ligases, lyases and hydrolases. Mn^{2+} is also an essential component of some metalloenzymes such as Mn superoxide dismutase (SOD2), glutamine synthetase (GS), and arginase (ARG) (Waldron, Rutherford, Ford, & Robinson, 2009). In biochemical processes, Mn^{2+} is very similar to Mg^{2+} in terms of the chemical properties. Previous work showed that Mn^{2+} is able to replace Mg^{2+} in almost half of Mg-dependent enzymes in vitro, in which the catalytic activity of the enzymes are often maintained (Wedler, 1993).

The gradients of Mn^{2+} across the membranes and the nonhomogeneous distribution of intracellular Mn^{2+}, similar to Ca^{2+}, are the biophysical foundation which endorses Mn^{2+} the possibility as a second messenger. In the resting state, most of the intracellular Mn^{2+} is kept in the mitochondria and the Golgi apparatus (Carmona, Roudeau, Perrin, Veronesi, & Ortega, 2014; Martinez-Finley, Gavin, Aschner, & Gunter, 2013), and excessive Mn^{2+} is stored as insoluble manganese phosphate or manganese carbonate in these organelles (Au, Benedetto, & Aschner, 2008; Bragadin, Pozzan, & Azzone, 1983; Gunter et al., 2013). Manganese is the only essential metal without a definite cellular homeostatic process. The detailed mechanism for the subcellular distribution of Mn^{2+} is still under investigation. Most of the known transporters involved in manganese transportation are nonexclusive, which also transport other essential metal ions. As such, the known aspect of the Mn transporter system cannot explain how the intracellular concentrations of Mn^{2+} are selectively maintained without simultaneously influencing the concentrations of other metal ions. To date, multiple ion transporters have shown permeability to Mn^{2+} and are able to mediate Mn^{2+} uptake, including divalent metal ion transporter-1 (DMT1) (Garrick et al., 2006; Salazar et al., 2008), the transferrin system (Aschner & Aschner, 1990; Davidsson, Lonnerdal, Sandstrom, Kunz, & Keen, 1989; Dickinson, Devenyi, & Connor, 1996; Gunter et al., 2013; Keefer, Barak, & Boyett, 1970), zinc transporters such as ZIP8/14 (Boycott et al., 2015; Park et al., 2015; Tuschl et al., 2016; Xin et al., 2017), calcium channels such as TRPM3/7 and store-operated calcium channels (Crossgrove & Yokel, 2005; Guilbert et al., 2009; Loutzenhiser & Loutzenhiser, 2000; Riccio et al., 2002; Xu et al., 2005). Besides, the zinc transporter ZnT10 (Chen, Bowman, Mukhopadhyay, & Aschner, 2015; Leyva-Illades et al., 2014; Quadri et al., 2012; Tuschl et al., 2012; Zaki et al., 2018; Zogzas, Aschner, & Mukhopadhyay, 2016), sodium-calcium exchanger NCX (Waghorn et al., 2009, 2011) and the iron transporter ferroportin (Madejczyk & Ballatori, 2012; Seo & Wessling-Resnick, 2015; Yin et al., 2010) are also involved in regulating the efflux of Mn^{2+}. Moreover, the specialized subcellular Mn^{2+} exchanger such as ATP13A2 on the endosome/lysosome (Schmidt, Wolfe, Stiller, & Pearce, 2009; Tan et al., 2011), SPCA1 and GPP130 on the Golgi membrane (Murin, Verleysdonk, Raeymaekers, Kaplan, & Lehotsky, 2006), the mitochondrial Ca^{2+} uniporter (Gavin, Gunter, & Gunter, 1999), the cytoplasm metallothioneins and calprotectin (Brophy & Nolan, 2015; Kobayashi et al., 2007) seem accountable for the intracellular mobility and organelle storage of manganese.

Mn^{2+} is indicated in regulating the immune responses, similar to Ca^{2+} and Zn^{2+}. The investigations of Mn^{2+} in the immune system largely focused on the nutritional immunity in the past, in which the immune system imposes manganese limitation, thus starving the invading pathogens (Kehl-Fie & Skaar, 2010). The requirement of manganese in the innate and adaptive immune responses has long been overlooked, possibly due to the rareness of Mn deficiency and other more prevalent symptoms in Mn dysregulation such as Mn-associated neurodegeneration (Haase, 2018). Based on numerous dietary sources for Mn, nutritional Mn deficiency is exceptionally rare in nonexperimental settings (Weekley & He, 2017). Under experimental conditions, inadequate dietary intake of Mn resulted in impaired growth, skeletal defects, abnormal glucose tolerance and altered lipid and carbohydrate metabolism (Horning et al., 2015; Keen et al., 1999; Rodriguez-Rodriguez, Bermejo, Lopez-Sobaler, & Ortega, 2011). So far, only a few studies reported genetic defects resulting in the deregulated manganese homeostasis. Mutations in *SLC39A8*, which encodes the Mn/Zn uptake transporter ZIP8, has been recognized to cause a severe manganese depletion syndrome associated with developmental delay and biochemical dysfunction of Mn-dependent enzymes such as the beta-1,4-glycosyltransferase involved in protein galactosylation (Boycott et al., 2015; Lin et al., 2017; Park et al., 2015). Recently, mutations in *SLC30A10* (ZnT10) (Leyva-Illades et al., 2014; Quadri et al., 2012; Tuschl et al., 2012; Zaki et al., 2018; Zogzas et al., 2016) or *SLC39A14* (ZIP14) (Tuschl et al., 2016; Xin et al., 2017) are found to cause inherited hypermanganesemia syndrome featured by dystonia, polycythemia and cirrhosis. The ZnT10 or ZIP14 deficiency damaged the normal serum replenishment (Chen, Bowman, et al., 2015; Zogzas et al., 2016) and the biliary excretion of Mn (Erikson, Thompson, Aschner, & Aschner, 2007; Santos et al., 2012), leading to the resultant circulatory Mn retention.

Unfortunately, the functional integrity of the immune system among the Mn dysregulated individuals has not been investigated, leaving the genetic evidence still inadequate for the requirement of Mn signaling in the regulation of the immune responses.

4.2 Mn^{2+} displays various immune stimulating properties

The application history of Mn^{2+} in regulating the immune response is not short, although the understanding of Mn^{2+} signaling is relatively undefined. Nearly 30 years ago, intraperitoneal injection of $MnCl_2$ showed an enhancement in the activity of murine natural killer cells, which appeared to be mediated by the production of type I interferons (IFNs) (Smialowicz, Riddle, Rogers, Luebke, & Burleson, 1988). Augmented humoral immune responses were also observed in the long-time $MnCl_2$-exposed mice (Srisuchart, Taylor, & Sharma, 1987). Additionally, Mn^{2+} has been demonstrated effective in the management of enterohemorrhagic *Shigella* infections (Mukhopadhyay & Linstedt, 2012). In recent years, Mn-containing nanostructures were found to be decomposed by the reaction with either H^+ or glutathione (GSH) within the tumor microenvironment. Tumor-specific release of Mn^{2+} was originally designed for the Mn^{2+}-enhanced T1-magnetic resonance imaging (MRI) for tumor detection (Fan et al., 2015; Zhang et al., 2015; Zhao et al., 2014). Unexpectedly, these Mn compounds were found to enhance the response of various cancer therapies such as chemotherapy, anti-PD-1 immunotherapy and photodynamic therapy (Chen et al., 2016; Fan et al., 2016; Prasad et al., 2014; Song, Liu, Shi, Zhang, & Chen, 2016; Yang et al., 2017). Besides, the released Mn^{2+} effectively shaped the immunosuppressive microenvironment to favor antitumor immunities, shifted tumor associated macrophage polarization from M2 to M1 phenotypes, and evaluated CTLs infiltration in the tumors (Chen et al., 2016; Fan et al., 2016; Prasad et al., 2014; Song et al., 2016; Yang et al., 2017). Although the precise mechanism of such Mn^{2+} enhanced antitumor activity remains unclear, the common observations in these studies like the provoking of antitumor immunity are nevertheless quite attractive.

The immune stimulating activity of Mn^{2+} was observed more than once in the past decades. Regrettably, the underlying mechanisms in Mn^{2+} signaling and the systematic application of Mn^{2+} have only burst on the scene very recently. The observations of Mn^{2+} mobilization during virus infection indicate the existence of a Mn^{2+}-induced signaling pathway. It is reported that, upon virus infection, stored Mn^{2+} was liberated from the mitochondria and/or Golgi apparatus, leading to the increase of cytosolic free Mn^{2+} reaching at approximate 20 μM in concentration. Consistently, extracellular Mn^{2+} was also observed to accumulate from both alive and pyroptotic virus-infected cells. In fact, the increased Mn^{2+} contents in bronchoalveolar lavage fluid, white blood cells, and alveolar macrophages in virus-infected mice confirmed the physiological relevance of the extracellular release of Mn^{2+}. Meanwhile, the liberated Mn^{2+} was able to induce type I-IFN production and antiviral gene expressions in the absence of infection (Wang et al., 2018), consisting with the observations that the astrocytes were capable of releasing inflammatory cytokines such as IL-6, IL-1β and TNF-α in response to Mn^{2+} exposure alone (Filipov, Seegal, & Lawrence, 2005; Liu et al., 2009; Wang et al., 2018). Hence, the release of Mn^{2+} can deliver danger signals and establish an antiviral state transcellularly in the uninfected bystander cells. Taking the inductive mobility and immune stimulation properties of Mn^{2+} together, it is possible that Mn^{2+} serves as a kind of signal transducers as danger-associated molecular patterns (DAMPs) or alarmins in vivo.

The immune stimulating properties of Mn^{2+} can be explained in several ways. Firstly, Mn^{2+} enhanced the sensitivity of cGAS to double-stranded DNA (dsDNA) and its enzymatic activity, enabling cGAS to produce the second messenger cGAMP in the presence of ultralow levels of dsDNA that would otherwise be non-stimulatory (Wang et al., 2018). Mn^{2+} also enhanced the activity of STING by augmenting the mammalian 2′3′-cGAMP-STING binding affinity, a phenomenon also observed in the Mn^{2+}-enhanced STING detection of pathogen derived cyclic-dinucleotides, such as c-di-GMP and 3′3′-cGAMP (Roembke et al., 2014; Stelitano et al., 2013). Taken together, Mn^{2+} provokes the hyper-activation of the cGAS-STING pathway under which the slightest DNA stimulation or even "perturbation" would lead to the production of type I interferons. Considering the observations that nuclear localized cGAS surveilled the micronuclei resulting from genome instability (Mackenzie et al., 2017) and that there was a steady dsDNA supply in the cytosol escaped from the nuclei, mitochondria or lysosomes, or taken up from dying surrounding cells (Dombrowski et al., 2011; Lan, Londono, Bouley, Rooney, & Hacohen, 2014; West et al., 2015), it is almost certain that the elevated intracellular Mn^{2+} could activate cGAS by the "normal" level of nuclear/cytosolic dsDNA. Such activation was further boosted by the enhanced Mn^{2+}-cGAMP-STING affinity. This might explain the fact that Mn^{2+} signal alarmed the uninfected cells with antiviral gene expressions. Secondly, the Mn^{2+} activated NLRP3 inflammasome may contribute to the immune stimulating activity of Mn^{2+}. Two groups successively reported that Mn^{2+} exposure activated the NLRP3 inflammasome and promoted the maturation of IL-1β, exacerbating the neuroinflammation in vitro and in vivo (Harischandra et al., 2019; Sarkar et al., 2019; Wang et al., 2017). Interestingly, the release of exosomes containing the inflammasome adaptor protein ASC is detected in the Mn^{2+} exposed cells, which mediated the cell-to-cell ASC transmission and the propagated NLRP3 inflammasome activation (Franklin et al., 2014). The microglial cells primed by the Mn^{2+}-induced ASC-containing exosomes became more sensitive to LPS stimulation, and produce a higher level of IL-1β. Consistently, the serum exosomes and serum from occupational manganese-exposed population through welding, mining, or smelting were found with a higher load of ASC and proinflammatory cytokines, respectively (Harischandra et al., 2019; Sarkar et al., 2019). Mn^{2+}-induced inflammasome activation and exosomal ASC release indicate another mechanism through which Mn^{2+} alarms cells and delivers danger signals. Thirdly, Mn^{2+} was reported to activate the ATM-p53 signaling pathway. During the detection of dsDNA breaks, Mre11 within the DNA damage sensor complex MRN required Mn^{2+} dependent exonuclease activity, which was indispensable and could not be substituted by Mg^{2+} or Ca^{2+} (Hopfner et al., 2001; Paull & Gellert, 1998; Trujillo, Yuan, Lee, & Sung, 1998). Mn^{2+} was also required by activated Ataxia telangiectasia mutated (ATM) which was a Mn-activated kinase that recruited by the MRN complex to phosphorylate downstream effector proteins, including the histone H2AX and the transcription factor p53 (Banin et al., 1998; Canman et al., 1998; Chan et al., 2000). Like ATM, ATR/FRP-1 also phosphorylated p53 in a Mn^{2+}-dependent manner (Canman et al., 1998). The phosphorylated ATM and p53 were directly detected in response to Mn^{2+} at physiologically relevant concentrations in the primary cells, and inhibitors of ATM kinase suppressed Mn^{2+} induced p53 phosphorylation. Analysis of gene expression changes revealed a prominent role of p53 in Mn^{2+} induced transcriptome alterations (Guilarte, 2010; Guilarte et al., 2008; Shi, Zhao, Yang, et al., 2015), providing further evidence of ATM-p53 as a Mn^{2+} homeostatic response pathway (Tidball et al., 2015). Under the supraphysiological concentrations, usually above 1 mM, Mn^{2+} exhibited catalase-like activity and induced apoptosis through the activation of either caspase-8 or caspase-12 pathway (El Mchichi, Hadji, Vazquez, & Leca, 2007; Oubrahim, Chock, & Stadtman, 2002; Oubrahim, Stadtman, & Chock, 2001). Thereby, Mn^{2+} seems to deliver danger signals which alarm the cells through the ultrasensitive ATM-p53 pathway, trigger protective apoptosis, and facilitate the incoming immune responses (Yoon et al., 2015). Additionally, Mn^{2+} was reported to stabilize the high-affinity conformation of integrins LFA-1 to ICAM-1 (Meijne et al., 1994; Petit et al., 2016; Takagi, Petre, Walz, & Springer, 2002) which are indispensably required for the migration of phagocytes toward infection and T cell adhesion to antigen-presenting cells.

4.3 Mn^{2+} functions as a damage-associated molecular pattern (DAMP)

Based on the above mentioned observations about the activities of Mn^{2+} during inflammation, the role of Mn^{2+} as a DAMP or alarmin is becoming intriguingly clear. On the one side, the intracellular distribution of Mn^{2+} is highly diverse. The clamp of insoluble manganese salts and the maintenance of Mn^{2+} gradients across the organelle membranes are energy consumption processes that need continuous energy input. Thereby, the free cytoplasmic Mn^{2+} might function as a trigger factor in the intracellular immunosurveillance system. The successful acute infections of intracellular pathogens are unexceptionally featured by hijacking the cellular metabolic system which is dispensable for the maintenance of the Mn^{2+} gradients. Further, the metabolic burden resulted from pathogen replications, the mitochondrial permeability transition and organelle disintegration as a part of the cytopathogenic effect make the restraint of Mn^{2+} even more difficult, let alone the releasing process of intracellular pathogens which would culminate the Mn^{2+} efflux to its epilogue (Salameh, Sheth, & Shukla, 2012). On the other side, the liberated Mn^{2+} is a multifunctional immunostimulant. The infection-induced Mn^{2+} efflux generates Mn^{2+} chemogradient surrounding the center of infection. In other words, the Mn^{2+} signal intensity is proportional to the distance from the infection, somehow similar to the alarm calls, the harsher it sounds, the more dangerous it represents. In cells most adjacent to infections, the high-level Mn^{2+} exposure (1 mM, equivalent to 1 mM of Mn^{2+} stimulation in culture dishes, hereinafter) could induce the caspase cascades and resultant apoptosis, which are prophylactic cell death pathways as if creating firebreaks in the forest of cells to prevent the spread of the infectious fire. As a result of Mn^{2+} diffusion, the slightly less strong Mn^{2+} signal (0.5–1 mM) then alters the ATM-p53 and the NLRP3-CASP1 signaling pathway in neighboring cells. Through the upregulated sensing sensitivity of dsDNA breaks and the disassembly of the trans-Golgi network (Chen & Chen, 2018) characterized as the early biochemistry events in the infection, the Mn^{2+} signal alarms cells to commit apoptosis and/or pyroptosis even under the mildest infections, thus blocking the secondary spread of pathogens to uninfected cells. As the Mn^{2+} diffusion goes on, a step-lower concentration of Mn^{2+} stimulation (0.05–0.5 mM) leads to strong type I interferon production together with the expression of antiviral effector genes in the uninfected bystander cells, preparing in advance for the incoming spread of the infection. A 10-fold weaker Mn^{2+} signal (2–50 μM) is sufficient to fully charge the cGAS-STING pathway and to stabilize the LFA-1: ICAM-1 interactions, which significantly lowers the detection threshold of the intracellular pathogens and benefits the clamp of infection through warning more cells in the distal of the infection sites. Thereby, the Mn^{2+} signal can orchestrate the immune responses with a comprehensive set of strategies (Fig. 3).

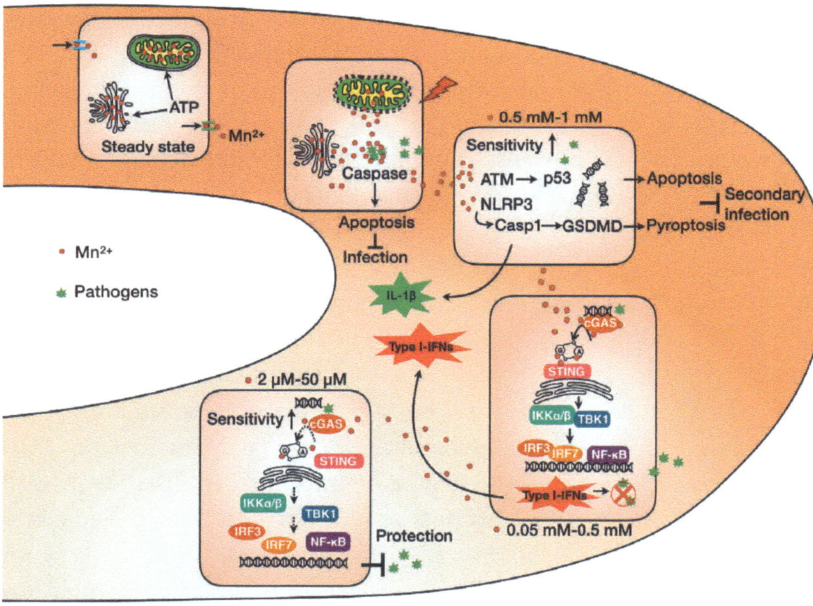

Fig. 3 Mn^{2+} functions as a damage-associated molecular pattern (DAMP). The highly diversified intracellular Mn^{2+} distribution relies on the integrality of the healthy cells. Damage or infection disrupts the restraint of intracellular Mn^{2+}, resulting in Mn^{2+} release and the establishment of Mn^{2+} chemogradient. The free Mn^{2+} is a kind of DAMPs: the strongest Mn^{2+} signal promotes prophylactic cell death; the less-stronger Mn^{2+} signal sensitizes the ATM-p53 and the NLRP3-caspase-1 pathway, increasing the potential of apoptosis or pyroptosis with the maturation of IL-1β; the moderate Mn^{2+} signal provokes the self-activated cGAS-STING pathway to produce type I-IFNs and other proinflammatory cytokines; the weakest Mn^{2+} signal lowers the threshold of the cGAS-STING activation. Mn^{2+} from the center of infection, together with the ASC-exosomes, cytokines including IL-1β/-18, chemokines, and type I-IFNs, generate the information stream that delivers danger signal to cells in the distal site of infection.

From the view of energy economizing, the hypothesis of Mn^{2+} as a DAMP or an alarmin in host defense against infection is also sensible. The strongest Mn^{2+} danger signal induces direct or prophylactic cell death which costs the most to ultimately cut off the transmission routes of the infection. The moderate Mn^{2+} signal enables the expression of anti-infection effector genes, featured by acute cell cycle arrest and additional biochemical synthesis. The weakest Mn^{2+} signal only alarms the housekeeping defense and thus may only raise affordable risk such as false positive errors. The beauty of this mechanism is that the storage of manganese is active but the release is passive. The release of Mn^{2+} does not rely on direct pathogen detections but is triggered by the loss of intracellular homeostasis or integrity. Considering that the diversity of pathogenic mechanisms has been practiced for subverting or escaping immune detection, the passive defense strategies, such as the Mn^{2+}-DAMPs signal, are valuable complements to the active defense system exemplified by the PAMP-PRR signals.

5. Iron (Fe)

Iron is an indispensable component for many enzymes, including hemoglobin, myoglobin and cytochromes (Muckenthaler, Rivella, Hentze, & Galy, 2017; Oexle, Gnaiger, & Weiss, 1999; Volani et al., 2017; Weinberg, 1978). An important function of iron is to act as a catalytic subunit, transferring electron and mediating redox reactions. Despite of the crucial roles iron may play, redundant iron is harmful as it induces the generation of toxic oxygen through *Fenton* reaction due to its great oxidizing ability. Dietary absorption and cellular recycling have been synergistically employed to achieve iron homeostasis (Andrews, Robinson, & Rodriguez-Quinones, 2003; Andrews & Schmidt, 2007; Breuer, Shvartsman, & Cabantchik, 2008). Intestinal absorption of iron is mediated by the H^+/divalent metal symporter DMT-1 (Hentze, Muckenthaler, & Andrews, 2004). The absorbed $Fe^{2+/3+}$ are transported via the transferrin cycles and then systematically distributed through the ubiquitously expressed transferrin receptor-1 (TfR1) and hepatocellular restricted transferrin receptor-2 (TfR2) (Cheng, Zak, Aisen, Harrison, & Walz, 2004). Besides, iron may also be taken up in other protein bound forms like acidic isoferritin or hemoglobin, which are mediated by the scavenger receptor CD163 (Meyron-Holtz et al., 1999). Owing to the fluctuating dietary iron intake, the absorption of iron is precisely controlled. Hepcidin, a hormone derived from liver, plays a crucial role in this process. In brief, the coding gene of hepcidin, *HAMP*, is transcriptionally activated by the increase of the level of iron. Hepcidin then induces the degradation of the iron exporter ferroportin, thus blocking dietary iron absorption and repressing the further rise of the plasma iron level. Reversely, when the iron level decreases, less hepcidin is produced and dietary iron absorption resumes (Ganz & Nemeth, 2015). Surplus iron can also be stored in hepatocytes and macrophages and return to the circulation during iron deprivation, thus stabilizing the iron homeostasis (Kristiansen et al., 2001).

The $Fe^{2+/3+}$-heme binding in hemoglobin takes up the majority of iron storage. During infection, the maintenance of iron homeostasis is challenged by the shortened red blood cell lifespan (Johnson & Wessling-Resnick, 2012). Accordingly, the infection related iron mobilization is initiated through hemolysis and phagocytosis of damaged erythrocytes. Moreover, the inflammatory signals such as IL-6 and activin B can cause hepatogenic hepcidin production and the resultant iron sequestration in macrophages (Kanamori et al., 2017; Latour et al., 2017; Nemeth et al., 2004; Verga Falzacappa et al., 2007). Without regard to extracellular iron limitation for microorganisms, the increased intracellular Fe^{2+} level seems to directly provoke immune responses. By catalyzing the formation of oxygen radicals via the *Fenton* reaction, labile Fe^{2+} stimulated NF-κB activity and HIF-1α stability and thus displayed pronounced proinflammatory properties (Koury & Haase, 2015; Nairz et al., 2018; Nizet & Johnson, 2009; Sonnweber et al., 2011). Moreover, free heme acted as a danger-associated molecular pattern (DAMP) and activated TLR4 in the extracellular space and the NLRP3 inflammasome in the intracellular space which might prevent the spreading of infection, but amplified the systemic inflammatory response in sepsis (Dutra et al., 2014; Figueiredo et al., 2007). Additionally, macrophage polarization is associated with the iron transporter repertoire involved in iron uptake, storage and release. M1 macrophages tend to store and deplete the irons in the microenvironment. Conversely, the metabolic profile of M2 macrophages sustains their propensities to take up, degrade heme and recirculate free irons (Cairo, Recalcati, Mantovani, & Locati, 2011).

Previous studies about the role of iron in immunity have always been focused on nutritional immunology. Since the term *Ferroptosis* was coined, increasing studies have revealed its participation in immune regulation, especially in the context of tumor immunology. Ferroptosis is an iron-dependent non-apoptotic form of regulated cell death defined in 2012, which is caused by lipid peroxidation and can be suppressed by iron chelators and lipid peroxidation inhibitors (Dixon et al., 2012). Thus, ferroptosis, to some extent, could be speculated as the result of iron homeostasis deregulation or even iron signal triggered active cell death. The induction of ferroptosis has already been found as an antitumor strategy. The depletion of intracellular iron pools and ferroptosis inhibitor suppressed the cytotoxic effects of sorafenib in hepatocellular carcinoma (HCC) cells (Louandre et al., 2013). Besides, in various different tumor types such as acute myeloid leukemia, diffuse large B cell lymphomas (DLBCLs) and renal cell carcinomas (RCCs), ferroptosis endowed higher sensitivity to chemotherapeutic agents (Yang et al., 2014; Yu et al., 2015). Although these studies clued on the benefits of ferroptosis in tumor suppression, there is more to find regarding the relevance between ferroptosis and the generation of antitumor immunity. Recently, $CD8^+$ T cells triggered ferroptosis was demonstrated to participate in the efficacy of the immune checkpoint therapy. During immunotherapy, activated $CD8^+$ T cells secreted IFNγ which activated the transcription factor STAT1 and inhibited the cystine/glutamate antiporter system X_c^- in the tumor cells, leading to lipid peroxide accumulation and ferroptosis. Suppression of ferroptosis could weaken the therapeutic effect (Wang et al., 2019). This might explain the phenotypes that the iron deficiency down-regulated acquired T cell responses in several experimental models (Grant, Wiesinger, Beard, & Cantorna, 2003; Kuvibidila & Porretta, 2003; Walker & Walker, 2000). Considering the observations that many cancer cells exhibit a greater demand for iron relative to their non-malignant counterparts (Torti & Torti, 2019), targeted regulation of iron and ferroptosis might benefit relevant cancer immunotherapy in the future.

6. Potassium (K)

In contrast to the divalent cations such as Ca^{2+}, Zn^{2+} and Mn^{2+} that function as second messengers, the monovalent cations such as Na^+ and K^+ mainly regulate the membrane potential, which indirectly controls other ionic signaling pathways. Potassium is an important element in the human body with the amount of about 50 mEq/kg. 98% of K^+ is found within cells, while only 2% is in the extracellular fluid. The balance between intracellular and extracellular fluid is maintained by the Na^+-K^+ ATPase (Cui & Xie, 2017), which pumps K^+ into and Na^+ out of cells. Different concentrations of K^+ and Na^+ across the membrane create the membrane potential, which is crucial for action potentials, muscle contractility and ion transportation. Human daily dietary contains about 120 mEq potassium. To keep the potassium homeostasis of the whole body, about 90% of the daily K^+ intake is excreted in the urine, whereas about 10% is excreted by the gastrointestinal tract (McDonough & Youn, 2017; Palmer & Clegg, 2016). In the immune system, the disorders of potassium homeostasis, such as hypokalemia and hyperkalemia, have been indicated as a determinant of the immune dysfunction.

Similar to the Ca^{2+} influx, the K^+ efflux is commonly detected in most agonist-stimulated NLRP3 inflammasome activation, including ATP, nigericin, gramicidin, $Al(OH)_3$, silica and calcium pyrophosphate crystals (Gong, Yang, Jin, Jiang, & Zhou, 2018; Munoz-Planillo et al., 2013; Petrilli et al., 2007). Additionally, the increased extracellular K^+ level inhibits agonist-induced NLRP3 inflammasome formation. The similar inhibitory effect of high extracellular K^+ is found in the lethal toxin (LT) induced NALP1 inflammasome activation (Petrilli et al., 2007). Consistently, the K^+-free medium was able to activate the NLRP3 inflammasome by straightforwardly triggering the K^+ efflux (Munoz-Planillo et al., 2013). However, the K^+ efflux might not be indispensably required for some other NLRP3 inflammasome activators, like GB111-NH2 (Sanman et al., 2016), imiquimod, and CL097 (Gross et al., 2016). The K^+ efflux is mediated by different channels in a context-dependent manner. P2X7 is found to be activated by extracellular ATP and then functions as the K^+ channel, which mediates the indispensable K^+ mobilization in the ATP-NLRP3 inflammasome activation (Mariathasan et al., 2006; North, 2002). A whole-genome RNAi screening showed that voltage-gated K^+ channels (*Kcna3* or *Kcnb2*) and K^+ inwardly-rectifying channel (*Kcnj3*) were involved in the parasite *Entamoeba histolytica* induced cell death (Marie, Verkerke, Theodorescu, & Petri, 2015). Inhibition of the voltage-gated K^+ channel of peripheral blood T lymphocytes decreased the activation of the NLRP3 inflammasome in hypertensive patients (Zhu et al., 2017).

The K^+ homeostasis pivots the function of the cGAS-STING pathway. The $Asc^{-/-}$, $Casp1^{-/-}Casp11^{-/-}$ and $Gsdmd^{-/-}$ gene-deficient bone marrow-derived macrophages (BMDMs) produced a significantly higher level of IFN-β during the *Francisella novicida* infection, indicative of a strengthened cGAS-STING activation (Banerjee et al., 2018). GSDMD is cleaved by activated caspase1/4/5/11, making the amino-terminal of GSDMD form membrane pores to induce the K^+ efflux and pyroptosis (Kayagaki et al., 2015; Shi, Zhao, Wang, et al., 2015). However, the treatment of inflammasome-deficient macrophages with K^+ ionophores weakened the production of cGAMP, which indicated that the K^+ efflux, but not pyroptosis, could inhibit the cGAS-STING pathway. Also, K^+-free medium reduced the production of IFN-β in the *F. novicida* infected BMDMs. In vitro assay showed that recombinant cGAS synthesized decreased cGAMP in the absence of K^+ (Banerjee et al., 2018). In conclusion, cytosolic K^+ is important for cGAS-dsDNA binding. Further, potassium was found to control a new immune checkpoint system—ionic checkpoint which was able to avoid excessive activation of immune responses (Chandy & Norton, 2016; Pardoll, 2012). Inspired by the relationship of tumor necrosis and bad prognosis, K^+ released by necrotic cells was found to suppress T cell activation. Elevated extracellular K^+ reduced TCR-induced Akt-mTOR signaling mediated by the serine/threonine phosphatase PP2A. However, how elevated K^+ activated PP2A was still unknown (Eil et al., 2016). Recent studies explored the impact of elevated K^+ on T cell stemness. Elevated extracellular K^+ reprogrammed the T cell metabolism without affecting their viability, switching the metabolic state from consumption of extracellular energy resources to autophagy and mitochondrial-driven energy production. As a result, the epigenetic states of the promoter and enhancer *loci* of T cell activation, exhaustion or stemness-associated genes were changed in high K^+ environment, which restricted effector programs and maintained T cell stemness (Vodnala et al., 2019). Based on observations of tumor-infiltrating lymphocytes, the overabundant extracellular K^+ in tumor interstitial fluid has two paradoxically different functions: inhibiting terminal T cell effector differentiation and function; while maintaining T cell stemness to enhance cancer immunotherapy.

7. Immunity controlled by unessential metal ions

Metal cation–ligand interactions define a great part of the chemical space commonly explored for drug design (Meggers, 2007; Mjos & Orvig, 2014; Riccardi, Genna, & De Vivo, 2018). Additionally, the successes in metallodrugs also inspire the exploiting of unessential minerals in the regulation of the immune responses. The clinical application of aluminum-containing compounds as the immune adjuvants in the vaccines is one of the most famous examples. The immune enhancement effect of antigen precipitation with insoluble aluminum salts was first reported in 1926 (Glenny, Pope, Waddington, & Wallace, 1926). Since then, aluminum adjuvants, mainly referring to the aluminum hydroxide and aluminum phosphate, have been incorporated into billions of doses of licensed vaccines and administered annually to millions of people. The success can be attributed to the fact that aluminum adjuvants are effective and inexpensive and have an excellent safety profile with minimal reactogenicity (Hogenesch, 2012; HogenEsch, O'Hagan, & Fox, 2018; Lindblad, 2004). The mechanism through which aluminum adjuvants enhance the immune responses remains not fully understood and even controversial. The physical depot effects of the aluminum-adjuvanted antigens seem indisputable for the increase of vaccine immunogenicity, which have made soluble antigens particulate, thus retaining antigens at the injection site (Calabro et al., 2011; de Veer, Kemp, Chatelier, Elhay, & Meeusen, 2010; Lu & Hogenesch, 2013), targeting (Ghimire, Benson, Garside, & Brewer, 2012; Rimaniol et al., 2004; Sokolovska, Hem, & HogenEsch, 2007) and enhancing (Mannhalter, Neychev, Zlabinger, Ahmad, & Eibl, 1985; Morefield et al., 2005) the uptake through phagocytosis by antigen-presenting cells. Besides, aluminum adjuvants are reported to simultaneously activate several pathways which might redundantly contribute to the adjuvant effect (HogenEsch et al., 2018): (1) Aluminum adjuvants activate the NLRP3 inflammasome, resulting in the secretion of IL-1β, which induces the differentiation of monocytes into mature dendritic cells (Seubert, Monaci, Pizza, O'Hagan, & Wack, 2008; Ulanova, Tarkowski, Hahn-Zoric, & Hanson, 2001) with more efficient antigen presentation (Ghimire et al., 2012; Li, Nookala, & Re, 2007). (2) The aluminum-adjuvanted vaccines induce necrosis and/or pyroptosis of tissue cells at the site of injection, which might lead to the release of DAMPs, including DNA, uric acid, ATP and IL-33 for immune activation (Kool, Soullie, et al., 2008; Li, Willingham, Ting, & Re, 2008; Marichal et al., 2011; McKee et al., 2013; Riteau et al., 2012; Rose, Okragly, Patel, & Benschop, 2015). (3) Aluminum adjuvants can activate the Syk-NFAT pathway with the inductive expression of IL-2 (Flach et al., 2011; Khameneh et al., 2017). (4) Aluminum adjuvants activate the complement cascade with the formation of the membrane attack complex which plays a critical role in the humoral immune responses (Guven, Duus, Laursen, Hojrup, & Houen, 2013). Aluminum adjuvants are successful but not perfect, in that they mainly induce TH_2 cell responses through NLPR3 inflammasome activation (Eisenbarth, Colegio, O'Connor, Sutterwala, & Flavell, 2008; Kool, Petrilli, et al., 2008; Li et al., 2008), but not TH_1 or CTL responses (Marrack, McKee, & Munks, 2009; Petrovsky & Aguilar, 2004). Therefore, aluminum adjuvants are thought unable to elicit cellular immune responses that are essential for virus or tumor vaccines. Moreover, both aluminum hydroxide and aluminum phosphate are sensitive to freeze and require cold-chain temperature control (Chen et al., 2009; Clapp, Munks, Trivedi, Kompella, & Braun, 2014; Zapata, Feldkamp, Peck, White, & Hem, 1984), pressuring the cost of aluminum-adjuvanted vaccines especially in the undeveloped countries.

cis-Diamminedichloroplatinum (II) (cisplatin) is one of the most commonly used chemotherapeutic agents in the treatment of a variety of solid tumors. Arsenic trioxide (As_2O_3) has been used for more than 20 years in patients with acute promyelocytic leukemia. The effectiveness of tumor-specific cytotoxicity of these metallodrugs is primarily based on ligand exchange reactions to generate drug-target covalent bonds, which causes structural lesions at the targeted nucleic acids and protein residues, ultimately leading to cellular apoptosis (Arriagada et al., 2004; Jamieson & Lippard, 1999; Messori & Merlino, 2016; Zhang et al., 2010). However, the cytotoxic activity alone is not enough to explain the successes of cisplatin and arsenic trioxide. In fact, it is the immune-dependent antineoplastic effects that feature these two metallodrugs such outstanding. The augmented CTLs-mediated antitumor immunity was usually observed in the cisplatin-responsive tumor treatments (Aranda et al., 2015; Merritt, Mahtabifard, Yamada, Crystal, & Korst, 2003). Accordingly, further atomistic understanding of the metal-ligand interactions, especially the artificial intervention of ion signals during the immune responses, seems to be promising in fostering the future design of metallodrugs and metalloenzyme inhibitors.

8. Concluding remarks

It is intriguing that the study on some metal ions which has been suspended for some time is now being restarted or reactivated. The comprehensive understanding of the Ca^{2+} signaling together with its roles in manifesting the immune responses provides an impetus to search for novel metal ion signaling pathway. Given the simple definition of a second messenger as a small chemical entity transmitting signals and modulating cells' activity, not only Ca^{2+}, but also Zn^{2+} and Mn^{2+} all seem to fit this description to some extent. In this respect, although the existence of free metal ions with the potential to alternate among different redox states is generally considered dangerous, as seen for iron in the Fenton reaction, Mn^{2+} seems to promote antioxidant defense at moderate concentrations (Haase, 2018). Learning the lessons from the Ca^{2+} signal research, good tools are essential in the studies of these ions. As the high sensitive calcium fluorescence probes enable seeing-is-believing super-resolution images of the Ca^{2+} signal, the fluorescence probe for specific metal ion detection would be the most powerful "weapon" for the appreciation of other ions as the second messenger. Understandably, more effectual chemical tools, such as high-specific metal ion chelators or metal ion channel agonists, are equally valuable in exploiting the boundary of our understandings on metal ion signals. With the ever-evolving gene-sequencing technology, it is predictable that more metal ion signal related-gene deficient animal models will be identified or generated. Moreover, tissue-specific metal ion transporter deficient animals would be necessary to provide deeper insights into their regulatory functions, in that the metal ion signals are not limited to the immune responses only. Besides, the opensource diets comprised of purified ingredients allow the selective removal of certain mineral nutrients and the establishment of malnutrition animal models, which facilitate the understanding of the metal ion signal malfunction during nutrient deficiency with a physiological relevance. In the scenario of the foreseeable technological advances, our understandings of the metalloimmunology, the metal ion-controlled immunity, would play a prominent role in the exploration, expansion and exploitation of novel therapeutic applications, including but not limited to metallodrugs and metalloimmunotherapies. In particular, we hope that the Mn^{2+}-DAMP hypothesis proposed by our studies shall open up the gate to future application of Mn^{2+}-containing compounds as immunostimulant vaccines or drugs in clinic trials.

Acknowledgments

We thank Dr. X. Zhou for critical reading of the manuscript. This work was supported by National Natural Science Foundation of China (31830022 and 81621001) and the Chinese Ministry of Science and Technology (2015CB943203).

References

Ablasser, A., & Chen, Z. J. (2019). cGAS in action: Expanding roles in immunity and inflammation. *Science*, *363*, eaat8657.

Ackland, M. L., & Michalczyk, A. (2006). Zinc deficiency and its inherited disorders—A review. *Genes & Nutrition*, *1*, 41–49.

Agostini, L., Martinon, F., Burns, K., McDermott, M. F., Hawkins, P. N., & Tschopp, J. (2004). NALP3 forms an IL-1beta-processing inflammasome with increased activity in Muckle-Wells autoinflammatory disorder. *Immunity*, *20*, 319–325.

Aifantis, I., Gounari, F., Scorrano, L., Borowski, C., & von Boehmer, H. (2001). Constitutive pre-TCR signaling promotes differentiation through Ca2+ mobilization and activation of NF-kappaB and NFAT. *Nature Immunology*, *2*, 403–409.

Allam, R., Lawlor, K. E., Yu, E. C., Mildenhall, A. L., Moujalled, D. M., Lewis, R. S., et al. (2014). Mitochondrial apoptosis is dispensable for NLRP3 inflammasome activation but non-apoptotic caspase-8 is required for inflammasome priming. *EMBO Reports*, *15*, 982–990.

Andreini, C., Bertini, I., & Rosato, A. (2009). Metalloproteomes: A bioinformatic approach. *Accounts of Chemical Research*, *42*, 1471–1479.

Andrews, S. C., Robinson, A. K., & Rodriguez-Quinones, F. (2003). Bacterial iron homeostasis. *FEMS Microbiology Reviews*, *27*, 215–237.

Andrews, N. C., & Schmidt, P. J. (2007). Iron homeostasis. *Annual Review of Physiology*, *69*, 69–85.

Anzilotti, C., Swan, D. J., Boisson, B., Deobagkar-Lele, M., Oliveira, C., Chabosseau, P., et al. (2019). An essential role for the Zn(2+) transporter ZIP7 in B cell development. *Nature Immunology*, *20*, 350–361.

Aranda, F., Bloy, N., Pesquet, J., Petit, B., Chaba, K., Sauvat, A., et al. (2015). Immune-dependent antineoplastic effects of cisplatin plus pyridoxine in non-small-cell lung cancer. *Oncogene*, *34*, 3053–3062.

Arriagada, R., Bergman, B., Dunant, A., Le Chevalier, T., Pignon, J. P., Vansteenkiste, J., et al. (2004). Cisplatin-based adjuvant chemotherapy in patients with completely resected non-small-cell lung cancer. *The New England Journal of Medicine*, *350*, 351–360.

Aschner, M., & Aschner, J. L. (1990). Manganese transport across the blood-brain barrier: Relationship to iron homeostasis. *Brain Research Bulletin*, *24*, 857–860.

Aschner, J. L., & Aschner, M. (2005). Nutritional aspects of manganese homeostasis. *Molecular Aspects of Medicine*, *26*, 353–362.

Au, C., Benedetto, A., & Aschner, M. (2008). Manganese transport in eukaryotes: The role of DMT1. *Neurotoxicology*, *29*, 569–576.

Aydemir, T. B., Liuzzi, J. P., McClellan, S., & Cousins, R. J. (2009). Zinc transporter ZIP8 (SLC39A8) and zinc influence IFN-gamma expression in activated human T cells. *Journal of Leukocyte Biology*, *86*, 337–348.

Baba, Y., Nishida, K., Fujii, Y., Hirano, T., Hikida, M., & Kurosaki, T. (2008). Essential function for the calcium sensor STIM1 in mast cell activation and anaphylactic responses. *Nature Immunology*, *9*, 81–88.

Banerjee, I., Behl, B., Mendonca, M., Shrivastava, G., Russo, A. J., Menoret, A., et al. (2018). Gasdermin D restrains type I interferon response to cytosolic DNA by disrupting ionic homeostasis. *Immunity*, *49*, 413–426.e5.

Banin, S., Moyal, L., Shieh, S., Taya, Y., Anderson, C. W., Chessa, L., et al. (1998). Enhanced phosphorylation of p53 by ATM in response to DNA damage. *Science*, *281*, 1674–1677.

Bao, S., Liu, M. J., Lee, B., Besecker, B., Lai, J. P., Guttridge, D. C., et al. (2010). Zinc modulates the innate immune response in vivo to polymicrobial sepsis through regulation of NF-kappaB. *American Journal of Physiology Lung Cellular and Molecular Physiology*, *298*, L744–L754.

Bao, B., Prasad, A. S., Beck, F. W., Bao, G. W., Singh, T., Ali, S., et al. (2011). Intracellular free zinc up-regulates IFN-gamma and T-bet essential for Th1 differentiation in Con-A stimulated HUT-78 cells. *Biochemical and Biophysical Research Communications*, *407*, 703–707.

Baumgart, D. C., Macdonald, J. K., & Feagan, B. (2008). Tacrolimus (FK506) for induction of remission in refractory ulcerative colitis. *The Cochrane Database of Systematic Reviews*, *3*, CD007216.

Baumgart, D. C., Pintoffl, J. P., Sturm, A., Wiedenmann, B., & Dignass, A. U. (2006). Tacrolimus is safe and effective in patients with severe steroid-refractory or steroid-dependent inflammatory bowel disease—A long-term follow-up. *The American Journal of Gastroenterology*, *101*, 1048–1056.

Bauquet, A. T., Jin, H., Paterson, A. M., Mitsdoerffer, M., Ho, I. C., Sharpe, A. H., et al. (2009). The costimulatory molecule ICOS regulates the expression of c-Maf and IL-21 in the development of follicular T helper cells and TH-17 cells. *Nature Immunology, 10,* 167–175.

Beck, F. W., Prasad, A. S., Kaplan, J., Fitzgerald, J. T., & Brewer, G. J. (1997). Changes in cytokine production and T cell subpopulations in experimentally induced zinc-deficient humans. *The American Journal of Physiology, 272,* E1002–E1007.

Besecker, B. Y., Exline, M. C., Hollyfield, J., Phillips, G., Disilvestro, R. A., Wewers, M. D., et al. (2011). A comparison of zinc metabolism, inflammation, and disease severity in critically ill infected and noninfected adults early after intensive care unit admission. *The American Journal of Clinical Nutrition, 93,* 1356–1364.

Bhakta, N. R., Oh, D. Y., & Lewis, R. S. (2005). Calcium oscillations regulate thymocyte motility during positive selection in the three-dimensional thymic environment. *Nature Immunology, 6,* 143–151.

Bopp, T., Palmetshofer, A., Serfling, E., Heib, V., Schmitt, S., Richter, C., et al. (2005). NFATc2 and NFATc3 transcription factors play a crucial role in suppression of CD4+ T lymphocytes by CD4+ CD25+ regulatory T cells. *The Journal of Experimental Medicine, 201,* 181–187.

Bose, T., Cieslar-Pobuda, A., & Wiechec, E. (2015). Role of ion channels in regulating Ca(2)(+) homeostasis during the interplay between immune and cancer cells. *Cell Death & Disease, 6,* e1648.

Bosse, M., Audette, M., Ferland, C., Pelletier, G., Chu, H. W., Dakhama, A., et al. (1996). Gene expression of interleukin-2 in purified human peripheral blood eosinophils. *Immunology, 87,* 149–154.

Boycott, K. M., Beaulieu, C. L., Kernohan, K. D., Gebril, O. H., Mhanni, A., Chudley, A. E., et al. (2015). Autosomal-recessive intellectual disability with cerebellar atrophy syndrome caused by mutation of the manganese and zinc transporter gene SLC39A8. *American Journal of Human Genetics, 97,* 886–893.

Bragadin, M., Pozzan, T., & Azzone, G. F. (1983). The nature of the electron spin resonance signal during aerobic uptake of Mn2+ in mitochondria from rat liver. *European Journal of Biochemistry, 134,* 385–390.

Brazao, V., Caetano, L. C., Del Vecchio Filipin, M., Paula Alonso Toldo, M., Caetano, L. N., & do Prado, J. C., Jr. (2008). Zinc supplementation increases resistance to experimental infection by Trypanosoma cruzi. *Veterinary Parasitology, 154,* 32–37.

Breuer, W., Shvartsman, M., & Cabantchik, Z. I. (2008). Intracellular labile iron. *The International Journal of Biochemistry & Cell Biology, 40,* 350–354.

Brieger, A., Rink, L., & Haase, H. (2013). Differential regulation of TLR-dependent MyD88 and TRIF signaling pathways by free zinc ions. *Journal of Immunology, 191,* 1808–1817.

Brophy, M. B., & Nolan, E. M. (2015). Manganese and microbial pathogenesis: Sequestration by the Mammalian immune system and utilization by microorganisms. *ACS Chemical Biology, 10,* 641–651.

Brough, D., Le Feuvre, R. A., Wheeler, R. D., Solovyova, N., Hilfiker, S., Rothwell, N. J., et al. (2003). Ca2+ stores and Ca2+ entry differentially contribute to the release of IL-1 beta and IL-1 alpha from murine macrophages. *Journal of Immunology, 170,* 3029–3036.

Brylinski, M., & Skolnick, J. (2011). FINDSITE-metal: Integrating evolutionary information and machine learning for structure-based metal-binding site prediction at the proteome level. *Proteins, 79,* 735–751.

Bueno, O. F., Brandt, E. B., Rothenberg, M. E., & Molkentin, J. D. (2002). Defective T cell development and function in calcineurin A beta-deficient mice. *Proceedings of the National Academy of Sciences of the United States of America, 99,* 9398–9403.

Byun, M., Abhyankar, A., Lelarge, V., Plancoulaine, S., Palanduz, A., Telhan, L., et al. (2010). Whole-exome sequencing-based discovery of STIM1 deficiency in a child with fatal classic Kaposi sarcoma. *The Journal of Experimental Medicine, 207,* 2307–2312.

Cabral, M. D., Paulet, P. E., Robert, V., Gomes, B., Renoud, M. L., Savignac, M., et al. (2010). Knocking down Cav1 calcium channels implicated in Th2 cell activation prevents experimental asthma. *American Journal of Respiratory and Critical Care Medicine, 181*, 1310–1317.

Cairo, G., Recalcati, S., Mantovani, A., & Locati, M. (2011). Iron trafficking and metabolism in macrophages: Contribution to the polarized phenotype. *Trends in Immunology, 32*, 241–247.

Calabro, S., Tortoli, M., Baudner, B. C., Pacitto, A., Cortese, M., O'Hagan, D. T., et al. (2011). Vaccine adjuvants alum and MF59 induce rapid recruitment of neutrophils and monocytes that participate in antigen transport to draining lymph nodes. *Vaccine, 29*, 1812–1823.

Camello-Almaraz, C., Gomez-Pinilla, P. J., Pozo, M. J., & Camello, P. J. (2006). Mitochondrial reactive oxygen species and Ca2+ signaling. *American Journal of Physiology Cell Physiology, 291*, C1082–C1088.

Canman, C. E., Lim, D. S., Cimprich, K. A., Taya, Y., Tamai, K., Sakaguchi, K., et al. (1998). Activation of the ATM kinase by ionizing radiation and phosphorylation of p53. *Science, 281*, 1677–1679.

Carmona, A., Roudeau, S., Perrin, L., Veronesi, G., & Ortega, R. (2014). Environmental manganese compounds accumulate as Mn(II) within the Golgi apparatus of dopamine cells: Relationship between speciation, subcellular distribution, and cytotoxicity. *Metallomics: Integrated Biometal Science, 6*, 822–832.

Casciano, J. C., Duchemin, N. J., Lamontagne, R. J., Steel, L. F., & Bouchard, M. J. (2017). Hepatitis B virus modulates store-operated calcium entry to enhance viral replication in primary hepatocytes. *PLoS One, 12*, e0168328.

Chan, D. W., Son, S. C., Block, W., Ye, R., Khanna, K. K., Wold, M. S., et al. (2000). Purification and characterization of ATM from human placenta. A manganese-dependent, wortmannin-sensitive serine/threonine protein kinase. *The Journal of Biological Chemistry, 275*, 7803–7810.

Chandy, K. G., & Norton, R. S. (2016). Immunology: Channelling potassium to fight cancer. *Nature, 537*, 497–499.

Chavakis, T., May, A. E., Preissner, K. T., & Kanse, S. M. (1999). Molecular mechanisms of zinc-dependent leukocyte adhesion involving the urokinase receptor and beta2-integrins. *Blood, 93*, 2976–2983.

Chen, P., Bowman, A. B., Mukhopadhyay, S., & Aschner, M. (2015). SLC30A10: A novel manganese transporter. *Worm, 4* e1042648.

Chen, J., & Chen, Z. J. (2018). PtdIns4P on dispersed trans-Golgi network mediates NLRP3 inflammasome activation. *Nature, 564*, 71–76.

Chen, B. C., Chou, C. F., & Lin, W. W. (1998). Pyrimidinoceptor-mediated potentiation of inducible nitric-oxide synthase induction in J774 macrophages. Role of intracellular calcium. *The Journal of Biological Chemistry, 273*, 29754–29763.

Chen, Q., Feng, L., Liu, J., Zhu, W., Dong, Z., Wu, Y., et al. (2016). Intelligent albumin-MnO_2 nanoparticles as pH-/H_2 O_2-responsive dissociable nanocarriers to modulate tumor hypoxia for effective combination therapy. *Advanced Materials, 28*, 7129–7136.

Chen, R., Ji, G., Ma, T., Huang, X., Ren, H., & Xi, L. (2015). Role of intracellular free calcium in killing Penicillium marneffei within human macrophages. *Microbial Pathogenesis, 83-84*, 29–34.

Chen, H., Sun, H., You, F., Sun, W., Zhou, X., Chen, L., et al. (2011). Activation of STAT6 by STING is critical for antiviral innate immunity. *Cell, 147*, 436–446.

Chen, D., Tyagi, A., Carpenter, J., Perkins, S., Sylvester, D., Guy, M., et al. (2009). Characterization of the freeze sensitivity of a hepatitis B vaccine. *Human Vaccines, 5*, 26–32.

Cheng, Y., Zak, O., Aisen, P., Harrison, S. C., & Walz, T. (2004). Structure of the human transferrin receptor-transferrin complex. *Cell, 116*, 565–576.

Cheshenko, N., Del Rosario, B., Woda, C., Marcellino, D., Satlin, L. M., & Herold, B. C. (2003). Herpes simplex virus triggers activation of calcium-signaling pathways. *The Journal of Cell Biology*, *163*, 283–293.

Chimienti, F., Aouffen, M., Favier, A., & Seve, M. (2003). Zinc homeostasis-regulating proteins: New drug targets for triggering cell fate. *Current Drug Targets*, *4*, 323–338.

Chowanadisai, W., Lonnerdal, B., & Kelleher, S. L. (2006). Identification of a mutation in SLC30A2 (ZnT-2) in women with low milk zinc concentration that results in transient neonatal zinc deficiency. *The Journal of Biological Chemistry*, *281*, 39699–39707.

Chu, J., Thomas, L. M., Watkins, S. C., Franchi, L., Nunez, G., & Salter, R. D. (2009). Cholesterol-dependent cytolysins induce rapid release of mature IL-1beta from murine macrophages in a NLRP3 inflammasome and cathepsin B-dependent manner. *Journal of Leukocyte Biology*, *86*, 1227–1238.

Clapp, T., Munks, M. W., Trivedi, R., Kompella, U. B., & Braun, L. J. (2014). Freeze-thaw stress of Alhydrogel (R) alone is sufficient to reduce the immunogenicity of a recombinant hepatitis B vaccine containing native antigen. *Vaccine*, *32*, 3765–3771.

Cousins, R. J., Liuzzi, J. P., & Lichten, L. A. (2006). Mammalian zinc transport, trafficking, and signals. *The Journal of Biological Chemistry*, *281*, 24085–24089.

Crabtree, G. R., & Olson, E. N. (2002). NFAT signaling: Choreographing the social lives of cells. *Cell*, *109*(Suppl), S67–S79.

Crossgrove, J. S., & Yokel, R. A. (2005). Manganese distribution across the blood-brain barrier. IV. Evidence for brain influx through store-operated calcium channels. *Neurotoxicology*, *26*, 297–307.

Cui, X., & Xie, Z. (2017). Protein interaction and Na/K-ATPase-mediated signal transduction. *Molecules*, *22*, 990.

Daniels, M. A., Teixeiro, E., Gill, J., Hausmann, B., Roubaty, D., Holmberg, K., et al. (2006). Thymic selection threshold defined by compartmentalization of Ras/MAPK signalling. *Nature*, *444*, 724–729.

Davidsson, L., Lonnerdal, B., Sandstrom, B., Kunz, C., & Keen, C. L. (1989). Identification of transferrin as the major plasma carrier protein for manganese introduced orally or intravenously or after in vitro addition in the rat. *The Journal of Nutrition*, *119*, 1461–1464.

Davis, C. D., Zech, L., & Greger, J. L. (1993). Manganese metabolism in rats: An improved methodology for assessing gut endogenous losses. *Proceedings of the Society for Experimental Biology and Medicine Society for Experimental Biology and Medicine*, *202*, 103–108.

de Veer, M., Kemp, J., Chatelier, J., Elhay, M. J., & Meeusen, E. N. (2010). The kinetics of soluble and particulate antigen trafficking in the afferent lymph, and its modulation by aluminum-based adjuvant. *Vaccine*, *28*, 6597–6602.

DePasquale-Jardieu, P., & Fraker, P. J. (1984). Interference in the development of a secondary immune response in mice by zinc deprivation: Persistence of effects. *The Journal of Nutrition*, *114*, 1762–1769.

Dickinson, T. K., Devenyi, A. G., & Connor, J. R. (1996). Distribution of injected iron 59 and manganese 54 in hypotransferrinemic mice. *The Journal of Laboratory and Clinical Medicine*, *128*, 270–278.

Dixon, S. J., Lemberg, K. M., Lamprecht, M. R., Skouta, R., Zaitsev, E. M., Gleason, C. E., et al. (2012). Ferroptosis: An iron-dependent form of nonapoptotic cell death. *Cell*, *149*, 1060–1072.

Dombrowski, Y., Peric, M., Koglin, S., Kammerbauer, C., Goss, C., Anz, D., et al. (2011). Cytosolic DNA triggers inflammasome activation in keratinocytes in psoriatic lesions. *Science Translational Medicine*, *3*, 82ra38.

Dowd, P. S., Kelleher, J., & Guillou, P. J. (1986). T-lymphocyte subsets and interleukin-2 production in zinc-deficient rats. *The British Journal of Nutrition*, *55*, 59–69.

Driessen, C., Hirv, K., Rink, L., & Kirchner, H. (1994). Induction of cytokines by zinc ions in human peripheral blood mononuclear cells and separated monocytes. *Lymphokine and Cytokine Research*, *13*, 15–20.
Du, M., & Chen, Z. J. (2018). DNA-induced liquid phase condensation of cGAS activates innate immune signaling. *Science*, *361*, 704–709.
Dubben, S., Honscheid, A., Winkler, K., Rink, L., & Haase, H. (2010). Cellular zinc homeostasis is a regulator in monocyte differentiation of HL-60 cells by 1 alpha,25-dihydroxyvitamin D3. *Journal of Leukocyte Biology*, *87*, 833–844.
Dufner-Beattie, J., Huang, Z. L., Geiser, J., Xu, W., & Andrews, G. K. (2005). Generation and characterization of mice lacking the zinc uptake transporter ZIP3. *Molecular and Cellular Biology*, *25*, 5607–5615.
Dutra, F. F., Alves, L. S., Rodrigues, D., Fernandez, P. L., de Oliveira, R. B., Golenbock, D. T., et al. (2014). Hemolysis-induced lethality involves inflammasome activation by heme. *Proceedings of the National Academy of Sciences of the United States of America*, *111*, E4110–E4118.
Eide, D. J. (2006). Zinc transporters and the cellular trafficking of zinc. *Biochimica et Biophysica Acta*, *1763*, 711–722.
Eil, R., Vodnala, S. K., Clever, D., Klebanoff, C. A., Sukumar, M., Pan, J. H., et al. (2016). Ionic immune suppression within the tumour microenvironment limits T cell effector function. *Nature*, *537*, 539–543.
Eisenbarth, S. C., Colegio, O. R., O'Connor, W., Sutterwala, F. S., & Flavell, R. A. (2008). Crucial role for the Nalp3 inflammasome in the immunostimulatory properties of aluminium adjuvants. *Nature*, *453*, 1122–1126.
El Mchichi, B., Hadji, A., Vazquez, A., & Leca, G. (2007). p38 MAPK and MSK1 mediate caspase-8 activation in manganese-induced mitochondria-dependent cell death. *Cell Death and Differentiation*, *14*, 1826–1836.
Erikson, K. M., Thompson, K., Aschner, J., & Aschner, M. (2007). Manganese neurotoxicity: A focus on the neonate. *Pharmacology & Therapeutics*, *113*, 369–377.
Faber, C., Gabriel, P., Ibs, K. H., & Rink, L. (2004). Zinc in pharmacological doses suppresses allogeneic reaction without affecting the antigenic response. *Bone Marrow Transplantation*, *33*, 1241–1246.
Fan, W., Bu, W., Shen, B., He, Q., Cui, Z., Liu, Y., et al. (2015). Intelligent MnO2 nanosheets anchored with upconversion nanoprobes for concurrent pH-/H_2O_2-responsive UCL imaging and oxygen-elevated synergetic therapy. *Advanced Materials*, *27*, 4155–4161.
Fan, H., Yan, G., Zhao, Z., Hu, X., Zhang, W., Liu, H., et al. (2016). A smart photosensitizer-manganese dioxide nanosystem for enhanced photodynamic therapy by reducing glutathione levels in cancer cells. *Angewandte Chemie*, *55*, 5477–5482.
Fang, R., Wang, C., Jiang, Q., Lv, M., Gao, P., Yu, X., et al. (2017). NEMO-IKKbeta are essential for IRF3 and NF-kappaB activation in the cGAS-STING pathway. *Journal of Immunology*, *199*, 3222–3233.
Fanger, C. M., Neben, A. L., & Cahalan, M. D. (2000). Differential Ca2+ influx, KCa channel activity, and Ca2+ clearance distinguish Th1 and Th2 lymphocytes. *Journal of Immunology*, *164*, 1153–1160.
Feldmeyer, L., Keller, M., Niklaus, G., Hohl, D., Werner, S., & Beer, H. D. (2007). The inflammasome mediates UVB-induced activation and secretion of interleukin-1beta by keratinocytes. *Current Biology: CB*, *17*, 1140–1145.
Ferrari, D., Pizzirani, C., Adinolfi, E., Lemoli, R. M., Curti, A., Idzko, M., et al. (2006). The P2X7 receptor: a key player in IL-1 processing and release. *Journal of Immunology*, *176*, 3877–3883.
Feske, S., Draeger, R., Peter, H. H., Eichmann, K., & Rao, A. (2000). The duration of nuclear residence of NFAT determines the pattern of cytokine expression in human SCID T cells. *Journal of Immunology*, *165*, 297–305.

Feske, S., Giltnane, J., Dolmetsch, R., Staudt, L. M., & Rao, A. (2001). Gene regulation mediated by calcium signals in T lymphocytes. *Nature Immunology*, *2*, 316–324.

Feske, S., Gwack, Y., Prakriya, M., Srikanth, S., Puppel, S. H., Tanasa, B., et al. (2006). A mutation in Orai1 causes immune deficiency by abrogating CRAC channel function. *Nature*, *441*, 179–185.

Figueiredo, R. T., Fernandez, P. L., Mourao-Sa, D. S., Porto, B. N., Dutra, F. F., Alves, L. S., et al. (2007). Characterization of heme as activator of Toll-like receptor 4. *The Journal of Biological Chemistry*, *282*, 20221–20229.

Filipov, N. M., Seegal, R. F., & Lawrence, D. A. (2005). Manganese potentiates in vitro production of proinflammatory cytokines and nitric oxide by microglia through a nuclear factor kappa B-dependent mechanism. *Toxicological Sciences: An Official Journal of the Society of Toxicology*, *84*, 139–148.

Finley, J. W., Johnson, P. E., & Johnson, L. K. (1994). Sex affects manganese absorption and retention by humans from a diet adequate in manganese. *The American Journal of Clinical Nutrition*, *60*, 949–955.

Flach, T. L., Ng, G., Hari, A., Desrosiers, M. D., Zhang, P., Ward, S. M., et al. (2011). Alum interaction with dendritic cell membrane lipids is essential for its adjuvanticity. *Nature Medicine*, *17*, 479–487.

Fraker, P. J., DePasquale-Jardieu, P., Zwickl, C. M., & Luecke, R. W. (1978). Regeneration of T-cell helper function in zinc-deficient adult mice. *Proceedings of the National Academy of Sciences of the United States of America*, *75*, 5660–5664.

Fraker, P. J., & King, L. E. (2004). Reprogramming of the immune system during zinc deficiency. *Annual Review of Nutrition*, *24*, 277–298.

Franciszkiewicz, K., Le Floc'h, A., Boutet, M., Vergnon, I., Schmitt, A., & Mami-Chouaib, F. (2013). CD103 or LFA-1 engagement at the immune synapse between cytotoxic T cells and tumor cells promotes maturation and regulates T-cell effector functions. *Cancer Research*, *73*, 617–628.

Franklin, B. S., Bossaller, L., De Nardo, D., Ratter, J. M., Stutz, A., Engels, G., et al. (2014). The adaptor ASC has extracellular and 'prionoid' activities that propagate inflammation. *Nature Immunology*, *15*, 727–737.

Fuchs, S., Rensing-Ehl, A., Speckmann, C., Bengsch, B., Schmitt-Graeff, A., Bondzio, I., et al. (2012). Antiviral and regulatory T cell immunity in a patient with stromal interaction molecule 1 deficiency. *Journal of Immunology*, *188*, 1523–1533.

Fukada, T., & Kambe, T. (2011). Molecular and genetic features of zinc transporters in physiology and pathogenesis. *Metallomics: Integrated Biometal Science*, *3*, 662–674.

Ganz, T., & Nemeth, E. (2015). Iron homeostasis in host defence and inflammation. *Nature Reviews Immunology*, *15*, 500–510.

Gao, E. K., Lo, D., Cheney, R., Kanagawa, O., & Sprent, J. (1988). Abnormal differentiation of thymocytes in mice treated with cyclosporin A. *Nature*, *336*, 176–179.

Garrick, M. D., Singleton, S. T., Vargas, F., Kuo, H. C., Zhao, L., Knopfel, M., et al. (2006). DMT1: Which metals does it transport? *Biological Research*, *39*, 79–85.

Gavin, C. E., Gunter, K. K., & Gunter, T. E. (1999). Manganese and calcium transport in mitochondria: Implications for manganese toxicity. *Neurotoxicology*, *20*, 445–453.

Geiser, J., Venken, K. J., De Lisle, R. C., & Andrews, G. K. (2012). A mouse model of acrodermatitis enteropathica: Loss of intestine zinc transporter ZIP4 (Slc39a4) disrupts the stem cell niche and intestine integrity. *PLoS Genetics*, *8*, e1002766.

Ghimire, T. R., Benson, R. A., Garside, P., & Brewer, J. M. (2012). Alum increases antigen uptake, reduces antigen degradation and sustains antigen presentation by DCs in vitro. *Immunology Letters*, *147*, 55–62.

Ghosh, S., Koralov, S. B., Stevanovic, I., Sundrud, M. S., Sasaki, Y., Rajewsky, K., et al. (2010). Hyperactivation of nuclear factor of activated T cells 1 (NFAT1) in T cells

attenuates severity of murine autoimmune encephalomyelitis. *Proceedings of the National Academy of Sciences of the United States of America*, *107*, 15169–15174.
Glenny, A. T., Pope, C. G., Waddington, H., & Wallace, U. (1926). Immunological notes. XVII–XXIV. *The Journal of Pathology and Bacteriology*, *29*, 31–40.
Gomez-Rodriguez, J., Sahu, N., Handon, R., Davidson, T. S., Anderson, S. M., Kirby, M. R., et al. (2009). Differential expression of interleukin-17A and -17F is coupled to T cell receptor signaling via inducible T cell kinase. *Immunity*, *31*, 587–597.
Gong, T., Yang, Y., Jin, T., Jiang, W., & Zhou, R. (2018). Orchestration of NLRP3 inflammasome activation by ion fluxes. *Trends in Immunology*, *39*, 393–406.
Goodridge, H. S., Simmons, R. M., & Underhill, D. M. (2007). Dectin-1 stimulation by *Candida albicans* yeast or zymosan triggers NFAT activation in macrophages and dendritic cells. *Journal of Immunology*, *178*, 3107–3115.
Grant, S. M., Wiesinger, J. A., Beard, J. L., & Cantorna, M. T. (2003). Iron-deficient mice fail to develop autoimmune encephalomyelitis. *The Journal of Nutrition*, *133*, 2635–2638.
Granucci, F., & Zanoni, I. (2009). The dendritic cell life cycle. *Cell Cycle*, *8*, 3816–3821.
Greenblatt, M. B., Aliprantis, A., Hu, B., & Glimcher, L. H. (2010). Calcineurin regulates innate antifungal immunity in neutrophils. *The Journal of Experimental Medicine*, *207*, 923–931.
Greger, J. L. (1998). Dietary standards for manganese: Overlap between nutritional and toxicological studies. *The Journal of Nutrition*, *128*, 368S–371S.
Gremese, E., & Ferraccioli, G. F. (2004). Benefit/risk of cyclosporine in rheumatoid arthritis. *Clinical and Experimental Rheumatology*, *22*, S101–S107.
Griffiths, B., & Emery, P. (2001). The treatment of lupus with cyclosporin A. *Lupus*, *10*, 165–170.
Gross, C. J., Mishra, R., Schneider, K. S., Medard, G., Wettmarshausen, J., Dittlein, D. C., et al. (2016). K(+) efflux-independent NLRP3 inflammasome activation by small molecules targeting mitochondria. *Immunity*, *45*, 761–773.
Guilarte, T. R. (2010). APLP1, Alzheimer's-like pathology and neurodegeneration in the frontal cortex of manganese-exposed non-human primates. *Neurotoxicology*, *31*, 572–574.
Guilarte, T. R., Burton, N. C., Verina, T., Prabhu, V. V., Becker, K. G., Syversen, T., et al. (2008). Increased APLP1 expression and neurodegeneration in the frontal cortex of manganese-exposed non-human primates. *Journal of Neurochemistry*, *105*, 1948–1959.
Guilbert, A., Gautier, M., Dhennin-Duthille, I., Haren, N., Sevestre, H., & Ouadid-Ahidouch, H. (2009). Evidence that TRPM7 is required for breast cancer cell proliferation. *American Journal of Physiology Cell Physiology*, *297*, C493–C502.
Gunter, T. E., Gerstner, B., Gunter, K. K., Malecki, J., Gelein, R., Valentine, W. M., et al. (2013). Manganese transport via the transferrin mechanism. *Neurotoxicology*, *34*, 118–127.
Guven, E., Duus, K., Laursen, I., Hojrup, P., & Houen, G. (2013). Aluminum hydroxide adjuvant differentially activates the three complement pathways with major involvement of the alternative pathway. *PLoS One*, *8*, e74445.
Haase, H. (2018). Innate immune cells speak manganese. *Immunity*, *48*, 616–618.
Haase, H., Hebel, S., Engelhardt, G., & Rink, L. (2006). Flow cytometric measurement of labile zinc in peripheral blood mononuclear cells. *Analytical Biochemistry*, *352*, 222–230.
Haase, H., & Maret, W. (2003). Intracellular zinc fluctuations modulate protein tyrosine phosphatase activity in insulin/insulin-like growth factor-1 signaling. *Experimental Cell Research*, *291*, 289–298.
Haase, H., Ober-Blobaum, J. L., Engelhardt, G., Hebel, S., Heit, A., Heine, H., et al. (2008). Zinc signals are essential for lipopolysaccharide-induced signal transduction in monocytes. *Journal of Immunology*, *181*, 6491–6502.

Haase, H., & Rink, L. (2014a). Multiple impacts of zinc on immune function. *Metallomics: Integrated Biometal Science*, *6*, 1175–1180.

Haase, H., & Rink, L. (2014b). Zinc signals and immune function. *BioFactors*, *40*, 27–40.

Hare, D. N., Collins, S. E., Mukherjee, S., Loo, Y. M., Gale, M., Jr., Janssen, L. J., et al. (2015). Membrane perturbation-associated Ca2 + signaling and incoming genome sensing are required for the host response to low-level enveloped virus particle entry. *Journal of Virology*, *90*, 3018–3027.

Harischandra, D. S., Rokad, D., Neal, M. L., Ghaisas, S., Manne, S., Sarkar, S., et al. (2019). Manganese promotes the aggregation and prion-like cell-to-cell exosomal transmission of alpha-synuclein. *Science Signaling*, *12*, eaau4543.

Harris, W. R., & Chen, Y. (1994). Electron paramagnetic resonance and difference ultraviolet studies of Mn2+ binding to serum transferrin. *Journal of Inorganic Biochemistry*, *54*, 1–19.

Hasan, R., Rink, L., & Haase, H. (2013). Zinc signals in neutrophil granulocytes are required for the formation of neutrophil extracellular traps. *Innate Immunity*, *19*, 253–264.

Heissmeyer, V., Macian, F., Im, S. H., Varma, R., Feske, S., Venuprasad, K., et al. (2004). Calcineurin imposes T cell unresponsiveness through targeted proteolysis of signaling proteins. *Nature Immunology*, *5*, 255–265.

Hentze, M. W., Muckenthaler, M. U., & Andrews, N. C. (2004). Balancing acts: Molecular control of mammalian iron metabolism. *Cell*, *117*, 285–297.

Hess, S. D., Oortgiesen, M., & Cahalan, M. D. (1993). Calcium oscillations in human T and natural killer cells depend upon membrane potential and calcium influx. *Journal of Immunology*, *150*, 2620–2633.

Heyland, D. K., Jones, N., Cvijanovich, N. Z., & Wong, H. (2008). Zinc supplementation in critically ill patients: A key pharmaconutrient? *JPEN Journal of Parenteral and Enteral Nutrition*, *32*, 509–519.

Hiramine, C., Hojo, K., & Matsumoto, H. (1988). Abnormal distribution of T cell subsets in the thymus of cyclosporin A (CsA)-treated mice. *Thymus*, *11*, 243–252.

Hogan, P. G., Chen, L., Nardone, J., & Rao, A. (2003). Transcriptional regulation by calcium, calcineurin, and NFAT. *Genes & Development*, *17*, 2205–2232.

Hogenesch, H. (2012). Mechanism of immunopotentiation and safety of aluminum adjuvants. *Frontiers in Immunology*, *3*, 406.

HogenEsch, H., O'Hagan, D. T., & Fox, C. B. (2018). Optimizing the utilization of aluminum adjuvants in vaccines: You might just get what you want. *NPJ Vaccines*, *3*, 51.

Hojyo, S., & Fukada, T. (2016). Roles of zinc signaling in the immune system. *Journal of Immunology Research*, *2016*, 6762343.

Hojyo, S., Miyai, T., Fujishiro, H., Kawamura, M., Yasuda, T., Hijikata, A., et al. (2014). Zinc transporter SLC39A10/ZIP10 controls humoral immunity by modulating B-cell receptor signal strength. *Proceedings of the National Academy of Sciences of the United States of America*, *111*, 11786–11791.

Hood, M. I., & Skaar, E. P. (2012). Nutritional immunity: Transition metals at the pathogen-host interface. *Nature Reviews Microbiology*, *10*, 525–537.

Hopfner, K. P., Karcher, A., Craig, L., Woo, T. T., Carney, J. P., & Tainer, J. A. (2001). Structural biochemistry and interaction architecture of the DNA double-strand break repair Mre11 nuclease and Rad50-ATPase. *Cell*, *105*, 473–485.

Horng, T. (2014). Calcium signaling and mitochondrial destabilization in the triggering of the NLRP3 inflammasome. *Trends in Immunology*, *35*, 253–261.

Horning, K. J., Caito, S. W., Tipps, K. G., Bowman, A. B., & Aschner, M. (2015). Manganese is essential for neuronal health. *Annual Review of Nutrition*, *35*, 71–108.

Hsiao, H. W., Liu, W. H., Wang, C. J., Lo, Y. H., Wu, Y. H., Jiang, S. T., et al. (2009). Deltex1 is a target of the transcription factor NFAT that promotes T cell anergy. *Immunity*, *31*, 72–83.

Huang, L., & Gitschier, J. (1997). A novel gene involved in zinc transport is deficient in the lethal milk mouse. *Nature Genetics*, *17*, 292–297.
Huse, M., Eck, M. J., & Harrison, S. C. (1998). A Zn2+ ion links the cytoplasmic tail of CD4 and the N-terminal region of Lck. *The Journal of Biological Chemistry*, *273*, 18729–18733.
Ibs, K. H., & Rink, L. (2003). Zinc-altered immune function. *The Journal of Nutrition*, *133*, 1452S–1456S.
Ishikawa, H., & Barber, G. N. (2008). STING is an endoplasmic reticulum adaptor that facilitates innate immune signalling. *Nature*, *455*, 674–678.
Itoh, N., Shibayama, H., Kanekiyo, M., Namphung, D., Nakanishi, T., Matsuyama, A., et al. (2005). Reduced bactericidal activity and nitric oxide production in metallothionein-deficient macrophages in response to lipopolysaccharide stimulation. *Toxicology*, *216*, 188–196.
Itsumura, N., Inamo, Y., Okazaki, F., Teranishi, F., Narita, H., Kambe, T., et al. (2013). Compound heterozygous mutations in SLC30A2/ZnT2 results in low milk zinc concentrations: A novel mechanism for zinc deficiency in a breast-fed infant. *PLoS One*, *8*, e64045.
Iwashima, M., Irving, B. A., van Oers, N. S., Chan, A. C., & Weiss, A. (2014). Pillars article: Sequential interactions of the TCR with two distinct cytoplasmic tyrosine kinases. Science. 1994. 263: 1136–1139. *Journal of Immunology*, *193*, 4279–4282.
Jamieson, E. R., & Lippard, S. J. (1999). Structure, recognition, and processing of cisplatin-DNA adducts. *Chemical Reviews*, *99*, 2467–2498.
Jenkins, M. K., Schwartz, R. H., & Pardoll, D. M. (1988). Effects of cyclosporine A on T cell development and clonal deletion. *Science*, *241*, 1655–1658.
Jin, S., Chin, J., Kitson, C., Woods, J., Majmudar, R., Carvajal, V., et al. (2013). Natural regulatory T cells are resistant to calcium release-activated calcium (CRAC/ORAI) channel inhibition. *International Immunology*, *25*, 497–506.
Johnson, E. E., & Wessling-Resnick, M. (2012). Iron metabolism and the innate immune response to infection. *Microbes and Infection*, *14*, 207–216.
Jung, D., Giallourakis, C., Mostoslavsky, R., & Alt, F. W. (2006). Mechanism and control of V(D)J recombination at the immunoglobulin heavy chain locus. *Annual Review of Immunology*, *24*, 541–570.
Kabu, K., Yamasaki, S., Kamimura, D., Ito, Y., Hasegawa, A., Sato, E., et al. (2006). Zinc is required for Fc epsilon RI-mediated mast cell activation. *Journal of Immunology*, *177*, 1296–1305.
Kaltenberg, J., Plum, L. M., Ober-Blobaum, J. L., Honscheid, A., Rink, L., & Haase, H. (2010). Zinc signals promote IL-2-dependent proliferation of T cells. *European Journal of Immunology*, *40*, 1496–1503.
Kambe, T., Fukue, K., Ishida, R., & Miyazaki, S. (2015). Overview of inherited zinc deficiency in infants and children. *Journal of Nutritional Science and Vitaminology*, *61*(Suppl), S44–S46.
Kambe, T., Weaver, B. P., & Andrews, G. K. (2008). The genetics of essential metal homeostasis during development. *Genesis*, *46*, 214–228.
Kanamori, Y., Murakami, M., Sugiyama, M., Hashimoto, O., Matsui, T., & Funaba, M. (2017). Interleukin-1beta (IL-1beta) transcriptionally activates hepcidin by inducing CCAAT enhancer-binding protein delta (C/EBPdelta) expression in hepatocytes. *The Journal of Biological Chemistry*, *292*, 10275–10287.
Kayagaki, N., Stowe, I. B., Lee, B. L., O'Rourke, K., Anderson, K., Warming, S., et al. (2015). Caspase-11 cleaves gasdermin D for non-canonical inflammasome signalling. *Nature*, *526*, 666–671.
Keefer, R. C., Barak, A. J., & Boyett, J. D. (1970). Binding of manganese and transferrin in rat serum. *Biochimica et Biophysica Acta*, *221*, 390–393.

Keen, C. L., Ensunsa, J. L., Watson, M. H., Baly, D. L., Donovan, S. M., Monaco, M. H., et al. (1999). Nutritional aspects of manganese from experimental studies. *Neurotoxicology*, *20*, 213–223.

Kehl-Fie, T. E., & Skaar, E. P. (2010). Nutritional immunity beyond iron: A role for manganese and zinc. *Current Opinion in Chemical Biology*, *14*, 218–224.

Khameneh, H. J., Ho, A. W., Spreafico, R., Derks, H., Quek, H. Q., & Mortellaro, A. (2017). The Syk-NFAT-IL-2 pathway in dendritic cells is required for optimal sterile immunity elicited by alum adjuvants. *Journal of Immunology*, *198*, 196–204.

Kim, K. D., Srikanth, S., Tan, Y. V., Yee, M. K., Jew, M., Damoiseaux, R., et al. (2014). Calcium signaling via Orai1 is essential for induction of the nuclear orphan receptor pathway to drive Th17 differentiation. *Journal of Immunology*, *192*, 110–122.

King, L. E., Frentzel, J. W., Mann, J. J., & Fraker, P. J. (2005). Chronic zinc deficiency in mice disrupted T cell lymphopoiesis and erythropoiesis while B cell lymphopoiesis and myelopoiesis were maintained. *Journal of the American College of Nutrition*, *24*, 494–502.

Kitamura, H., Morikawa, H., Kamon, H., Iguchi, M., Hojyo, S., Fukada, T., et al. (2006). Toll-like receptor-mediated regulation of zinc homeostasis influences dendritic cell function. *Nature Immunology*, *7*, 971–977.

Klein, M., Klein-Hessling, S., Palmetshofer, A., Serfling, E., Tertilt, C., Bopp, T., et al. (2006). Specific and redundant roles for NFAT transcription factors in the expression of mast cell-derived cytokines. *Journal of Immunology*, *177*, 6667–6674.

Knoell, D. L., Julian, M. W., Bao, S., Besecker, B., Macre, J. E., Leikauf, G. D., et al. (2009). Zinc deficiency increases organ damage and mortality in a murine model of polymicrobial sepsis. *Critical Care Medicine*, *37*, 1380–1388.

Knoell, D. L., & Liu, M. J. (2010). Impact of zinc metabolism on innate immune function in the setting of sepsis. *International Journal for Vitamin and Nutrition Research*, *80*, 271–277.

Kobayashi, K., Kuroda, J., Shibata, N., Hasegawa, T., Seko, Y., Satoh, M., et al. (2007). Induction of metallothionein by manganese is completely dependent on interleukin-6 production. *The Journal of Pharmacology and Experimental Therapeutics*, *320*, 721–727.

Kojima, C., Kawakami, A., Takei, T., Nitta, K., & Yoshida, M. (2007). Angiotensin-converting enzyme inhibitor attenuates monocyte adhesion to vascular endothelium through modulation of intracellular zinc. *The Journal of Pharmacology and Experimental Therapeutics*, *323*, 855–860.

Kool, M., Petrilli, V., De Smedt, T., Rolaz, A., Hammad, H., van Nimwegen, M., et al. (2008). Cutting edge: Alum adjuvant stimulates inflammatory dendritic cells through activation of the NALP3 inflammasome. *Journal of Immunology*, *181*, 3755–3759.

Kool, M., Soullie, T., van Nimwegen, M., Willart, M. A., Muskens, F., Jung, S., et al. (2008). Alum adjuvant boosts adaptive immunity by inducing uric acid and activating inflammatory dendritic cells. *The Journal of Experimental Medicine*, *205*, 869–882.

Koury, M. J., & Haase, V. H. (2015). Anaemia in kidney disease: Harnessing hypoxia responses for therapy. *Nature Reviews Nephrology*, *11*, 394–410.

Krezel, A., & Maret, W. (2007). Dual nanomolar and picomolar Zn(II) binding properties of metallothionein. *Journal of the American Chemical Society*, *129*, 10911–10921.

Kristiansen, M., Graversen, J. H., Jacobsen, C., Sonne, O., Hoffman, H. J., Law, S. K., et al. (2001). Identification of the haemoglobin scavenger receptor. *Nature*, *409*, 198–201.

Kunsleben, N., Rudrich, U., Gehring, M., Novak, N., Kapp, A., & Raap, U. (2015). IL-31 induces chemotaxis, calcium mobilization, release of reactive oxygen species, and CCL26 in eosinophils, which are capable to release IL-31. *The Journal of Investigative Dermatology*, *135*, 1908–1911.

Kury, S., Dreno, B., Bezieau, S., Giraudet, S., Kharfi, M., Kamoun, R., et al. (2002). Identification of SLC39A4, a gene involved in acrodermatitis enteropathica. *Nature Genetics*, *31*, 239–240.

Kuvibidila, S. R., & Porretta, C. (2003). Iron deficiency and in vitro iron chelation reduce the expression of cluster of differentiation molecule (CD)28 but not CD3 receptors on murine thymocytes and spleen cells. *The British Journal of Nutrition*, *90*, 179–189.

Laity, J. H., & Andrews, G. K. (2007). Understanding the mechanisms of zinc-sensing by metal-response element binding transcription factor-1 (MTF-1). *Archives of Biochemistry and Biophysics*, *463*, 201–210.

Lan, Y. Y., Londono, D., Bouley, R., Rooney, M. S., & Hacohen, N. (2014). Dnase2a deficiency uncovers lysosomal clearance of damaged nuclear DNA via autophagy. *Cell Reports*, *9*, 180–192.

Lasry, I., Seo, Y. A., Ityel, H., Shalva, N., Pode-Shakked, B., Glaser, F., et al. (2012). A dominant negative heterozygous G87R mutation in the zinc transporter, ZnT-2 (SLC30A2), results in transient neonatal zinc deficiency. *The Journal of Biological Chemistry*, *287*, 29348–29361.

Latour, C., Besson-Fournier, C., Gourbeyre, O., Meynard, D., Roth, M. P., & Coppin, H. (2017). Deletion of BMP6 worsens the phenotype of HJV-deficient mice and attenuates hepcidin levels reached after LPS challenge. *Blood*, *130*, 2339–2343.

Laudisi, F., Spreafico, R., Evrard, M., Hughes, T. R., Mandriani, B., Kandasamy, M., et al. (2013). Cutting edge: The NLRP3 inflammasome links complement-mediated inflammation and IL-1beta release. *Journal of Immunology*, *191*, 1006–1010.

Lazarczyk, M., Dalard, C., Hayder, M., Dupre, L., Pignolet, B., Majewski, S., et al. (2012). EVER proteins, key elements of the natural anti-human papillomavirus barrier, are regulated upon T-cell activation. *PLoS One*, *7*, e39995.

Lazarczyk, M., Pons, C., Mendoza, J. A., Cassonnet, P., Jacob, Y., & Favre, M. (2008). Regulation of cellular zinc balance as a potential mechanism of EVER-mediated protection against pathogenesis by cutaneous oncogenic human papillomaviruses. *The Journal of Experimental Medicine*, *205*, 35–42.

Lee, G. S., Subramanian, N., Kim, A. I., Aksentijevich, I., Goldbach-Mansky, R., Sacks, D. B., et al. (2012). The calcium-sensing receptor regulates the NLRP3 inflammasome through Ca2+ and cAMP. *Nature*, *492*, 123–127.

Leibbrandt, M. E., & Koropatnick, J. (1994). Activation of human monocytes with lipopolysaccharide induces metallothionein expression and is diminished by zinc. *Toxicology and Applied Pharmacology*, *124*, 72–81.

Leyva-Illades, D., Chen, P., Zogzas, C. E., Hutchens, S., Mercado, J. M., Swaim, C. D., et al. (2014). SLC30A10 is a cell surface-localized manganese efflux transporter, and parkinsonism-causing mutations block its intracellular trafficking and efflux activity. *The Journal of Neuroscience: The Official Journal of the Society for Neuroscience*, *34*, 14079–14095.

Li, H., Nookala, S., & Re, F. (2007). Aluminum hydroxide adjuvants activate caspase-1 and induce IL-1beta and IL-18 release. *Journal of Immunology*, *178*, 5271–5276.

Li, H., Willingham, S. B., Ting, J. P., & Re, F. (2008). Cutting edge: Inflammasome activation by alum and alum's adjuvant effect are mediated by NLRP3. *Journal of Immunology*, *181*, 17–21.

Li, J., Zheng, P., Zhao, J., Chen, P. R., & Guo, Z. (2019). Metal-mediated immune regulations and interventions: Prospects of the emerging field of metalloimmunology. *Scientia Sinica Chimica*, *49*, 1037.

Lian, J., Cuk, M., Kahlfuss, S., Kozhaya, L., Vaeth, M., Rieux-Laucat, F., et al. (2018). ORAI1 mutations abolishing store-operated Ca(2+) entry cause anhidrotic ectodermal dysplasia with immunodeficiency. *The Journal of Allergy and Clinical Immunology*, *142*, 1297–1310.e1211.

Lichten, L. A., & Cousins, R. J. (2009). Mammalian zinc transporters: Nutritional and physiologic regulation. *Annual Review of Nutrition*, *29*, 153–176.

Lichten, L. A., Ryu, M. S., Guo, L., Embury, J., & Cousins, R. J. (2011). MTF-1-mediated repression of the zinc transporter Zip10 is alleviated by zinc restriction. *PLoS One*, *6*, e21526.

Lin, R. S., Rodriguez, C., Veillette, A., & Lodish, H. F. (1998). Zinc is essential for binding of p56(lck) to CD4 and CD8alpha. *The Journal of Biological Chemistry*, *273*, 32878–32882.

Lin, W., Vann, D. R., Doulias, P. T., Wang, T., Landesberg, G., Li, X., et al. (2017). Hepatic metal ion transporter ZIP8 regulates manganese homeostasis and manganese-dependent enzyme activity. *The Journal of Clinical Investigation*, *127*, 2407–2417.

Lindblad, E. B. (2004). Aluminium compounds for use in vaccines. *Immunology and Cell Biology*, *82*, 497–505.

Liu, M. J., Bao, S., Galvez-Peralta, M., Pyle, C. J., Rudawsky, A. C., Pavlovicz, R. E., et al. (2013). ZIP8 regulates host defense through zinc-mediated inhibition of NF-kappaB. *Cell Reports*, *3*, 386–400.

Liu, M., Cai, T., Zhao, F., Zheng, G., Wang, Q., Chen, Y., et al. (2009). Effect of microglia activation on dopaminergic neuronal injury induced by manganese, and its possible mechanism. *Neurotoxicity Research*, *16*, 42–49.

Liu, J., Farmer, J. D., Jr., Lane, W. S., Friedman, J., Weissman, I., & Schreiber, S. L. (1991). Calcineurin is a common target of cyclophilin-cyclosporin A and FKBP-FK506 complexes. *Cell*, *66*, 807–815.

Liu, Y. P., Zeng, L., Tian, A., Bomkamp, A., Rivera, D., Gutman, D., et al. (2012). Endoplasmic reticulum stress regulates the innate immunity critical transcription factor IRF3. *Journal of Immunology*, *189*, 4630–4639.

Lopez-Castejon, G., Theaker, J., Pelegrin, P., Clifton, A. D., Braddock, M., & Surprenant, A. (2010). P2X(7) receptor-mediated release of cathepsins from macrophages is a cytokine-independent mechanism potentially involved in joint diseases. *Journal of Immunology*, *185*, 2611–2619.

Louandre, C., Ezzoukhry, Z., Godin, C., Barbare, J. C., Maziere, J. C., Chauffert, B., et al. (2013). Iron-dependent cell death of hepatocellular carcinoma cells exposed to sorafenib. *International Journal of Cancer*, *133*, 1732–1742.

Loutzenhiser, K., & Loutzenhiser, R. (2000). Angiotensin II-induced Ca(2+) influx in renal afferent and efferent arterioles: Differing roles of voltage-gated and store-operated Ca(2+) entry. *Circulation Research*, *87*, 551–557.

Lu, F., & Hogenesch, H. (2013). Kinetics of the inflammatory response following intramuscular injection of aluminum adjuvant. *Vaccine*, *31*, 3979–3986.

Lupfer, C., Thomas, P. G., Anand, P. K., Vogel, P., Milasta, S., Martinez, J., et al. (2013). Receptor interacting protein kinase 2-mediated mitophagy regulates inflammasome activation during virus infection. *Nature Immunology*, *14*, 480–488.

Ma, J., McCarl, C. A., Khalil, S., Luthy, K., & Feske, S. (2010). T-cell-specific deletion of STIM1 and STIM2 protects mice from EAE by impairing the effector functions of Th1 and Th17 cells. *European Journal of Immunology*, *40*, 3028–3042.

MacGlashan, D., Jr., & Guo, C. B. (1991). Oscillations in free cytosolic calcium during IgE-mediated stimulation distinguish human basophils from human mast cells. *Journal of Immunology*, *147*, 2259–2269.

Macian, F. (2005). NFAT proteins: Key regulators of T-cell development and function. *Nature Reviews Immunology*, *5*, 472–484.

Mackenzie, K. J., Carroll, P., Martin, C. A., Murina, O., Fluteau, A., Simpson, D. J., et al. (2017). cGAS surveillance of micronuclei links genome instability to innate immunity. *Nature*, *548*, 461–465.

MacLennan, I. C., Gotch, F. M., & Golstein, P. (1980). Limited specific T-cell mediated cytolysis in the absence of extracellular Ca2+. *Immunology*, *39*, 109–117.

Madejczyk, M. S., & Ballatori, N. (2012). The iron transporter ferroportin can also function as a manganese exporter. *Biochimica et Biophysica Acta*, *1818*, 651–657.

Mannhalter, J. W., Neychev, H. O., Zlabinger, G. J., Ahmad, R., & Eibl, M. M. (1985). Modulation of the human immune response by the non-toxic and non-pyrogenic adjuvant aluminium hydroxide: Effect on antigen uptake and antigen presentation. *Clinical and Experimental Immunology*, *61*, 143–151.

Marchan, R., Cadenas, C., & Bolt, H. M. (2012). Zinc as a multipurpose trace element. *Archives of Toxicology*, *86*, 519–520.

Maret, W. (2003). Cellular zinc and redox states converge in the metallothionein/thionein pair. *The Journal of Nutrition*, *133*, 1460S–1462S.

Maret, W., & Li, Y. (2009). Coordination dynamics of zinc in proteins. *Chemical Reviews*, *109*, 4682–4707.

Maret, W., & Sandstead, H. H. (2006). Zinc requirements and the risks and benefits of zinc supplementation. *Journal of Trace Elements in Medicine and Biology: Organ of the Society for Minerals and Trace Elements*, *20*, 3–18.

Mariathasan, S., Weiss, D. S., Newton, K., McBride, J., O'Rourke, K., Roose-Girma, M., et al. (2006). Cryopyrin activates the inflammasome in response to toxins and ATP. *Nature*, *440*, 228–232.

Marichal, T., Ohata, K., Bedoret, D., Mesnil, C., Sabatel, C., Kobiyama, K., et al. (2011). DNA released from dying host cells mediates aluminum adjuvant activity. *Nature Medicine*, *17*, 996–1002.

Marie, C., Verkerke, H. P., Theodorescu, D., & Petri, W. A. (2015). A whole-genome RNAi screen uncovers a novel role for human potassium channels in cell killing by the parasite Entamoeba histolytica. *Scientific Reports*, *5*, 13613.

Marrack, P., McKee, A. S., & Munks, M. W. (2009). Towards an understanding of the adjuvant action of aluminium. *Nature Reviews Immunology*, *9*, 287–293.

Martinez-Finley, E. J., Gavin, C. E., Aschner, M., & Gunter, T. E. (2013). Manganese neurotoxicity and the role of reactive oxygen species. *Free Radical Biology & Medicine*, *62*, 65–75.

Matsumoto, M., Fujii, Y., Baba, A., Hikida, M., Kurosaki, T., & Baba, Y. (2011). The calcium sensors STIM1 and STIM2 control B cell regulatory function through interleukin-10 production. *Immunity*, *34*, 703–714.

Maul-Pavicic, A., Chiang, S. C., Rensing-Ehl, A., Jessen, B., Fauriat, C., Wood, S. M., et al. (2011). ORAI1-mediated calcium influx is required for human cytotoxic lymphocyte degranulation and target cell lysis. *Proceedings of the National Academy of Sciences of the United States of America*, *108*, 3324–3329.

Maus, M., Cuk, M., Patel, B., Lian, J., Ouimet, M., Kaufmann, U., et al. (2017). Store-operated Ca(2+) entry controls induction of lipolysis and the transcriptional reprogramming to lipid metabolism. *Cell Metabolism*, *25*, 698–712.

Maus, M., Jairaman, A., Stathopulos, P. B., Muik, M., Fahrner, M., Weidinger, C., et al. (2015). Missense mutation in immunodeficient patients shows the multifunctional roles of coiled-coil domain 3 (CC3) in STIM1 activation. *Proceedings of the National Academy of Sciences of the United States of America*, *112*, 6206–6211.

McCarl, C. A., Picard, C., Khalil, S., Kawasaki, T., Rother, J., Papolos, A., et al. (2009). ORAI1 deficiency and lack of store-operated Ca2+ entry cause immunodeficiency, myopathy, and ectodermal dysplasia. *The Journal of allergy and clinical immunology*, *124*, 1311–1318.e1317.

McDonough, A. A., & Youn, J. H. (2017). Potassium homeostasis: The knowns, the unknowns, and the health benefits. *Physiology*, *32*, 100–111.

McKee, A. S., Burchill, M. A., Munks, M. W., Jin, L., Kappler, J. W., Friedman, R. S., et al. (2013). Host DNA released in response to aluminum adjuvant enhances MHC class II-mediated antigen presentation and prolongs CD4 T-cell interactions with dendritic cells. *Proceedings of the National Academy of Sciences of the United States of America*, *110*, E1122–E1131.

Meggers, E. (2007). Exploring biologically relevant chemical space with metal complexes. *Current Opinion in Chemical Biology*, *11*, 287–292.
Meijne, A. M., Driessens, M. H., La Riviere, G., Casey, D., Feltkamp, C. A., & Roos, E. (1994). LFA-1 integrin redistribution during T-cell hybridoma invasion of hepatocyte cultures and manganese-induced adhesion to ICAM-1. *Journal of Cell Science*, *107*(Pt. 9), 2557–2566.
Meng, Q., Ying, S., Corrigan, C. J., Wakelin, M., Assoufi, B., Moqbel, R., et al. (1997). Effects of rapamycin, cyclosporin A, and dexamethasone on interleukin 5-induced eosinophil degranulation and prolonged survival. *Allergy*, *52*, 1095–1101.
Merritt, R. E., Mahtabifard, A., Yamada, R. E., Crystal, R. G., & Korst, R. J. (2003). Cisplatin augments cytotoxic T-lymphocyte-mediated antitumor immunity in poorly immunogenic murine lung cancer. *The Journal of Thoracic and Cardiovascular Surgery*, *126*, 1609–1617.
Messori, L., & Merlino, A. (2016). Cisplatin binding to proteins: A structural perspective. *Coordination Chemistry Reviews*, *315*, 67–89.
Meyron-Holtz, E. G., Vaisman, B., Cabantchik, Z. I., Fibach, E., Rouault, T. A., Hershko, C., et al. (1999). Regulation of intracellular iron metabolism in human erythroid precursors by internalized extracellular ferritin. *Blood*, *94*, 3205–3211.
Miyai, T., Hojyo, S., Ikawa, T., Kawamura, M., Irie, T., Ogura, H., et al. (2014). Zinc transporter SLC39A10/ZIP10 facilitates antiapoptotic signaling during early B-cell development. *Proceedings of the National Academy of Sciences of the United States of America*, *111*, 11780–11785.
Mjos, K. D., & Orvig, C. (2014). Metallodrugs in medicinal inorganic chemistry. *Chemical Reviews*, *114*, 4540–4563.
Morefield, G. L., Sokolovska, A., Jiang, D., HogenEsch, H., Robinson, J. P., & Hem, S. L. (2005). Role of aluminum-containing adjuvants in antigen internalization by dendritic cells in vitro. *Vaccine*, *23*, 1588–1595.
Moynahan, E. J. (1975). Letter: Zinc deficiency and cellular immune deficiency in acrodermatitis enteropathica in man and zinc deficiency with thymic hypoplasia in fresian calves: A possible genetic link. *Lancet*, *2*, 710.
Muckenthaler, M. U., Rivella, S., Hentze, M. W., & Galy, B. (2017). A red carpet for iron metabolism. *Cell*, *168*, 344–361.
Mukherjee, S., & Mukherjee, U. (2009). A comprehensive review of immunosuppression used for liver transplantation. *Journal of Transplantation*, *2009*, 701464.
Mukhopadhyay, S., & Linstedt, A. D. (2012). Manganese blocks intracellular trafficking of Shiga toxin and protects against Shiga toxicosis. *Science*, *335*, 332–335.
Munoz-Planillo, R., Kuffa, P., Martinez-Colon, G., Smith, B. L., Rajendiran, T. M., & Nunez, G. (2013). K(+) efflux is the common trigger of NLRP3 inflammasome activation by bacterial toxins and particulate matter. *Immunity*, *38*, 1142–1153.
Murakami, T., Ockinger, J., Yu, J., Byles, V., McColl, A., Hofer, A. M., et al. (2012). Critical role for calcium mobilization in activation of the NLRP3 inflammasome. *Proceedings of the National Academy of Sciences of the United States of America*, *109*, 11282–11287.
Murin, R., Verleysdonk, S., Raeymaekers, L., Kaplan, P., & Lehotsky, J. (2006). Distribution of secretory pathway Ca2+ ATPase (SPCA1) in neuronal and glial cell cultures. *Cellular and Molecular Neurobiology*, *26*, 1355–1365.
Muzzioli, M., Stecconi, R., Donnini, A., Re, F., & Provinciali, M. (2007). Zinc improves the development of human CD34+ cell progenitors towards Natural Killer cells and induces the expression of GATA-3 transcription factor. *The International Journal of Biochemistry & Cell Biology*, *39*, 955–965.
Nairz, M., Dichtl, S., Schroll, A., Haschka, D., Tymoszuk, P., Theurl, I., et al. (2018). Iron and innate antimicrobial immunity-depriving the pathogen, defending the host. *Journal of*

Trace Elements in Medicine and Biology: Organ of the Society for Minerals and Trace Elements, 48, 118–133.

Neilson, J. R., Winslow, M. M., Hur, E. M., & Crabtree, G. R. (2004). Calcineurin B1 is essential for positive but not negative selection during thymocyte development. *Immunity, 20*, 255–266.

Nemeth, E., Rivera, S., Gabayan, V., Keller, C., Taudorf, S., Pedersen, B. K., et al. (2004). IL-6 mediates hypoferremia of inflammation by inducing the synthesis of the iron regulatory hormone hepcidin. *The Journal of Clinical Investigation, 113*, 1271–1276.

Nischwitz, V., Berthele, A., & Michalke, B. (2008). Speciation analysis of selected metals and determination of their total contents in paired serum and cerebrospinal fluid samples: An approach to investigate the permeability of the human blood-cerebrospinal fluid-barrier. *Analytica Chimica Acta, 627*, 258–269.

Nishida, K., Hasegawa, A., Nakae, S., Oboki, K., Saito, H., Yamasaki, S., et al. (2009). Zinc transporter Znt5/Slc30a5 is required for the mast cell-mediated delayed-type allergic reaction but not the immediate-type reaction. *The Journal of Experimental Medicine, 206*, 1351–1364.

Nizet, V., & Johnson, R. S. (2009). Interdependence of hypoxic and innate immune responses. *Nature Reviews Immunology, 9*, 609–617.

North, R. A. (2002). Molecular physiology of P2X receptors. *Physiological Reviews, 82*, 1013–1067.

Nowak, J. E., Harmon, K., Caldwell, C. C., & Wong, H. R. (2012). Prophylactic zinc supplementation reduces bacterial load and improves survival in a murine model of sepsis. *Pediatric Critical Care Medicine: A Journal of the Society of Critical Care Medicine and the World Federation of Pediatric Intensive and Critical Care Societies, 13*, e323–e329.

Oexle, H., Gnaiger, E., & Weiss, G. (1999). Iron-dependent changes in cellular energy metabolism: Influence on citric acid cycle and oxidative phosphorylation. *Biochimica et Biophysica Acta, 1413*, 99–107.

O'Grady, J. G., Burroughs, A., Hardy, P., Elbourne, D., Truesdale, A., & UK and Republic of Ireland Liver Transplant Study Group. (2002). Tacrolimus versus microemulsified ciclosporin in liver transplantation: The TMC randomised controlled trial. *Lancet, 360*, 1119–1125.

Oh-Hora, M., Yamashita, M., Hogan, P. G., Sharma, S., Lamperti, E., Chung, W., et al. (2008). Dual functions for the endoplasmic reticulum calcium sensors STIM1 and STIM2 in T cell activation and tolerance. *Nature Immunology, 9*, 432–443.

Orrenius, S., Gogvadze, V., & Zhivotovsky, B. (2015). Calcium and mitochondria in the regulation of cell death. *Biochemical and Biophysical Research Communications, 460*, 72–81.

Oubrahim, H., Chock, P. B., & Stadtman, E. R. (2002). Manganese(II) induces apoptotic cell death in NIH3T3 cells via a caspase-12-dependent pathway. *The Journal of Biological Chemistry, 277*, 20135–20138.

Oubrahim, H., Stadtman, E. R., & Chock, P. B. (2001). Mitochondria play no roles in Mn(II)-induced apoptosis in HeLa cells. *Proceedings of the National Academy of Sciences of the United States of America, 98*, 9505–9510.

Palmer, B. F., & Clegg, D. J. (2016). Physiology and pathophysiology of potassium homeostasis. *Advances in Physiology Education, 40*, 480–490.

Pardoll, D. M. (2012). The blockade of immune checkpoints in cancer immunotherapy. *Nature Reviews Cancer, 12*, 252–264.

Park, J. H., Hogrebe, M., Gruneberg, M., DuChesne, I., von der Heiden, A. L., Reunert, J., et al. (2015). SLC39A8 deficiency: A disorder of manganese transport and glycosylation. *American Journal of Human Genetics, 97*, 894–903.

Paull, T. T., & Gellert, M. (1998). The 3' to 5' exonuclease activity of Mre 11 facilitates repair of DNA double-strand breaks. *Molecular Cell, 1*, 969–979.

Petit, A. E., Demotte, N., Scheid, B., Wildmann, C., Bigirimana, R., Gordon-Alonso, M., et al. (2016). A major secretory defect of tumour-infiltrating T lymphocytes due to galectin impairing LFA-1-mediated synapse completion. *Nature Communications*, *7*, 12242.

Petrilli, V., Papin, S., Dostert, C., Mayor, A., Martinon, F., & Tschopp, J. (2007). Activation of the NALP3 inflammasome is triggered by low intracellular potassium concentration. *Cell Death and Differentiation*, *14*, 1583–1589.

Petrovsky, N., & Aguilar, J. C. (2004). Vaccine adjuvants: Current state and future trends. *Immunology and Cell Biology*, *82*, 488–496.

Picard, C., McCarl, C. A., Papolos, A., Khalil, S., Luthy, K., Hivroz, C., et al. (2009). STIM1 mutation associated with a syndrome of immunodeficiency and autoimmunity. *The New England Journal of Medicine*, *360*, 1971–1980.

Plum, L. M., Rink, L., & Haase, H. (2010). The essential toxin: Impact of zinc on human health. *International Journal of Environmental Research and Public Health*, *7*, 1342–1365.

Pores-Fernando, A. T., & Zweifach, A. (2009). Calcium influx and signaling in cytotoxic T-lymphocyte lytic granule exocytosis. *Immunological Reviews*, *231*, 160–173.

Pradeu, T., & Vivier, E. (2016). The discontinuity theory of immunity. *Science Immunology*, *1*, aag0479.

Prasad, A. S. (2000). Effects of zinc deficiency on Th1 and Th2 cytokine shifts. *The Journal of Infectious Diseases*, *182*(Suppl. 1), S62–S68.

Prasad, A. S. (2012). Discovery of human zinc deficiency: 50 years later. *Journal of Trace Elements in Medicine and Biology: Organ of the Society for Minerals and Trace Elements*, *26*, 66–69.

Prasad, P., Gordijo, C. R., Abbasi, A. Z., Maeda, A., Ip, A., Rauth, A. M., et al. (2014). Multifunctional albumin-MnO(2) nanoparticles modulate solid tumor microenvironment by attenuating hypoxia, acidosis, vascular endothelial growth factor and enhance radiation response. *ACS Nano*, *8*, 3202–3212.

Prasad, A. S., Meftah, S., Abdallah, J., Kaplan, J., Brewer, G. J., Bach, J. F., et al. (1988). Serum thymulin in human zinc deficiency. *The Journal of Clinical Investigation*, *82*, 1202–1210.

Qi, X., Nishida, J., Chaves, L., Ohmori, K., & Huang, H. (2011). CCAAT/enhancer-binding protein alpha (C/EBPalpha) is critical for interleukin-4 expression in response to FcepsilonRI receptor cross-linking. *The Journal of Biological Chemistry*, *286*, 16063–16073.

Quadri, M., Federico, A., Zhao, T., Breedveld, G. J., Battisti, C., Delnooz, C., et al. (2012). Mutations in SLC30A10 cause parkinsonism and dystonia with hypermanganesemia, polycythemia, and chronic liver disease. *American Journal of Human Genetics*, *90*, 467–477.

Quintana, A., Pasche, M., Junker, C., Al-Ansary, D., Rieger, H., Kummerow, C., et al. (2011). Calcium microdomains at the immunological synapse: How ORAI channels, mitochondria and calcium pumps generate local calcium signals for efficient T-cell activation. *The EMBO Journal*, *30*, 3895–3912.

Rajagopalan, S., & Long, E. O. (1998). Zinc bound to the killer cell-inhibitory receptor modulates the negative signal in human NK cells. *Journal of Immunology*, *161*, 1299–1305.

Rajagopalan, S., Winter, C. C., Wagtmann, N., & Long, E. O. (1995). The Ig-related killer cell inhibitory receptor binds zinc and requires zinc for recognition of HLA-C on target cells. *Journal of Immunology*, *155*, 4143–4146.

Riccardi, L., Genna, V., & De Vivo, M. (2018). Metal-ligand interactions in drug design. *Nature Reviews Chemistry*, *2*, 100–112.

Riccio, A., Mattei, C., Kelsell, R. E., Medhurst, A. D., Calver, A. R., Randall, A. D., et al. (2002). Cloning and functional expression of human short TRP7, a candidate protein for store-operated Ca2+ influx. *The Journal of Biological Chemistry*, *277*, 12302–12309.

Rimaniol, A. C., Gras, G., Verdier, F., Capel, F., Grigoriev, V. B., Porcheray, F., et al. (2004). Aluminum hydroxide adjuvant induces macrophage differentiation towards a specialized antigen-presenting cell type. *Vaccine*, *22*, 3127–3135.
Rink, L., & Gabriel, P. (2000). Zinc and the immune system. *The Proceedings of the Nutrition Society*, *59*, 541–552.
Rink, L., & Haase, H. (2007). Zinc homeostasis and immunity. *Trends in Immunology*, *28*, 1–4.
Rink, L., & Kirchner, H. (2000). Zinc-altered immune function and cytokine production. *The Journal of Nutrition*, *130*, 1407S–1411S.
Riteau, N., Baron, L., Villeret, B., Guillou, N., Savigny, F., Ryffel, B., et al. (2012). ATP release and purinergic signaling: A common pathway for particle-mediated inflammasome activation. *Cell Death & Disease*, *3*, e403.
Robert, V., Triffaux, E., Paulet, P. E., Guery, J. C., Pelletier, L., & Savignac, M. (2014). Protein kinase C-dependent activation of CaV1.2 channels selectively controls human TH2-lymphocyte functions. *The Journal of Allergy and Clinical Immunology*, *133*, 1175–1183.
Robinson, L. C., & Marchant, J. S. (2008). Enhanced Ca2+ leak from ER Ca2+ stores induced by hepatitis C NS5A protein. *Biochemical and Biophysical Research Communications*, *368*, 593–599.
Rodriguez-Rodriguez, E., Bermejo, L. M., Lopez-Sobaler, A. M., & Ortega, R. M. (2011). An inadequate intake of manganese may favour insulin resistance in girls. *Nutrición Hospitalaria*, *26*, 965–970.
Roembke, B. T., Zhou, J., Zheng, Y., Sayre, D., Lizardo, A., Bernard, L., et al. (2014). A cyclic dinucleotide containing 2-aminopurine is a general fluorescent sensor for c-di-GMP and 3',3'-cGAMP. *Molecular Biosystems*, *10*, 1568–1575.
Rogers, N. C., Slack, E. C., Edwards, A. D., Nolte, M. A., Schulz, O., Schweighoffer, E., et al. (2005). Syk-dependent cytokine induction by Dectin-1 reveals a novel pattern recognition pathway for C type lectins. *Immunity*, *22*, 507–517.
Rose, W. A., 2nd, Okragly, A. J., Patel, C. N., & Benschop, R. J. (2015). IL-33 released by alum is responsible for early cytokine production and has adjuvant properties. *Scientific Reports*, *5*, 13146.
Rossol, M., Pierer, M., Raulien, N., Quandt, D., Meusch, U., Rothe, K., et al. (2012). Extracellular Ca2+ is a danger signal activating the NLRP3 inflammasome through G protein-coupled calcium sensing receptors. *Nature Communications*, *3*, 1329.
Rukgauer, M., Klein, J., & Kruse-Jarres, J. D. (1997). Reference values for the trace elements copper, manganese, selenium, and zinc in the serum/plasma of children, adolescents, and adults. *Journal of Trace Elements in Medicine and Biology: Organ of the Society for Minerals and Trace Elements*, *11*, 92–98.
Ryu, M. S., Langkamp-Henken, B., Chang, S. M., Shankar, M. N., & Cousins, R. J. (2011). Genomic analysis, cytokine expression, and microRNA profiling reveal biomarkers of human dietary zinc depletion and homeostasis. *Proceedings of the National Academy of Sciences of the United States of America*, *108*, 20970–20975.
Salameh, S., Sheth, U., & Shukla, D. (2012). Early events in herpes simplex virus lifecycle with implications for an infection of lifetime. *The Open Virology Journal*, *6*, 1–6.
Salas, M., & Kirchner, H. (1987). Induction of interferon-gamma in human leukocyte cultures stimulated by Zn2+. *Clinical Immunology and Immunopathology*, *45*, 139–142.
Salazar, J., Mena, N., Hunot, S., Prigent, A., Alvarez-Fischer, D., Arredondo, M., et al. (2008). Divalent metal transporter 1 (DMT1) contributes to neurodegeneration in animal models of Parkinson's disease. *Proceedings of the National Academy of Sciences of the United States of America*, *105*, 18578–18583.
Salmon, M. D., & Ahluwalia, J. (2011). Pharmacology of receptor operated calcium entry in human neutrophils. *International Immunopharmacology*, *11*, 145–148.

Sanman, L. E., Qian, Y., Eisele, N. A., Ng, T. M., van der Linden, W. A., Monack, D. M., et al. (2016). Disruption of glycolytic flux is a signal for inflammasome signaling and pyroptotic cell death. *eLife*, *5*, e13663.
Santos, D., Batoreu, M. C., Almeida, I., Ramos, R., Sidoryk-Wegrzynowicz, M., Aschner, M., et al. (2012). Manganese alters rat brain amino acids levels. *Biological Trace Element Research*, *150*, 337–341.
Sarkar, S., Rokad, D., Malovic, E., Luo, J., Harischandra, D. S., Jin, H., et al. (2019). Manganese activates NLRP3 inflammasome signaling and propagates exosomal release of ASC in microglial cells. *Science Signaling*, *12*, eaat9900.
Sayadi, A., Nguyen, A. T., Bard, F. A., & Bard-Chapeau, E. A. (2013). Zip14 expression induced by lipopolysaccharides in macrophages attenuates inflammatory response. *Inflammation Research: Official Journal of the European Histamine Research Society*, *62*, 133–143.
Schaff, U. Y., Dixit, N., Procyk, E., Yamayoshi, I., Tse, T., & Simon, S. I. (2010). Orai1 regulates intracellular calcium, arrest, and shape polarization during neutrophil recruitment in shear flow. *Blood*, *115*, 657–666.
Schenk, U., Frascoli, M., Proietti, M., Geffers, R., Traggiai, E., Buer, J., et al. (2011). ATP inhibits the generation and function of regulatory T cells through the activation of purinergic P2X receptors. *Science Signaling*, *4*, ra12.
Schmidt, K., Wolfe, D. M., Stiller, B., & Pearce, D. A. (2009). Cd2+, Mn2+, Ni2+ and Se2+ toxicity to Saccharomyces cerevisiae lacking YPK9p the orthologue of human ATP13A2. *Biochemical and Biophysical Research Communications*, *383*, 198–202.
Schroeder, H. A., Balassa, J. J., & Tipton, I. H. (1966). Essential trace metals in man: Manganese. A study in homeostasis. *Journal of Chronic Diseases*, *19*, 545–571.
Schwarz, E. C., Qu, B., & Hoth, M. (2013). Calcium, cancer and killing: The role of calcium in killing cancer cells by cytotoxic T lymphocytes and natural killer cells. *Biochimica et Biophysica Acta*, *1833*, 1603–1611.
Scott, B. J., & Bradwell, A. R. (1983). Identification of the serum binding proteins for iron, zinc, cadmium, nickel, and calcium. *Clinical Chemistry*, *29*, 629–633.
Scuderi, P. (1990). Differential effects of copper and zinc on human peripheral blood monocyte cytokine secretion. *Cellular Immunology*, *126*, 391–405.
Seo, Y. A., & Wessling-Resnick, M. (2015). Ferroportin deficiency impairs manganese metabolism in flatiron mice. *FASEB Journal: Official Publication of the Federation of American Societies for Experimental Biology*, *29*, 2726–2733.
Seubert, A., Monaci, E., Pizza, M., O'Hagan, D. T., & Wack, A. (2008). The adjuvants aluminum hydroxide and MF59 induce monocyte and granulocyte chemoattractants and enhance monocyte differentiation toward dendritic cells. *Journal of Immunology*, *180*, 5402–5412.
Shankar, A. H., & Prasad, A. S. (1998). Zinc and immune function: The biological basis of altered resistance to infection. *The American Journal of Clinical Nutrition*, *68*, 447S–463S.
Shaw, P. J., Weidinger, C., Vaeth, M., Luethy, K., Kaech, S. M., & Feske, S. (2014). CD4(+) and CD8(+) T cell-dependent antiviral immunity requires STIM1 and STIM2. *The Journal of Clinical Investigation*, *124*, 4549–4563.
Sheikh, A., Shamsuzzaman, S., Ahmad, S. M., Nasrin, D., Nahar, S., Alam, M. M., et al. (2010). Zinc influences innate immune responses in children with enterotoxigenic Escherichia coli-induced diarrhea. *The Journal of Nutrition*, *140*, 1049–1056.
Shi, J., Zhao, Y., Wang, K., Shi, X., Wang, Y., Huang, H., et al. (2015). Cleavage of GSDMD by inflammatory caspases determines pyroptotic cell death. *Nature*, *526*, 660–665.
Shi, S., Zhao, J., Yang, L., Nie, X., Han, J., Ma, X., et al. (2015). KHSRP participates in manganese-induced neurotoxicity in rat striatum and PC12 cells. *Journal of Molecular Neuroscience: MN*, *55*, 454–465.

Shimada, K., Crother, T. R., Karlin, J., Dagvadorj, J., Chiba, N., Chen, S., et al. (2012). Oxidized mitochondrial DNA activates the NLRP3 inflammasome during apoptosis. *Immunity*, *36*, 401–414.

Smialowicz, R. J., Riddle, M. M., Rogers, R. R., Luebke, R. W., & Burleson, G. R. (1988). Enhancement of natural killer cell activity and interferon production by manganese in young mice. *Immunopharmacology and Immunotoxicology*, *10*, 93–107.

Sokolovska, A., Hem, S. L., & HogenEsch, H. (2007). Activation of dendritic cells and induction of CD4(+) T cell differentiation by aluminum-containing adjuvants. *Vaccine*, *25*, 4575–4585.

Solle, M., Labasi, J., Perregaux, D. G., Stam, E., Petrushova, N., Koller, B. H., et al. (2001). Altered cytokine production in mice lacking P2X(7) receptors. *The Journal of Biological Chemistry*, *276*, 125–132.

Song, M., Liu, T., Shi, C., Zhang, X., & Chen, X. (2016). Bioconjugated manganese dioxide nanoparticles enhance chemotherapy response by priming tumor-associated macrophages toward M1-like phenotype and attenuating tumor hypoxia. *ACS Nano*, *10*, 633–647.

Sonnweber, T., Theurl, I., Seifert, M., Schroll, A., Eder, S., Mayer, G., et al. (2011). Impact of iron treatment on immune effector function and cellular iron status of circulating monocytes in dialysis patients. *Nephrology, Dialysis, Transplantation: Official Publication of the European Dialysis and Transplant Association—European Renal Association*, *26*, 977–987.

Srikanth, S., Woo, J. S., Wu, B., El-Sherbiny, Y. M., Leung, J., Chupradit, K., et al. (2019). The Ca(2+) sensor STIM1 regulates the type I interferon response by retaining the signaling adaptor STING at the endoplasmic reticulum. *Nature Immunology*, *20*, 152–162.

Srisuchart, B., Taylor, M. J., & Sharma, R. P. (1987). Alteration of humoral and cellular immunity in manganese chloride-treated mice. *Journal of Toxicology and Environmental Health*, *22*, 91–99.

Stefanidou, M., Maravelias, C., Dona, A., & Spiliopoulou, C. (2006). Zinc: A multipurpose trace element. *Archives of Toxicology*, *80*, 1–9.

Steinckwich, N., Schenten, V., Melchior, C., Brechard, S., & Tschirhart, E. J. (2011). An essential role of STIM1, Orai1, and S100A8-A9 proteins for Ca2+ signaling and FcgammaR-mediated phagosomal oxidative activity. *Journal of Immunology*, *186*, 2182–2191.

Stelitano, V., Brandt, A., Fernicola, S., Franceschini, S., Giardina, G., Pica, A., et al. (2013). Probing the activity of diguanylate cyclases and c-di-GMP phosphodiesterases in real-time by CD spectroscopy. *Nucleic Acids Research*, *41*, e79.

Stoye, D., Schubert, C., Goihl, A., Guttek, K., Reinhold, A., Brocke, S., et al. (2012). Zinc aspartate suppresses T cell activation in vitro and relapsing experimental autoimmune encephalomyelitis in SJL/J mice. *Biometals: An International Journal on the Role of Metal Ions in Biology, Biochemistry, and Medicine*, *25*, 529–539.

Sugiura, T., Kuroda, E., & Yamashita, U. (2004). Dysfunction of macrophages in metallothionein-knock out mice. *Journal of UOEH*, *26*, 193–205.

Sun, W., Li, Y., Chen, L., Chen, H., You, F., Zhou, X., et al. (2009). ERIS, an endoplasmic reticulum IFN stimulator, activates innate immune signaling through dimerization. *Proceedings of the National Academy of Sciences of the United States of America*, *106*, 8653–8658.

Sun, L., Wu, J., Du, F., Chen, X., & Chen, Z. J. (2013). Cyclic GMP-AMP synthase is a cytosolic DNA sensor that activates the type I interferon pathway. *Science*, *339*, 786–791.

Suzuki, Y., Inoue, T., & Ra, C. (2012). Calcium signaling in mast cells: Focusing on L-type calcium channels. *Advances in Experimental Medicine and Biology*, *740*, 955–977.

Takagi, J., Petre, B. M., Walz, T., & Springer, T. A. (2002). Global conformational rearrangements in integrin extracellular domains in outside-in and inside-out signaling. *Cell*, *110*, 599–611.

Takayama, H., & Sitkovsky, M. V. (1987). Antigen receptor-regulated exocytosis in cytotoxic T lymphocytes. *The Journal of Experimental Medicine*, *166*, 725–743.

Tan, J., Zhang, T., Jiang, L., Chi, J., Hu, D., Pan, Q., et al. (2011). Regulation of intracellular manganese homeostasis by Kufor-Rakeb syndrome-associated ATP13A2 protein. *The Journal of Biological Chemistry*, *286*, 29654–29662.

Tanaka, Y., Shiozawa, S., Morimoto, I., & Fujita, T. (1989). Zinc inhibits pokeweed mitogen-induced development of immunoglobulin-secreting cells through augmentation of both CD4 and CD8 cells. *International Journal of Immunopharmacology*, *11*, 673–679.

Tapiero, H., & Tew, K. D. (2003). Trace elements in human physiology and pathology: Zinc and metallothioneins. *Biomedicine & Pharmacotherapy = Biomedecine & Pharmacotherapie*, *57*, 399–411.

Tassi, I., Cella, M., Presti, R., Colucci, A., Gilfillan, S., Littman, D. R., et al. (2008). NK cell-activating receptors require PKC-theta for sustained signaling, transcriptional activation, and IFN-gamma secretion. *Blood*, *112*, 4109–4116.

Taylor, K. M., Vichova, P., Jordan, N., Hiscox, S., Hendley, R., & Nicholson, R. I. (2008). ZIP7-mediated intracellular zinc transport contributes to aberrant growth factor signaling in antihormone-resistant breast cancer cells. *Endocrinology*, *149*, 4912–4920.

Thyssen, J. P., & Menne, T. (2010). Metal allergy—A review on exposures, penetration, genetics, prevalence, and clinical implications. *Chemical Research in Toxicology*, *23*, 309–318.

Tidball, A. M., Bryan, M. R., Uhouse, M. A., Kumar, K. K., Aboud, A. A., Feist, J. E., et al. (2015). A novel manganese-dependent ATM-p53 signaling pathway is selectively impaired in patient-based neuroprogenitor and murine striatal models of Huntington's disease. *Human Molecular Genetics*, *24*, 1929–1944.

Tone, Y., Furuuchi, K., Kojima, Y., Tykocinski, M. L., Greene, M. I., & Tone, M. (2008). Smad3 and NFAT cooperate to induce Foxp3 expression through its enhancer. *Nature Immunology*, *9*, 194–202.

Torti, S. V., & Torti, F. M. (2019). Winning the war with iron. *Nature Nanotechnology*, *14*, 499–500.

Triantafilou, K., Hughes, T. R., Triantafilou, M., & Morgan, B. P. (2013). The complement membrane attack complex triggers intracellular Ca2+ fluxes leading to NLRP3 inflammasome activation. *Journal of Cell Science*, *126*, 2903–2913.

Trujillo, K. M., Yuan, S. S., Lee, E. Y., & Sung, P. (1998). Nuclease activities in a complex of human recombination and DNA repair factors Rad50, Mre11, and p95. *The Journal of Biological Chemistry*, *273*, 21447–21450.

Trumbo, P., Yates, A. A., Schlicker, S., & Poos, M. (2001). Dietary reference intakes: Vitamin A, vitamin K, arsenic, boron, chromium, copper, iodine, iron, manganese, molybdenum, nickel, silicon, vanadium, and zinc. *Journal of the American Dietetic Association*, *101*, 294–301.

Tuschl, K., Clayton, P. T., Gospe, S. M., Jr., Gulab, S., Ibrahim, S., Singhi, P., et al. (2012). Syndrome of hepatic cirrhosis, dystonia, polycythemia, and hypermanganesemia caused by mutations in SLC30A10, a manganese transporter in man. *American Journal of Human Genetics*, *90*, 457–466.

Tuschl, K., Meyer, E., Valdivia, L. E., Zhao, N., Dadswell, C., Abdul-Sada, A., et al. (2016). Mutations in SLC39A14 disrupt manganese homeostasis and cause childhood-onset parkinsonism-dystonia. *Nature Communications*, 7, 11601.

Ulanova, M., Tarkowski, A., Hahn-Zoric, M., & Hanson, L. A. (2001). The common vaccine adjuvant aluminum hydroxide up-regulates accessory properties of human monocytes via an interleukin-4-dependent mechanism. *Infection and Immunity*, *69*, 1151–1159.

Ulleras, E., Karlberg, M., Moller Westerberg, C., Alfredsson, J., Gerondakis, S., Strasser, A., et al. (2008). NFAT but not NF-kappaB is critical for transcriptional induction of the prosurvival gene A1 after IgE receptor activation in mast cells. *Blood*, *111*, 3081–3089.

Vaeth, M., Eckstein, M., Shaw, P. J., Kozhaya, L., Yang, J., Berberich-Siebelt, F., et al. (2016). Store-operated Ca(2+) entry in follicular T Cells controls humoral immune responses and autoimmunity. *Immunity*, *44*, 1350–1364.

Vaeth, M., & Feske, S. (2018a). Ion channelopathies of the immune system. *Current Opinion in Immunology*, *52*, 39–50.

Vaeth, M., & Feske, S. (2018b). NFAT control of immune function: New frontiers for an abiding trooper. *F1000Research*, *7*, 260.

Vaeth, M., Maus, M., Klein-Hessling, S., Freinkman, E., Yang, J., Eckstein, M., et al. (2017). Store-operated Ca(2+) entry controls clonal expansion of T cells through metabolic reprogramming. *Immunity*, *47*, 664–679.e666.

Vallee, B. L., & Falchuk, K. H. (1993). The biochemical basis of zinc physiology. *Physiological Reviews*, *73*, 79–118.

Verga Falzacappa, M. V., Vujic Spasic, M., Kessler, R., Stolte, J., Hentze, M. W., & Muckenthaler, M. U. (2007). STAT3 mediates hepatic hepcidin expression and its inflammatory stimulation. *Blood*, *109*, 353–358.

Vig, M., Peinelt, C., Beck, A., Koomoa, D. L., Rabah, D., Koblan-Huberson, M., et al. (2006). CRACM1 is a plasma membrane protein essential for store-operated Ca2+ entry. *Science*, *312*, 1220–1223.

Vodnala, S. K., Eil, R., Kishton, R. J., Sukumar, M., Yamamoto, T. N., Ha, N. H., et al. (2019). T cell stemness and dysfunction in tumors are triggered by a common mechanism. *Science*, *363*, eaau0135.

Volani, C., Doerrier, C., Demetz, E., Haschka, D., Paglia, G., Lavdas, A. A., et al. (2017). Dietary iron loading negatively affects liver mitochondrial function. *Metallomics: Integrated Biometal Science*, *9*, 1634–1644.

von Bulow, V., Rink, L., & Haase, H. (2005). Zinc-mediated inhibition of cyclic nucleotide phosphodiesterase activity and expression suppresses TNF-alpha and IL-1 beta production in monocytes by elevation of guanosine 3',5'-cyclic monophosphate. *Journal of Immunology*, *175*, 4697–4705.

Vukcevic, M., Zorzato, F., Spagnoli, G., & Treves, S. (2010). Frequent calcium oscillations lead to NFAT activation in human immature dendritic cells. *The Journal of Biological Chemistry*, *285*, 16003–16011.

Waghorn, B., Schumacher, A., Liu, J., Jacobs, S., Baba, A., Matsuda, T., et al. (2011). Indirectly probing Ca(2+) handling alterations following myocardial infarction in a murine model using T(1)-mapping manganese-enhanced magnetic resonance imaging. *Magnetic Resonance in Medicine*, *65*, 239–249.

Waghorn, B., Yang, Y., Baba, A., Matsuda, T., Schumacher, A., Yanasak, N., et al. (2009). Assessing manganese efflux using SEA0400 and cardiac T1-mapping manganese-enhanced MRI in a murine model. *NMR in Biomedicine*, *22*, 874–881.

Walczak-Drzewiecka, A., Ratajewski, M., Wagner, W., & Dastych, J. (2008). HIF-1α is up-regulated in activated mast cells by a process that involves calcineurin and NFAT. *Journal of Immunology*, *181*, 1665–1672.

Waldron, K. J., Rutherford, J. C., Ford, D., & Robinson, N. J. (2009). Metalloproteins and metal sensing. *Nature*, *460*, 823–830.

Walker, E. M., Jr., & Walker, S. M. (2000). Effects of iron overload on the immune system. *Annals of Clinical and Laboratory Science*, *30*, 354–365.

Wang, W., Green, M., Choi, J. E., Gijon, M., Kennedy, P. D., Johnson, J. K., et al. (2019). CD8(+) T cells regulate tumour ferroptosis during cancer immunotherapy. *Nature*, *569*, 270–274.

Wang, H., Grzywacz, B., Sukovich, D., McCullar, V., Cao, Q., Lee, A. B., et al. (2007). The unexpected effect of cyclosporin A on CD56+CD16− and CD56+CD16+ natural killer cell subpopulations. *Blood*, *110*, 1530–1539.

Wang, C., Guan, Y., Lv, M., Zhang, R., Guo, Z., Wei, X., et al. (2018). Manganese increases the sensitivity of the cGAS-STING pathway for double-stranded DNA and is required for the host defense against DNA viruses. *Immunity, 48*, 675–687.e677.

Wang, D., Zhang, J., Jiang, W., Cao, Z., Zhao, F., Cai, T., et al. (2017). The role of NLRP3-CASP1 in inflammasome-mediated neuroinflammation and autophagy dysfunction in manganese-induced, hippocampal-dependent impairment of learning and memory ability. *Autophagy, 13*, 914–927.

Wang, K., Zhou, B., Kuo, Y. M., Zemansky, J., & Gitschier, J. (2002). A novel member of a zinc transporter family is defective in acrodermatitis enteropathica. *American Journal of Human Genetics, 71*, 66–73.

Wastney, M. E., Aamodt, R. L., Rumble, W. F., & Henkin, R. I. (1986). Kinetic analysis of zinc metabolism and its regulation in normal humans. *The American Journal of Physiology, 251*, R398–R408.

Watanabe, N., Suzuki, J., & Kobayashi, Y. (1996). Role of calcium in tumor necrosis factor-alpha production by activated macrophages. *Journal of Biochemistry, 120*, 1190–1195.

Weber, K. S., Hildner, K., Murphy, K. M., & Allen, P. M. (2010). Trpm4 differentially regulates Th1 and Th2 function by altering calcium signaling and NFAT localization. *Journal of Immunology, 185*, 2836–2846.

Wedler, F. C. (1993). Biological significance of manganese in mammalian systems. *Progress in Medicinal Chemistry, 30*, 89–133.

Weekley, C. M., & He, C. (2017). Developing drugs targeting transition metal homeostasis. *Current Opinion in Chemical Biology, 37*, 26–32.

Weidinger, C., Shaw, P. J., & Feske, S. (2013). STIM1 and STIM2-mediated Ca(2+) influx regulates antitumour immunity by CD8(+) T cells. *EMBO Molecular Medicine, 5*, 1311–1321.

Weinberg, E. D. (1978). Iron and infection. *Microbiological Reviews, 42*, 45–66.

Wellinghausen, N., Kirchner, H., & Rink, L. (1997). The immunobiology of zinc. *Immunology Today, 18*, 519–521.

Wellinghausen, N., & Rink, L. (1998). The significance of zinc for leukocyte biology. *Journal of Leukocyte Biology, 64*, 571–577.

West, A. P., Khoury-Hanold, W., Staron, M., Tal, M. C., Pineda, C. M., Lang, S. M., et al. (2015). Mitochondrial DNA stress primes the antiviral innate immune response. *Nature, 520*, 553–557.

Woodruff, G., Bouwkamp, C. G., de Vrij, F. M., Lovenberg, T., Bonaventure, P., Kushner, S. A., et al. (2018). The zinc transporter SLC39A7 (ZIP7) is essential for regulation of cytosolic zinc levels. *Molecular Pharmacology, 94*, 1092–1100.

Wu, J., Sun, L., Chen, X., Du, F., Shi, H., Chen, C., et al. (2013). Cyclic GMP-AMP is an endogenous second messenger in innate immune signaling by cytosolic DNA. *Science, 339*, 826–830.

Xin, Y., Gao, H., Wang, J., Qiang, Y., Imam, M. U., Li, Y., et al. (2017). Manganese transporter Slc39a14 deficiency revealed its key role in maintaining manganese homeostasis in mice. *Cell Discovery, 3*, 17025.

Xu, S. Z., Zeng, F., Boulay, G., Grimm, C., Harteneck, C., & Beech, D. J. (2005). Block of TRPC5 channels by 2-aminoethoxydiphenyl borate: A differential, extracellular and voltage-dependent effect. *British Journal of Pharmacology, 145*, 405–414.

Yamasaki, S., Sakata-Sogawa, K., Hasegawa, A., Suzuki, T., Kabu, K., Sato, E., et al. (2007). Zinc is a novel intracellular second messenger. *The Journal of Cell Biology, 177*, 637–645.

Yang, W. S., SriRamaratnam, R., Welsch, M. E., Shimada, K., Skouta, R., Viswanathan, V. S., et al. (2014). Regulation of ferroptotic cancer cell death by GPX4. *Cell, 156*, 317–331.

Yang, G., Xu, L., Chao, Y., Xu, J., Sun, X., Wu, Y., et al. (2017). Hollow MnO_2 as a tumor-microenvironment-responsive biodegradable nano-platform for combination therapy favoring antitumor immune responses. *Nature Communications, 8*, 902.

Yin, Z., Jiang, H., Lee, E. S., Ni, M., Erikson, K. M., Milatovic, D., et al. (2010). Ferroportin is a manganese-responsive protein that decreases manganese cytotoxicity and accumulation. *Journal of Neurochemistry*, *112*, 1190–1198.

Yoon, K. W., Byun, S., Kwon, E., Hwang, S. Y., Chu, K., Hiraki, M., et al. (2015). Control of signaling-mediated clearance of apoptotic cells by the tumor suppressor p53. *Science*, *349*, 1261669.

Yu, M., Lee, W. W., Tomar, D., Pryshchep, S., Czesnikiewicz-Guzik, M., Lamar, D. L., et al. (2011). Regulation of T cell receptor signaling by activation-induced zinc influx. *The Journal of Experimental Medicine*, *208*, 775–785.

Yu, Y., Wang, D., Liu, C., Kaosaard, K., Semple, K., Anasetti, C., et al. (2011). Prevention of GVHD while sparing GVL effect by targeting Th1 and Th17 transcription factor T-bet and RORgammat in mice. *Blood*, *118*, 5011–5020.

Yu, Y., Xie, Y., Cao, L., Yang, L., Yang, M., Lotze, M. T., et al. (2015). The ferroptosis inducer erastin enhances sensitivity of acute myeloid leukemia cells to chemotherapeutic agents. *Molecular & Cellular Oncology*, *2*, e1054549.

Zaki, M. S., Issa, M. Y., Elbendary, H. M., El-Karaksy, H., Hosny, H., Ghobrial, C., et al. (2018). Hypermanganesemia with dystonia, polycythemia and cirrhosis in 10 patients: Six novel SLC30A10 mutations and further phenotype delineation. *Clinical Genetics*, *93*, 905–912.

Zanoni, I., Ostuni, R., Capuano, G., Collini, M., Caccia, M., Ronchi, A. E., et al. (2009). CD14 regulates the dendritic cell life cycle after LPS exposure through NFAT activation. *Nature*, *460*, 264–268.

Zapata, M. I., Feldkamp, J. R., Peck, G. E., White, J. L., & Hem, S. L. (1984). Mechanism of freeze-thaw instability of aluminum hydroxycarbonate and magnesium hydroxide gels. *Journal of Pharmaceutical Sciences*, *73*, 3–8.

Zhang, M., Cao, Y., Wang, L., Ma, Y., Tu, X., & Zhang, Z. (2015). Manganese doped iron oxide theranostic nanoparticles for combined T1 magnetic resonance imaging and photothermal therapy. *ACS Applied Materials & Interfaces*, *7*, 4650–4658.

Zhang, H., Clemens, R. A., Liu, F., Hu, Y., Baba, Y., Theodore, P., et al. (2014). STIM1 calcium sensor is required for activation of the phagocyte oxidase during inflammation and host defense. *Blood*, *123*, 2238–2249.

Zhang, X. W., Yan, X. J., Zhou, Z. R., Yang, F. F., Wu, Z. Y., Sun, H. B., et al. (2010). Arsenic trioxide controls the fate of the PML-RARalpha oncoprotein by directly binding PML. *Science*, *328*, 240–243.

Zhao, Z., Fan, H., Zhou, G., Bai, H., Liang, H., Wang, R., et al. (2014). Activatable fluorescence/MRI bimodal platform for tumor cell imaging via MnO_2 nanosheet-aptamer nanoprobe. *Journal of the American Chemical Society*, *136*, 11220–11223.

Zhong, B., Yang, Y., Li, S., Wang, Y. Y., Li, Y., Diao, F., et al. (2008). The adaptor protein MITA links virus-sensing receptors to IRF3 transcription factor activation. *Immunity*, *29*, 538–550.

Zhong, Z., Zhai, Y., Liang, S., Mori, Y., Han, R., Sutterwala, F. S., et al. (2013). TRPM2 links oxidative stress to NLRP3 inflammasome activation. *Nature Communications*, *4*, 1611.

Zhu, J., Yang, Y., Hu, S. G., Zhang, Q. B., Yu, J., & Zhang, Y. M. (2017). T-lymphocyte Kv1.3 channel activation triggers the NLRP3 inflammasome signaling pathway in hypertensive patients. *Experimental and Therapeutic Medicine*, *14*, 147–154.

Zogzas, C. E., Aschner, M., & Mukhopadhyay, S. (2016). Structural elements in the transmembrane and cytoplasmic domains of the metal transporter SLC30A10 are required for its manganese efflux activity. *The Journal of Biological Chemistry*, *291*, 15940–15957.

Zweifach, A. (2000). Target-cell contact activates a highly selective capacitative calcium entry pathway in cytotoxic T lymphocytes. *The Journal of Cell Biology*, *148*, 603–614.

FSC
www.fsc.org
MIX
Papier | Fördert gute Waldnutzung
FSC® C083411

Kolibri 360 GmbH
Ferdinand-Jühlke-Straße 7
99095 Erfurt, Deutschland
produktsicherheit@kolibri360.de